D1709415

# *Stereotactic Body Radiation Therapy*

# *Stereotactic Body Radiation Therapy*

EDITED BY

**Brian D. Kavanagh, M.D.,**

Associate Professor and Vice-Chair
Department of Radiation Oncology
University of Colorado Comprehensive Cancer Center
Anschutz Center for Advanced Medicine
Aurora, Colorado

**Robert D. Timmerman, M.D.**

Professor and Vice Chair
Department of Radiation Oncology
Director, Image Guided Stereotactic Radiation Therapeutics
University of Texas Southwestern Medical Center
Dallas, Texas

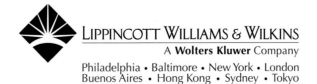

LIPPINCOTT WILLIAMS & WILKINS
A **Wolters Kluwer** Company

Philadelphia • Baltimore • New York • London
Buenos Aires • Hong Kong • Sydney • Tokyo

*Acquisitions Editor:* Jonathan Pine
*Developmental Editor:* Kevin C. Dietz
*Production Editor:* Dave Murphy
*Manufacturing Manager:* Ben Rivera
*Compositor:* Graphic World, Inc.
*Printer:* Quebecor-Kingsport

**© 2005 by LIPPINCOTT WILLIAMS & WILKINS**
**530 Walnut Street**
**Philadelphia, PA 19106 USA**
**LWW.com**

Printed in the USA

**Library of Congress Cataloging-in-Publication Data**

Stereotactic body radiation therapy / edited by Brian D. Kavanagh, Robert D. Timmerman.
    p. ; cm.
  Includes bibliographical references and index.
  ISBN 0-7817-5420-8 (alk. paper)
    1. Cancer--Radiotherapy. 2. Stereotaxtic techniques. 3. Radiography,
  Medical--Positioning. I. Kavanagh, Brian D. II. Timmerman, Robert D.
    [DNLM: 1. Radiotherapy--methods. 2. Neoplasms--radiotherapy. QZ 269 S838 2005]
  RC271.R3S747 2005
  616.99'46042--dc22

                                                                        2004048592

Care has been taken to confirm the accuracy of the information presented and to describe
generally accepted practices. However, the authors, editors, and publisher are not responsible for
errors or omissions or for any consequences from application of the information in this book
and make no warranty, expressed or implied, with respect to the currency, completeness, or
accuracy of the contents of the publication. Application of this information in a particular
situation remains the professional responsibility of the practitioner.

The authors, editors, and publisher have exerted every effort to ensure that drug selection
and dosage set forth in this text are in accordance with current recommendations and practice at
the time of publication. However, in view of ongoing research, changes in government
regulations, and the constant flow of information relating to drug therapy and drug reactions, the
reader is urged to check the package insert for each drug for any change in indications and
dosage and for added warnings and precautions. This is particularly important when the
recommended agent is a new or infrequently employed drug.

Some drugs and medical devices presented in this publication have Food and Drug
Administration (FDA) clearance for limited use in restricted research settings. It is the
responsibility of the health care provider to ascertain the FDA status of each drug or device
planned for use in their clinical practice.

                                    10 9 8 7 6 5 4 3 2 1

*To Julia, Thomas, and Clare Kavanagh*

*and*

*To Julie, Casey, Corey, Ramsey, and Riley Timmerman*

# CONTENTS

# CONTRIBUTING AUTHORS

**Scott Alleman, M.S.**
Instructor, Radiation Therapy Program
Willis-Knighton Cancer Center
2600 Kings Highway
Shreveport, Louisiana

**Tetsuya Aoki, M.D.**
Department of Therapeutic Radiology and Oncology
Graduate School of Medicine
Kyoto University
Sakyo, Kyoto, Japan

**Stanley H. Benedict, Ph.D.**
Associate Professor and Chief of Clinical Physics
Department of Radiation Oncology
Medical College of Virginia Hospitals
Virginia Commonwealth University
Richmond, Virginia

**Henric Blomgren, M.D., Ph.D.**
Associate Professor
Department of Oncology and Immunology
Karolinska University Hospital and Karolinska
    Institute
Stockolm, Sweden

**John M. Buatti, M.D.**
Professor and Head
Department of Radiation Oncology
Carver College of Medicine
University of Iowa
Iowa City, Iowa

**Robert M. Cardinale, M.D.**
Princeton Radiology Associates
Kendall Park, New Jersey

**Higinia R. Cardenes, M.D., Ph.D.**
Clinical Associate Professor
Department of Radiation Oncology
Indiana University School of Medicine
Indianapolis, Indiana

**Paul Dent, Ph.D.**
Associate Professor
Department of Radiation Oncology
Virginia Commonwealth University
Medical College of Virginia
Richmond, Virginia

**Laura Jeanne Esagui, C.M.D.**
Chief Dosimetrist
Section of Radiation Oncology
Virginia Mason Medical Center
Seattle, Washington

**Jack F. Fowler, D. Sc., Ph.D.**
Emeritus Professor
Department of Human Oncology
Radiobiologist
Department of Radiation Oncology
University of Wisconsin Medical Center
Madison, Wisconsin

**Martin Fuss, M.D.**
Associate Professor
Department of Radiation Oncology
The University of Texas Health Science Center
San Antonio, Texas

**James Galvin, D.Sc.**
Professor and Director
Medical Physics Division
Department of Radiation Oncology
Thomas Jefferson University
Philadelphia, Pennsylvania

**Steven Grant, M.D.**
Professor
Department of Medicine
Division of Hematology and Oncology
Virginia Commonwealth University
Richmond, Virginia

**Ulrich Haedinger, M.D.**
Chief Medical Physicist
Klinik fuer Strahlentherapie und Radiologische
    Onkologie
St. Vincentius-Kliniken
Karlsruhe
Germany

**Michael P. Hagan, M.D., Ph.D.**
Associate Professor
Department of Radiation Oncology
Virginia Commonwealth University
Medical College of Virginia
Richmond, Virginia

**Anna Hall, R.N.**
Tulane University Hospital and Clinic
New Orleans, Louisiana

**Klaus K. Herfarth, M.D.**
Department of Radiation Oncology
University of Heidelberg
Heidelberg, Germany

**William H. Hinson Ph.D.**
Assistant Professor
Department of Radiation Oncology
Wake Forest University School of Medicine
North Carolina Baptist Hospital
Winston-Salem, North Carolina

**Masahiro Hiraoka**
Professor
Department of Therapeutic Radiology and Oncology
Kyoto University Graduate School of Medicine
Sakyo, Kyoto, Japan

**Terese L. Howes, M.D.**
Resident Physician
Department of Radiation Oncology
Carver College of Medicine
University of Iowa
Iowa City, Iowa

**Geoffrey S. Ibbott Ph.D.**
Associate Professor
Department of Radiation Physics
The University of Texas MD Anderson Cancer Center
Houston, Texas

**Brian D. Kavanagh, M.D.**
Associate Professor and Vice-Chair
Department of Radiation Oncology
University of Colorado Comprehensive Cancer Center
Clinical Practice Director
Department of Radiation Oncology
University of Colorado Hospital
Aurora, Colorado

**Ingmar Lax, Ph.D.**
Associate Professor in Medical Radiation Physics
Department of Hospital Physics
Karolinska University Hospital and Karolinska
    Institute
Stockholm, Sweden

**Frank Lohr, M.D.**
Department of Radiation Oncology
Mannheim Medical Center
University of Heidelberg
Mannheim, Germany

**Michael Lovelock, M.D.**
Departments of Medical Physics and Radiation
    Oncology
Memorial Sloan-Kettering Cancer Center
New York, New York

**Berit L. Madsen, M.D.**
Radiation Oncologist
Section of Radiation Oncology
Virginia Mason Medical Center
Seattle, Washington

**Yukinori Matsuo, M.D.**
Department of Therapeutic Radiology and Oncology,
Graduate School of Medicine,
Kyoto University
Sakyo, Kyoto, Japan

**Ronald C. McGarry, M.D. Ph.D.**
Clinical Assistant Professor
Department of Radiation Oncology
Indiana University School of Medicine
Indianapolis, Indiana

**Sanford L. Meeks, Ph.D.**
Associate Professor, Director of Physics
Department of Radiation Oncology
Carver College of Medicine
University of Iowa
Iowa City, Iowa

**Takashi Mizowaki, M.D.**
Department of Radiology
Tenri Hospital
Nara, Japan

**Vadim Moskvin, M.D. Ph.D.**
Visiting Assistant Professor
Department of Radiation Oncology
Indiana University School of Medicine
Indianapolis, Indiana

**Yasushi Nagata, M.D.**
Associate Professor
Department of Therapeutic Radiology and Oncology
Kyoto University
Sakyo, Kyoto, Japan

**Lucien Nedzi, M.D.**
Assistant Professor
Department of Radiology
Tulane University
New Orleans, Louisiana

**Yoshitsugu Norihisa**
Department of Therapeutic Radiology and Oncology
Kyoto University
Sakyo, Kyoto, Japan

**Paul Okunieff, M.D.**
Chairman, Department of Radiation Oncology
Philip Rubin Professor of Radiation Oncology
Department of Radiation Oncology
University of Rochester School of Medicine and
    Dentistry
Rochester, New York

**Lech Papiez, M.D.**
Director of Radiation Physics
Department of Radiation Oncology
Indiana University School of Medicine
Indianapolis, Indiana

**Jack Rock, M.D.**
Co-Director, Surgical Neuro-Oncology Clinic
Henry Ford Hospital
Detroit, Michigan

**Samuel Ryu, M.D.**
Department of Radiation Oncology
Henry Ford Hospital
Detroit, Michigan

**Masato Sakamoto, M.D.**
Department of Therapeutic Radiology and Oncology
Graduate School of Medicine
Kyoto University
Sakyo, Kyoto, Japan

**Takashi Sakamoto, M.D.**
Department of Therapeutic Radiology and Oncology
Graduate School of Medicine
Kyoto University
Sakyo, Kyoto, Japan

**William Salter, Ph.D.**
Associate Director of Medical Physics
Cancer Therapy & Research Center
Assistant Professor
Department of Radiation Oncology
University of Texas Health Science Center
San Antonio, Texas

**Robert A. Sanford, M.D.**
Assistant Professor of Radiation Oncology
Tulane University Hospital and Clinic
New Orleans, Louisiana

**Tracey E. Schefter, M.D.**
Assistant Professor
Department of Radiation Oncology
University of Colorado Comprehensive Cancer Center
Aurora, Colorado

**Volker W. Stieber, M.D.**
Director of Stereotactic Body Radiotherapy
Assistant Professor
Department of Radiation Oncology
Wake Forest University School of Medicine
North Carolina Baptist Hospital
Winston-Salem, North Carolina

**Danny Y. Song, M.D.**
Assistant Professor
Department of Radiation Oncology and Molecular
    Radiation Sciences
The Sidney Kimmel Comprehensive Cancer Center
Johns Hopkins University
Baltimore, Maryland

**Kenji Takayama, M.D.**
Department of Therapeutic Radiology and Oncology,
Kyoto University
Sakyo, Kyoto, Japan

**Robert D. Timmerman, M.D.**
Professor and Vice Chair
Director, Image Guided Stereotactic Radiation
    Therapeutics
Department of Radiation Oncology
University of Texas Southwestern Medical Center
Dallas, Texas

**Wolfgang A. Tome Ph.D.**
Associate Professor
Department of Human Oncology
University of Wisconsin Medical School
Medical Physicist
Department of Radiation Oncology
University of Wisconsin Medical Center
Madison, Wisconsin

**Minoru Uematsu, M.D.**
Assistant Professor and Chief
Department of Radiation Oncology
National Defense Medical College
Tokorozawa Saitama
Japan

**James S. Welsh, M.S., M.D.**
Assistant Professor
Department of Human Oncology
University of Wisconsin Medical School
Madison, Wisconsin

**J. Peter Wersäll, M.D., Dr. Med. Sci.**
Associate Professor
Department of General Oncology
Radiumhemmet, Karolinska University Hospital and
    Karolinska Institute
Stockholm, Sweden

**Alichia White, MBA, CMD**
Tulane University Hospital and Clinic
New Orleans, Louisiana

**James R. Wong, M.D.**
Associate Clinical Professor
Department of Radiation Oncology
Columbia University College of Physicians
    & Surgeons
New York, New York
Chairman
Department of Radiation Oncology
Morristown Memorial Hospital
Morristown, New Jersey

**Jörn Wulf, M.D.**
Department of Radiotherapy
University of Würzburg
Würzburg
Germany

**Adly Yacoub, Ph.D.**
Departments of Radiation Oncology and Molecular
    Radiobiology
Virginia Commonwealth University School of
    Medicine
Richmond, Virginia

**Yoshiya Yamada, M.D. FRCPC**
Clinical Assistant Attending
Department of Radiation Oncology
Memorial Sloan Kettering Cancer Center
New York, New York

**Shinsuke Yano, R.T.T.**
Department of Therapeutic Radiology and Oncology,
Kyoto University
Sakyo, Kyoto, Japan

**Fang-Fang Yin, Ph.D.**
Medical Physicist
Department of Radiation Oncology
Henry Ford Hospital
Detroit, Michigan

**Elly Zakris, M.D.**
Associate Professor and Chief of Radiation Oncology
Tulane University Hospital and Clinic
New Orleans, Louisiana

# PREFACE

Stereotactic Body Radiation Therapy (SBRT) represents the newest plateau in the art and science of radiation oncology. Previously unimaginable radiation doses are administered precisely and non-invasively in an aggressive, decisive action to eradicate a discrete focus of cancer.

SBRT has evolved as a result of enormous technological advances in image-guided therapy. As the name implies, the technology involves the use of external fiducial markers referenced in 3-D space to internal targets, allowing *stereotactic* guidance of treatment to targets within the body. Previously applied monikers included the term "Stereotactic Radioablation," which conveyed the sense that the high-dose treatment is intended to ablate, or completely eradicate, targeted tumors. "Extracranial Radiosurgery" is another popular term, appealing insofar as it reflects the debt SBRT owes to cranial radiosurgery, through which the concept of stereotactic localization has been refined. However, as discussed in the book, "radiosurgery" generally implies a single fraction course of treatment, whereas SBRT is quite commonly administered in a hypofractioned regimen of 3-5 fractions.

Equally important for the development of SBRT have been the accomplishments in diagnostic imaging and systemic therapy during the last decade. High-quality CT, MRI, and PET scans can provide very accurate information about the exact locations of measurable deposits of tumor cells within a cancer patient's body. Newer chemotherapy combinations and novel growth factor-targeted drugs have achieved significant improvements in progression-free survival for many solid tumors. The complementary role of SBRT, then, is to provide directly cytotoxic treatment focally to the clinically evident disease sites that are unlikely to be cleared with systemic agents alone. Competing with SBRT in this regard are the numerous invasive methodologies for accomplishing this same goal, namely surgical resection and temperature-based therapies (radiofrequency ablation and cryosurgery). The advantage of SBRT in many cases is the greatly reduced toxicity profile, lack of invasiveness, and capacity to deliver the treatment entirely on an outpatient basis.

This book is partly constructed as an educational tool for all oncologists to promote understanding of the power and elegance of SBRT as a new and important weapon in the cancer-fighting arsenal. Modern multi-disciplinary management strategies mandate input from radiation, medical, and surgical oncologists—and we all need to keep sight of the expanding frontiers of each other's primary modalities.

At the same time that we acknowledge that SBRT is made possible by technological progress in medical physics, we must concede that SBRT will only be implemented safely and effectively with an appreciation of the underlying basic and clinical radiobiology. In their learned contribution to this book, Dr. Fowler and colleagues explain that to attain a high probability of actually killing off a tumor with radiation, it requires a biologically very potent dose—much more than is generally given with conventionally fractionated treatment.

Here is the catch: if you give the tumor a large dose of radiation, then some adjacent normal tissue will get a large dose as well. Fortunately, with careful attention to technique, it is frequently possible to steer the radiation toward the tumor from enough different directions that only a very small rim of normal tissue is affected noticeably. Just how much radiation can really be given with SBRT remains to be seen, and the radiation oncology community needs to continue careful clinical-biological-physics-inclusive translational research to establish where the reasonable safe limits really are. In seeking great success, we risk great failure, so we are compelled to work together.

The book is also, then, intended to be a primer for radiation oncologists, physicists, radiobiologists, dosimetrists, therapists, and other invaluable members of the team who wish to become comfortable with emerging techniques that raise radiotherapy to bold new heights.

*Brian Kavanagh, Robert Timmerman*

# The Clinical Transition from Intracranial to Extracranial Stereotactic Radiation Therapy

*Ingmar Lax and Henric Blomgren*

Local recurrence remains a problem in a relatively large fraction of patients after radical radiotherapy. Improved methods of radiotherapy, makes dose escalation possible, reflected in clinical trials worldwide, to improve local result after radiotherapy. One emerging method for dose escalation to improve local results is stereotactic body radiation therapy (SBRT), also known as extracranial stereotactic radiation therapy (ESRT). This method was introduced in clinical use at the Karolinska Hospital in 1991 and was significantly based on experience from intracranial stereotactic radiosurgery at the same hospital. This section describes the transition into SBRT, in terms of methodologic and clinical aspects and the early results.

## INTRACRANIAL STEREOTACTIC RADIATION DELIVERY

The field of intracranial stereotactic radiosurgery was developed during the 1950s to the 1970s (1,2). The treatment was given in a single session with doses aiming to kill all cells in the irradiated volume. The method was primarily intended for functional disorders in the brain, and the treatment was suggested as an alternative to neurosurgery. The term "radiosurgery" was coined by Leksell (1) for this type of treatment. Additionally the treatment method was based on the use of an external three-dimensional (3D) reference system (stereotactic system) for accurate localization of the target as well as for directing the radiation therapy. Thus, "stereotactic radiosurgery" was the term used for geometrically accurate delivery of very high doses, in a single session, to relatively small volumes in the

Karolinska University Hospital and Karolinska Institute, Stockholm, Sweden

brain. This treatment modality, which was pioneered at the Karolinska Hospital using the Gamma Knife since 1968, is now in widespread use throughout the world. The treatment is delivered using multiple beams spread in a large solid angle to minimize the dose and volume of normal tissue irradiated. Since the introduction, there has been a gradual change in indications toward treatment of localized malignant and benign tumors as well as arteriovenous malformations. The utility of this treatment modality is evidence based from worldwide experience for a number of different malignant and nonmalignant intracranial targets.

## STEREOTACTIC BODY RADIATION THERAPY

### Principles

Extracranial solid tumors are relatively often impossible to kill with conventional radiotherapy. This can be explained by the restrictions in target dose delivery imposed by the tolerance of the surrounding normal tissues. Limited geometric accuracy in the dose delivery in conventional radiotherapy necessitates a large margin of normal tissues outside of the tumor to receive nearly the same dose as the tumor. The large margins are consequences of the typical conduct of conventional radiotherapy whose attributes include (a) the use of setup methods based on anatomic reference systems, (b) geometric verification based on portal imaging, (c) homogeneous dose distribution throughout the target volume, and (d) about 2 Gy per fraction.

To circumvent the limitations of conventional radiotherapy, a program applying the stereotactic treatment principles to extracranial targets (mainly in the thoracic, abdominal, and pelvic regions) was initiated at the departments of Hospital Physics and Oncology, Karolinska Hospital in 1991 (3). The important prerequisites available at the time included (a) a long-term experience of intracranial stereotactic radiosurgery with high rates of local control for selected targets, (b) a 3D dose planning system in clinical use, and (c) a computed tomography (CT) scanner (intended to be used for geometric verification) available at the radiotherapy department. The missing hardware was a stereotactic frame for the body, which was subsequently developed (3).

The principal difference between the use of the stereotactic method for intracranial targets and extracranial targets is imposed by anatomy. In the intracranial application, a very firm relation is given between the diagnostic or treatment unit and the target of interest by the fixation of the stereotactic frame to the skull bone as shown in Fig. 1. For extracranial applications, no such conditions exist, and motion between the target in the stereotactic reference system is the rule rather than the exception. The task was to develop a stereotactic frame capable of allowing geometric verification of the position of soft-tissue tumors while simultaneously ensuring that the position of the target could be accurately reproduced (see "methods" below). The solution involved using the department's CT scanner for verification of the position of the tumor in the stereotactic coordinate system.

For extracranial treatment delivery, doses high enough to kill even large macroscopic tumors with central cores populated by radioresistant hypoxic cells needed to be given with acceptable toxicity. The solution to this was the introduction of considerably heterogeneous dose distributions throughout the tumor volume, with increasing dose to the center of the tumor. Finally, to make the treatment method clinically feasible and not too demanding for the patient, hypofractionation schedules with a few fractions of high doses were introduced.

Altogether, there were a number of new radiotherapy principles for stereotactic treatment of extracranial macroscopic solid tumors introduced with this method (3,4).

## Methods

Stereotactic radiotherapy differs from conventional radiotherapy in that no anatomically based patient reference system is needed (apart from the target-system) as illustrated in Fig. 2. The three coordinate systems used in conventional radiotherapy are T = target system, Anatom. = anatomic reference system, and Acc. = accelerator reference system. For stereotactic radiotherapy, the anatomic reference system is exchanged to the stereotactic reference system ( = Ster.). The accelerator system coordinates may be exchanged with CT, magnetic resonance imaging (MR), and other coordinate systems for the diagnostic localization procedure.

In conventional radiotherapy, there are two significant uncertainties relative to the accelerator and anatomy and subsequently relative to the anatomy and the target coordinate systems as indicated in Table 1. In contrast, for SBRT the stereotactic and accelerator systems are rigid mechanical systems. As such, these can be aligned with an uncertainty that, in this context, is nonsignificant (4). Improved geometric accuracy is derived from using no anatomically based reference system other than the target system and by striving for good fixation of the target in the stereotactic reference system.

### Geometric Verification

The principle problem with the verification method used in conventional radiotherapy is that projection images obtained in portal imaging give a contrast resolution that is unable to resolve almost all soft-tissue targets. Thus, portal imaging is indirect and based on the assumption that

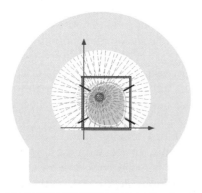 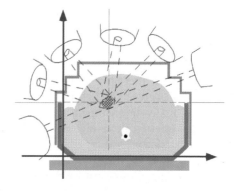

**FIGURE 1.** The left panel shows a schematic drawing of intracranial stereotactic radiosurgery with the Gamma Knife (Elekta). The stereotactic frame is fixed with screws into the skull. The right panel shows a schematic drawing of extracranial stereotactic radiation therapy with linear accelerator. The patient is fixed in the stereotactic body frame.

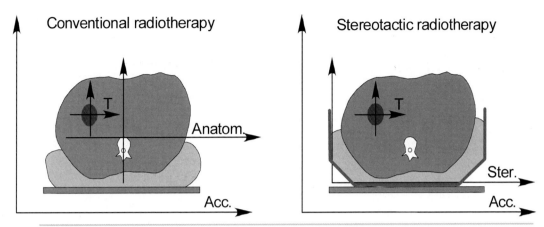

**FIGURE 2.** Illustration of coordinate systems used in conventional radiotherapy (**left**) and stereotactic body radiation therapy (**right**).

there is a reasonably stable relation between the bony structures and the target. This is a valid method when large margins between the clinical target volume (CTV) and the planning treatment volume (PTV) can be used in conjunction with relatively small, daily dose-per-fraction treatments accumulating to relatively modest total doses. If, however, solid macroscopic tumors are treated with the intention of local control, (very) high doses have to be prescribed, thus prohibiting large margins.

Ideally, the geometric verification procedure should have the same geometric and contrast resolution as that used for the definition of the target. Thus, CT was introduced from the start of SBRT in 1991 for the verification of the position of the target in the stereotactic system (3,4). Figure 3 illustrates the comparison between verification images and reference images (for definition of target) of the position of the target in stereotactic space. With the use of suitable software for image registration, the quantitative difference of the position of the target in stereotactic space between the two examinations can be determined in all directions.

Unless the geometric verification is done exactly at the same time as the dose is delivered, all verification procedures will give a probabilistic view of the reproducibility. Thus, probability measures based on this information will be used for the determination of the margin to be used between the CTV and PTV (3,4). The experience from

Karolinska Hospital showed that margins of 5 mm in transverse direction and 10 mm in longitudinal direction were generally sufficient to cover 95% of treatments (4). This was mainly based on the treatment of lung and liver tumors. To get these results, a standardized procedure to position the patient in the stereotactic frame was important.

## Dose Distribution

The paradigm in conventional radiation therapy of a homogeneous dose distribution in the target volume is essentially based on two presumptions. First, the tumor aspect follows from the fact that there is generally not enough information available regarding the tumor cell density and sensitivity to differentiate the dose throughout the target volume. Next, normal tissue within the planning target volume may be given doses exceeding the

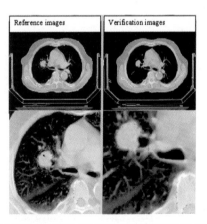

**FIGURE 3.** Comparison of target location in the stereotactic reference system in verification images (**right**) to reference images (**left**). Lower images shows magnified images illustrating the matching procedure between the two computed tomography examinations.

▶ **TABLE 1** Uncertainties Between Coordinate Systems (Shown in Fig. 2).

|  | Coordinate Systems | Uncertainty |
|---|---|---|
| Conventional radiation therapy | T—anatom. | Significant |
|  | Anatom.—acc. | Significant |
| Stereotactic radiation therapy | T—ster. | Significant |
|  | Ster.—acc. | Nonsignificant |

tolerance level and/or make predictions of side effects very difficult for heterogeneous dose distributions in the target volume. Solid tumors are in many cases impossible to control with conventional radiotherapy given with moderate homogeneous doses. It is generally considered that reduced radiosensitivity due to hypoxia in gross tumors may be an important cause of local failure in conventional radiotherapy.

For intracranial stereotactic radiosurgery of solid tumors, there is a long-term experience with high rates of local control using very heterogeneous dose distributions in the target volume. Analyses of these dose distributions (5) shows that 50% or even higher doses compared to the dose to the periphery can be given to the central parts of a macroscopic solid tumor with a very minor dose increase to the volume of normal tissue outside the solid tumor. This paradigm, which is valid for multiple convergent beams spread in a large solid angle, was also introduced from the start of SBRT at Karolinska Hospital in 1991 (3).

Figure 4 shows dose distributions that compare intratarget and extratarget dose distributions with different degrees of heterogeneity as well as a case with homogeneous dose distribution in the target. The calculations were made for a continuum of beams, incident from all directions (3). However, this is also relevant for a relatively few number of beams, as used in the clinical setting (4). The initial clinical trial with SBRT at Karolinska Hospital was started with dose distributions with a 50% higher dose to the central parts of the target compared to the prescription dose at the periphery of the PTV (3). The parallel between and experience from radiosurgery of intracranial metastasis and SBRT of lung and liver metastasis were partly used for this choice.

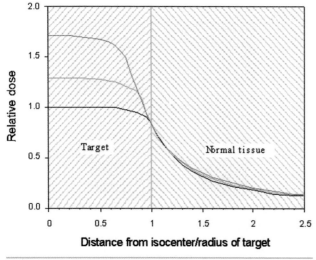

**FIGURE 4.** Relative dose distributions calculated for an isotropic beam geometry (3).

## Fractionation

In addition, with regard to fractionation, the comparison to intracranial radiosurgery was the obvious source of clinical experience and data. However, a single fraction was soon abandoned in lieu of a few fractions of very high doses-per-fraction treatments. This choice was pragmatically made to restrict the number of fractions to make the treatment more convenient for the patient and to be able to put more emphasis of geometric accuracy on few fractions rather than many. During the 12-year experience from the Karolinska Hospital, the treatments are generally given with three fractions, but depending on surrounding organs at risk, fewer or more fractions are given.

Data at hand today indicate that three fractions of about 15 Gy per fraction at the periphery of the PTV is necessary for a high rate of local control for many solid tumors. This corresponds to a total dose of 100 Gy or more converted to 2 Gy per fraction with $\alpha/\beta$ equals ten using biologically equivalent dose (BED) formalism.

## Equipment

As mentioned above, the driving force for the development of SBRT was primarily the experience and results from intracranial stereotactic radiosurgery. Otherwise, the SBRT method was based on standard radiotherapy equipment apart from the addition of a stereotactic frame for the body. A standard linear accelerator, initially without a multileaf collimator, was used at the time of clinical introduction. A 3D dose-planning system was also necessary, as well as the availability to a CT scanner for geometric verification. Furthermore, software for verification image matching and evaluation was available in the dose-planning system.

## Internal Organ Motion Control

Motion of the target with the breathing was dealt with by applying pressure on the abdomen of the patient during the diagnostic procedure and treatment (3,4). This technique forces the patients to more intercostal breathing while restricting the diaphragmatic motion. This method was introduced from the start of SBRT. The device for this is shown in Fig. 5. The pressure on the abdomen is used if the target is located so as it is affected by the diaphragmatic motion and that the motion of the diaphragm is more than ±5 mm as measured by fluoroscopy. This methodology was found to be simple and practical to apply in clinical practice.

## Stereotactic Body Frame

The intended use of the stereotactic body frame was for targets in the thorax, abdomen, and pelvic regions. The idea from the start was to use a low-density rigid frame,

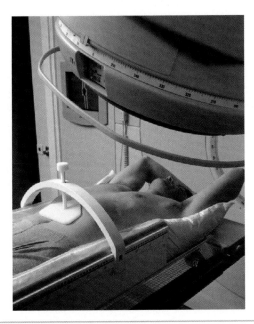

**FIGURE 5.** A patient positioned in the stereotactic body frame, with the abdominal pressure device applied to reduce diaphragmatic motion with the respiration.

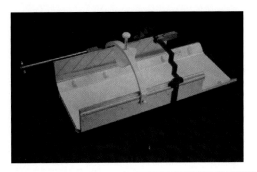

**FIGURE 6.** Stereotactic body frame with accessory devices.

with a vacuum pillow inside for fixation of the target (patient) in the stereotactic system as shown in Fig. 5 and Fig. 6 (3,4). The vacuum pillow makes a large contact area between the patient and the frame, which was designed with fiducials for CT and MRI (Fig. 6), defining the stereotactic reference system in the images. The frame was further designed with a material in the walls to make possible any direction of the incident beams (without collision with the gantry) with only a marginal attenuation when irradiating through the frame-wall.

## CLINICAL INTRODUCTION

### Fractionation

When we started SBRT in 1991 using a prototype of the stereotactic body frame, the intention was to be able to deliver one single tumor-ablative dose in analogy to that of Gamma Knife radiosurgery. We observed that dose escalation up to 20 Gy in the periphery of the PTV of metastases (5–10 mm margin between CTV and PTV) was well tolerated for patients with relatively small tumors. However, since the rate of local tumor control was not satisfactory, fractionated treatments were started. During the first years of learning and empirical development, the conclusion was reached that a few fractions of 8 to 20 Gy (prescribed doses, at the periphery of the PTV) could be given every second day, with acceptable toxicity and tumor control (6). However, there were several factors to consider when determining how to treat the tumor in-

cluding histopathologic type, its location in the body, previous conventional radiation therapy to the same anatomic site, previous chemotherapy, general medical condition, and age of the patient.

The treatment policy at the Karolinska Hospital, throughout the 12 years of clinical use of SBRT has been described in published reports (6,7). As a rule, small tumors (<3 cm) are treated with two to three fractions (15–20 Gy, prescribed dose) and large tumors with four to six fractions of 5 to 8 Gy. Most sarcomas, spinal gliomas, and adenocarcinomas of gastrointestinal or pulmonary origin seem to be the most resistant to SBRT requiring a high BED. These tumors' degree of radioresistance is followed by kidney cancer, melanoma, and thyroid cancer. All types of gynecologic cancers (including leiomyosarcoma uteri), primary hepatic cancer, cholangiocarcinomas, and squamous cell carcinomas seem to be relatively sensitive. Tumors that are located close to or at the hilus of the liver and lung are treated with low fraction sizes as are tumors growing close to organs such as the esophagus, myocardium, intestine, urinary bladder, and spinal cord. It is also our impression that tumors of patients who have been treated with some cytotoxic drugs display a reduced radiosensitivity. Relatively low fraction sizes are used in children.

Our most frequently used fraction schedule today is a prescribed dose of 15 Gy given on three occasions (for instance Monday, Wednesday, and Friday). Due to the inhomogeneity of the dose distribution, this gives a mean BED to the CTV (transformed into 2-Gy fractions and assuming an $\alpha/\beta$ of ten) of approximately 150 Gy. This treatment schedule is mainly used for radioablation of relatively small, peripherally located tumors in the liver and lungs.

## INDICATIONS FOR STEREOTACTIC BODY RADIATION THERAPY: YESTERDAY, TODAY, AND TOMORROW

During the first 5 years following the introduction of SBRT, very few patients were treated because of the developmental character of the method. SBRT was used pri-

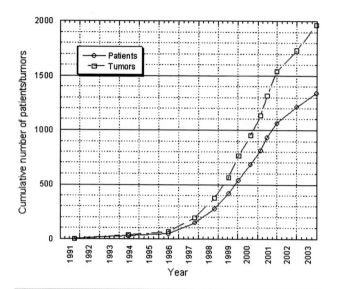

*FIGURE 7.* Diagram shows the cumulative number of patients and tumors treated during the years 1991 to 2003.

| Organ | No. Tumors |
|---|---|
| Lungs | 997 |
| Mediastinum | 78 |
| Liver | 484 |
| Pancreas | 149 |
| Suprarenal glands | 30 |
| Abdomen[a] | 118 |
| Skeleton | 25 |
| Miscellaneous[b] | 46 |

▶ TABLE 2 Anatomic Distribution of 1965 Tumors That Have Been Treated with Stereotactic Body Radiation Therapy at the Karolinska Hospital from 1991 to 2003.

[a]Mainly kidneys and para-aortic regions.
[b]Pelvic area, muscles, and so forth.

marily in patients in whom conventional treatment modalities had failed or who were considered nonapplicable. Among the referred patients, a large number could not be treated with this technique for several reasons including too many tumors, too-large tumors, and the tumors were invading radiosensitive organs. Most patients who were selected for treatment had one to four metastases in the liver or lungs. When the positive results on toxicity and local control after SBRT were summarized (6,7) the number of patients undergoing SBRT at the Karolinska Hospital increased (Fig. 7). This increase was mainly because some physicians started to use SBRT, rather than chemotherapy, as the first-line treatment of metastatic disease. Admittedly, there are still respected physicians trained in cancer surgery, chemotherapy, and conventional radiotherapy who hesitate to refer patients for SBRT.

As can be seen in Table 2, 1,965 tumors were treated during the 1991 to 2003. Fifty-five percent represented intrathoracic tumors (997 in the lungs and 78 in the mediastinum). The second most common site was the liver. Most tumors represented metastases from a variety of primary tumors.

Patients who have undergone SBRT at the Karolinska Hospital have been examined by CT at 3- to 4-month intervals after a treatment. The main reason for such frequent follow-up schedules is to treat new tumors (metastases) at an early stage with the same method. Thus, some patients have received SBRT of more than 20 tumors during observation periods of several years. The quality of life during this period has usually been very good because the side effects have been mild or absent, and the patients have not been hospitalized during the treatment periods. Eventually, however, many patients need chemotherapy because of the development of too many metastases.

It is likely that the role of SBRT in the management of cancer will increase in the future. Well-controlled prospective clinical trials will show whether this noninvasive, cost-effective treatment modality may replace surgery not only of some metastases but also of some primary tumors such as lung cancer and kidney cancer.

## REFERENCES

1. Leksell L. The stereotaxic method and radiosurgery of the brain. *Acta Chirurg Scand* 1951;102:316–319.
2. Leksell L. *Stereotaxis and radiosurgery*. Springfield, IL: Charles C. Thomas, 1971.
3. Lax I, Blomgren H, Nüslund I, et al. Stereotactic radiotherapy of malignancies in the abdomen: methodological aspects. *Acta Oncol* 1994;33:677–683.
4. Lax I, Blomgren H, Larson D, et al. Extracranial stereotactic radiosurgery of localized targets. *J Radiosurg* 1998;1:135-148.
5. Lax I. Target dose versus extratarget dose in stereotactic radiosurgery. *Acta Oncol* 1993;32:453–457.
6. Blomgren H, Lax I, Nüslund I, et al. Stereotactic high dose fraction radiation therapy of extracranial tumors using an accelerator. *Acta Oncol* 1995;34:861–870.
7. Blomgren H, Lax I, Göransson H, et al. Radiosurgery for tumors in the body: clinical experience using a new method. *J Radiosurg* 1998;1:63–74.

# The Radiobiology of Stereotactic Body Radiation Therapy (SBRT)

## Chapter 1

## Estimation of Required Doses in Stereotactic Body Radiation Therapy

*Jack F. Fowler, Wolfgang A. Tome, and \*James S. Welsh*

### INTRODUCTION

It has been established clinically that very high radiation doses can be given to patients with medically inoperable carcinomas of lung, using hypofractionated stereotactic body radiation therapy (SBRT) without serious acute or long-term normal-tissue reactions. Both lung and liver tumors have been safely treated in this manner (1–13). Certain dose and volume limitations are necessary, and their limits are still under discussion. The fractions (F) can be as large as 3F × 15 Gy or even 3F × 23 Gy, and our first

Department of Radiation Ocology, University of Wisconsin Medical Center; *Department of Human Oncology, University of Wisconsin Medical School, Madison, Wisconsin 53792

discussion is how large should these doses be from the point of view of eliminating non–small cell lung tumors? Will 3F × 15 Gy be sufficient (2), or do we need 3 × 20 Gy or more?

### THE RADIATION DOSE RESPONSE FOR TUMOR CONTROL

#### An Analysis for Non–Small Cell Lung Cancer

We first review briefly the evidence for dose-response relationships in non–small cell lung cancer (NSCLC) and discuss the prospects for large increases in long-term progression-free survival.

One of the best dose-response curves for NSCLC, in the sense of widest ranging in dose, is that published by Mary Martel and colleagues in 1999 (14). Their paper described the results of the University of Michigan (Ann Arbor) dose-escalation study in patients with inoperable NSCLC. They escalated doses to 103 Gy in 2-Gy fractions given at five fractions per week (abbreviated as normalized total dose in 2-Gy fractions, NTD). Their tumor results were summarized as a logistic dose-response curve with a $D_{50}$ of 84.5 Gy and a modest slope of gamma-50 equal to 1.5 (percent of local control per 1% increment of total dose) (Fig. 1.1). This curve explains why we are obtaining such dismal results with conventional doses of 60 or 70 Gy (as 2-Gy fractions in 6 or 7 weeks). They are predicted to yield 15% or 24%, respectively.

When investigators at the University of Michigan gave 95 Gy in conventional fractions, one in three patients recurred locally, in accordance with Fig.1.1. Although that level of success would be an enormous improvement on the 10% to 30% local recurrence-free survival currently

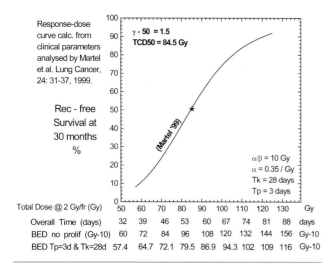

Response-dose curve calc. from clinical parameters analysed by Martel et al. Lung Cancer, 24: 31-37, 1999.

Rec - free Survival at 30 months %

| Total Dose @ 2 Gy/fr (Gy) | 50 | 60 | 70 | 80 | 90 | 100 | 110 | 120 | 130 | Gy |
|---|---|---|---|---|---|---|---|---|---|---|
| Overall Time (days) | 32 | 39 | 46 | 53 | 60 | 67 | 74 | 81 | 88 | days |
| BED no prolif (Gy-10) | 60 | 72 | 84 | 96 | 108 | 120 | 132 | 144 | 156 | Gy-10 |
| BED Tp=3d & Tk=28d | 57.4 | 64.7 | 72.1 | 79.5 | 86.9 | 94.3 | 102 | 109 | 116 | Gy-10 |

**FIGURE 1.1.** Recurrence-free survival percentage at 30 months, calculated from Martel's parameters (14). In addition to the doses in 2 Gy per fraction at 5 F per week, the ordinate values also show the overall time in days, the BED (Gy 10) if zero proliferation is assumed, and (*fourth* line) the BED if proliferation at a cell doubling time of 3 days, starting at Time to repopulation (Tk) = 28 days (34), is assumed.

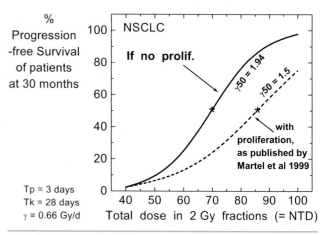

% Progression -free Survival of patients at 30 months

Tp = 3 days
Tk = 28 days
$\gamma$ = 0.66 Gy/d

**FIGURE 1.2.** Recurrence-free survival percentage at 30 months. Lower [(*dashed*) curve: as in Fig. 1.1 including repopulation with 2 Gy given five fractions per week]. Upper (*full*) curve: the same data after subtracting the effect of proliferation from the x-axis at 0.66 Gy per day from the 28th day after starting irradiation of NSCLC, assuming Tk = 28 days, potential doubling time (Tp) = 3 days, $\alpha$ = 0.35 ln/Gy, and $\alpha\beta$ = 10 Gy.

standard at 3 years, it is clear that doses up to 100 Gy (given at 2-Gy fractions five times a week) would be required to obtain success in the 90% region. However, the overall treatment time of 10 weeks would be unreasonably long for a patient, in contrast with SBRT, which is typically completed in 2 weeks or less. The total duration of SBRT is thus shorter than the starting time, $T_k$, of accelerated repopulation in tumors, believed to be 3 to 5 weeks in tumors with the same rate of repopulation (15–19). Therefore, proliferation at the equivalent rate in Gy/day must be subtracted from the dose scale in Fig. 1.1.

For this analysis a $T_k$ of 28 days was assumed, with a repopulation doubling time ($T_p$) of 3 days (20), the generic $\alpha$ value of 0.35 ln/Gy, and the $\alpha\beta$ ratio of 10 Gy (21,22). The result, assuming no repopulation occurring in the tumors, is shown in Fig. 1.2 as a full line to the left of the dashed line, which indicates the original Martel curve from Fig 1.1. The no-repopulation (full) curve is the one that is relevant for modeling results from SBRT. Its slope is steeper at a gamma-50 of 1.94, instead of 1.5 as in the original Martel curve (14), and its D50 is at 70 Gy, instead of at 84.5 Gy.

Table 1.1 shows the biologically equivalent doses (BEDs) for a range of SBRT schedules that are being currently used clinically, together with the 2-Gy–equivalent total doses (NTD). A 5-F × 12-Gy schedule is included as used by Gomi et al.(12) and in the Department of Human Oncology at the University of Wisconsin–Madison. It is assumed that no tumor cell repopulation occurs in the SBRT schedules. Also shown are two "standard" schedules of 6 and 7 weeks' duration. Allowance was made for

tumor repopulation in those two, with parameters listed above, resulting in a loss in BED of 7.2 and 11.9 Gy$_{10}$ respectively. All were calibrated with one or other of the two curves in Fig. 1.2. It is clear that some of these schedules yield an estimated progression-free survival at 30 months—abbreviated as tumor control probability (TCP) in subsequent discussion—close to 100%, *if the presence of radioresistant cells (due to hypoxia or phase of the cell cycle), or of cells missed by the irradiation, is ignored.*

## Why Might We Need Such High Doses?

Let us consider why we might need the upper range of such high tumor doses. Figure 1.3 illustrates one of the arguments on this point. If radioresistant hypoxic cells were present in the tumors, or cells in a resistant phase of the cell cycle, the doses required would be 2.5 to 3 times greater than if they were not. The steeper curve with closed circles represents the multifraction cell killing of a well-oxygenated tumor with 10 or 11 logs (to base 10) of viable cells, for example in a tumor of 1- to 10-g mass. A total dose of 75 to 80 Gy NTD would then give a good chance of reducing the tumor burden to approximately one viable cell on average, provided that all the cells were well-oxygenated or became so by reoxygenation early in the treatment.

If reoxygenation is incomplete so that only 1% of the tumor cells remain hypoxic, then many orders of magnitude (seven or eight) of resistant cells remain. Therefore, total doses two to three times greater than 60 or 70 Gy would be required to obtain a finite chance of eliminating malignant cells from the target. In particular, three fractions would have to be each as large as approximately

▶ **TABLE 1.1** For Typically Used Stereotactic Body Radiotherapy Schedules, the Tumor BEDs and NTDs Were Calculated by LQ with $\alpha\beta$ = 10 Gy. Then Progression-Free Survival of Patients with NSCLC at 30 months was Estimated from Martel (14) *with Proliferation Subtracted at Tp = 3days and Tk = 28 days (Fig. 1.2).* No Repopulation was Assumed to Occur in any SBRT Schedule, but it is Included in the 6- and 7-Week Standard Schedules

| Total Dose | Reference | BED Gy10 | NTD, Gy 2-Gy Fractions) | Estimated Progression-free Survival at 30 Mo. (Assuming No Hypoxia) |
|---|---|---|---|---|
| **Conventional fractionation** | — | (Fig. 1.8) | — | — |
| 60 Gy, 30 fractions | — | 72 | 60 | 15% |
| 70 Gy, 35 fractions | — | 84 | 70 | 24% |
| **SBRT** | — | (Fig. 1.9) | — | — |
| 48 Gy, 4 fractions | (6) | 106 | 63 | 34% |
| 45 Gy, 3 fractions | (2) | 113 | 94 | 95% |
| 48 Gy, 3 fractions | (2) | 125 | 104 | 99% |
| 60 Gy, 5 fractions | (12) | 132 | 110 | >99% |
| 60 Gy, 3 fractions | (3) | 180 | 150 | >99% |
| 69 Gy, 3 fractions | (33) | 228 | 190 | >99% |

BED, biologically equivalent dose; NTD, normalized total dose in 2-Gy fractions; SBRT, stereotactic body radiation therapy; NSCLC, non–small cell lung cancer; Tk, time to repopulation; Tp, potential doubling time; LQ, linear–quadratic.

23 Gy so as to reduce the viable tumor burden by the necessary factor of $10^{-10}$ or $10^{-11}$.

The time course of reoxygenation is highly variable in different types of tumor and cannot be reliably predicted (23). Although a large amount of reoxygenation can occur within 24 hours, it is not clear how often reoxygenation can reduce the proportion of hypoxic cells to the very small numbers—less than one surviving cell—that are necessary to avoid local recurrence. This is especially true when "acute" hypoxia, due to transient shutdown of capillary vessels is considered. The question about hypoxia

and reoxygenation might not be answered until measurements are routinely obtained after a few days of radiotherapy to image or to measure hypoxic cells remaining in a tumor. Thus, while the use of $3 \times 15$ Gy might be sufficient in patients who do reoxygenate their tumors rapidly and completely, the net has to be spread wider to cover the potential hypoxic-resistance problem. It therefore seems prudent to explore doses up to this level provided that they can be given without undue normal tissue injury, as clinical results indicate (1).

## DOSE INHOMOGENEITY AND INTRAFRACTION RADIATION REPAIR

### Cold Spots in the Isodose Distribution

The difficulties of resolving and describing dose inhomogeneity in clinical SBRT and addressing the overall time for individual treatments are revisited in Chapter 6, but let us first consider here certain important points. It has long been accepted that a "reduction of not more than 10% in tumor dose to not more than 10% of the tumor volume" leads to an acceptably small decrease in TCP (for example from 50% TCP to 40%–45%). We have published modeling that shows that this rule of thumb is very unsymmetrical (24), using an improved algorithm based on the one developed by Niemierko and Goitein 1993 (25). Figures 1.4 and 1.5 contain identical data, plotted in two different ways. It was assumed that a uniform dose of 30 fractions of 2 Gy would cause a TCP of 50% with a dose-response curve of average slope (i.e., having a gamma-50 of 2.0). Figure 1.4 shows that a fall of *10% in dose* (below

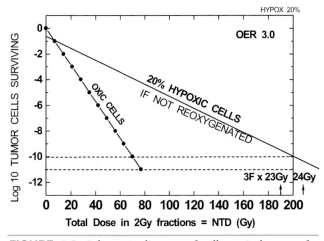

*FIGURE 1.3.* Schematic diagram of cell survival curves for well-oxygenated cells (*full line with filled circles*), with a line of less slope representing 20% hypoxic cells remaining hypoxic throughout radiotherapy with 2-Gy fractions. The oxygen enhancement ratio is assumed to be 3. To reduce the proportion of surviving cells to $10^{-11}$ would require three fractions of more than 24 Gy.

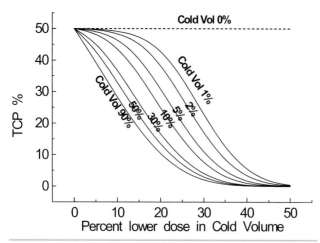

**FIGURE 1.4.** The decrease in TCP (tumor control probability), plotted against percent reduction in dose in each subvolume. Each curve is for a different tumor subvolume. It is assumed that a homogeneous treatment of 30×2 Gy = 60 Gy would yield TCP = 50%.

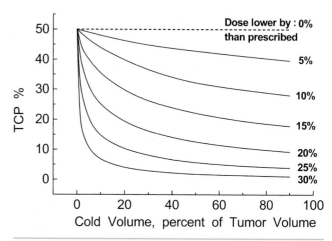

**FIGURE 1.5.** The same data as in Fig. 1.4 but plotted against percentage of tumor volume, each curve being for a different dose reduction. A 30% dose reduction in a 10% volume (*lowest curve*) gives a much lower tumor control probability (TCP) (8%) than a 10% dose reduction (*second curve down*) in 30% of the tumor subvolume (TCP, 37%).

the prescribed dose) delivered to *a 30% cold subvolume in the tumor* will cause a modest fall of TCP to 35% to 40% TCP. This occurs along the sloping curve for "30% cold volume" in Fig. 1.7.

However a fall of *30% in tumor dose to a 10% subvolume of tumor* leads to unacceptably low TCPs below 10%. This is shown in Fig. 1.5 by the drop from the second to the lowest curve down. (It can also be seen in Fig. 1.7 by tracing the "10% volume curve" along to a 30% lower dose as shown along the x-axis.). We explained that this is a particular hazard with dose-prescription for tumor dose in IMRT, where an apparently small-volume tail but of surprisingly low dose can appear on the DVH, unless a minimum tumor dose is specified (24). This problem can also be avoided if the effective uniform dose (EUD) is calculated (26) from the DVH of the target, and is not allowed to be less than the prescribed dose. This point has also been made in an editorial by Goitein and Niemierko (27), and the application of EUD for SBRT dosimetry is discussed additionally in Chapter 6.

## Loss of Biologic Efficiency with Prolonged Fraction Delivery

There is compelling evidence that radiation damage repair is not monophasic but consists of at least two components with different half-times, and possibly a range of half-times. Assuming the simplest interpretation of only two half-times, one of 0.2 to 0.4 hours and the other of 4 hours, our team has calculated the loss of biologic efficiency during continuous irradiation of various doses between 2 and 23 Gy with durations of up to 2 hours. The calculations were done by applying the Lea–Catcheside formula *G* for simultaneous buildup and decay of radia-

tion damage into the beta-containing term in the linear quadratic formulation for BED, $(1 + Gd/[\alpha\beta])$. Figure 1.6 shows the calculated results, which indicate biologically significant losses of effect in about an hour.

The loss of tumor bioeffective dose (BED in $Gy_{10}$, that is with $\alpha\beta = 10$ Gy) in 1 hour's duration of irradiation was calculated to be only about 5% for 2 Gy fractions, but was 10% to 15% for fraction sizes of 23 Gy. The effect on TCP however would be greater, by up to twice these percent-

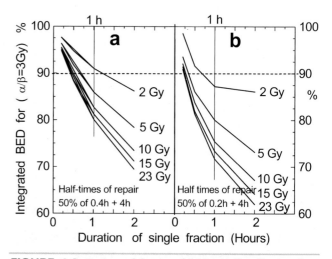

**FIGURE 1.6.** Estimated losses of biologically effective dose (BED) (for late effects, $\alpha\beta = 3$Gy) as a function of prolonged delivery times for fraction sizes of 2 to 23 Gy. Two monoexponential repair rates are assumed (30), with two equally weighted half-times of 0.4 hour +4.0 hours **(A)** and 0.2 hours +4.0 hours **(B).** The effect of faction size is illustrated. The longer half-life has a small effect up to 1 hour's duration. The loss of BED is approximately half as great for tumor effects ($\alpha\beta = 10$ Gy).

ages, because of the slope of the dose-response curve (Fig. 1.2). The effect on late complications was a loss of nearly 30% in BED $Gy_3$. This difference from the prescribed dose would have a significant effect in lowering the incidence of late complications. It is therefore suggested that for single fraction exposures of duration more than 20 or 30 minutes, careful records should be kept of these durations, for later correlation with clinical outcome.

## NORMAL TISSUE CONSIDERATIONS

### Reduction of the High-dose Target Volume and Limiting Normalized Total Doses

Simple considerations of small target volume show that if a 5-cm sphere has a margin of 0.5 cm reduced all round it, the diameter reduces from 5 to 4 cm *but the volume decreases to one half, from 66 to 34 cm³*. Since the probability of damaging molecules by ionizing radiation is proportional to the number at risk, approximately twice the dose could then be given, but somewhat less because the number of damaged molecules goes up with dose per fraction in the usual linear quadratic way. If another margin width of 0.5 cm is removed, the diameter is 3 cm, volume becomes 9.5 cm³, so very much greater doses can be given—*about five to seven times larger than in a 5-cm sphere of 66 cm³*, as far as the target volume is concerned. Such enormous increases in dose should sterilize all of the cells within the high-dose volume. This "ablation" may be feasible if the organ is a good approximation to a parallel organ so that the loss of such a small volume of functioning tissue is tolerated, and if it contains no particularly sensitive structures. This condition may be the case in peripheral lung tissues and is further discussed in Chapter 4, and techniques of arranging beams efficiently to ensure rapid dose fall-off in normal tissue are discussed in Chapter 8.

There is, of course, no way that the incoming beamlets that contribute to the dose within the target volume can avoid contributing also to the buildup of mean dose within the surrounding tissues, so these three doses (the within-GTV dose; the dose just outside the PTV; and the whole-lung-minus-GTV mean lung NTD) cannot be completely independent. It has been suggested that the mean lung dose should be kept below the range of 18 to 22 Gy (in 2-Gy–fraction equivalents) to assure that the risk of grade 2 or higher pneumonitis remains acceptably low (28–30).

When the volume index $n$ equals 1 in the Lyman–Kutcher–Burman model of complication incidence (31,32), as in lung as a parallel tissue or liver, mean lung dose is easy to compute and is identical to $NTD_{mean}$ for the last-mentioned limitation with respect to pneumonitis. Then the Veff becomes the proportion of the irradiated organ obtained by the ratio of mean lung dose

(NTD) divided by the mean dose in the target volume NTD.

## Classical Radiobiology Does Not Contradict These High Doses to Small Volumes in "Parallel" Tissues

Figure 1.7 shows log-log plots ("tolerance dose" vs. partial volume) for the original Emami et al. (1991) data (33), and subsequent modeling from Ann Arbor (34,35), Stockholm and Amsterdam (36), to predict doses to keep the incidence of pneumonitis grade 2 and above at or below the stated percentages, from 5% to 50%. The resulting curves were approximately straight lines of slope 1:1, indicating a linear relationship between tolerance dose and Veff. This would be expected for an organ that is close to a "parallel-type" tissue, and conforms to the concept of "a little dose to a lot of volume has the same effect as a lot to a little," at least for radiation pneumonitis.

Figure 1.8 shows in more detail that the Amsterdam data fit this curve and that the Ann Arbor data, up to 103 Gy in 2 Gy fractions, suggested that the tolerance doses were still somewhat underestimated by this modeling, especially for the smaller volumes (34,35). Both these groups have suggested the use of mean lung dose as a correlate with incidence of pneumonitis. Data from Stockholm also fit the same plot, although using the relative seriality algorithm instead of the Lyman–Kutcher–Burman one (36).

We next propose an extrapolation, whose predictions must be regarded as speculative until further clinical information is available. Some of this information appears to be available already from the SBRT data reported by Timmerman et al. (1,37). Figure 1.9 shows our extrapola-

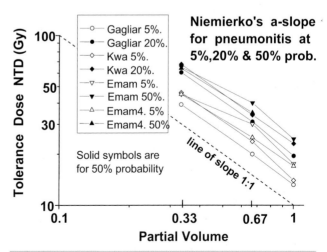

**FIGURE 1.7.** Log tolerance dose versus partial volume of lung irradiated, for 5%, 20%, and 50% incidence of pneumonitis. The curves are not inconsistent with a linear–linear relationship (27–31).

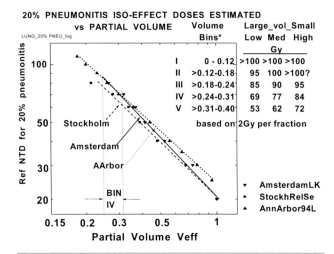

FIGURE 1.8. Log tolerance dose versus log volume of lung tissue, for an estimated 20% incidence of not greater than grade 2 pneumonitis. Predictions from the Karolinska Radiumhemmet at Stockholm, the Netherlands Cancer Institute at Amsterdam, and the University of Michigan at Ann Arbor. All are consistent with a linear–linear slope, that is a "parallel organ" volume exponent of $n = 1$.

tion from Fig. 1.8 to smaller volumes and higher doses, assuming the linear–linear dose-volume relationship illustrated above, and with the BED dose scale computed assuming that the linear–quadratic (LQ) formula remains true up to doses per faction of 23 Gy [as indeed found by Douglas and Fowler in 1976 (22)].

We emphasize that the accuracy of any particular volume-dose relationship suggested in Fig. 1.9 requires more detailed experimental verification in the future.

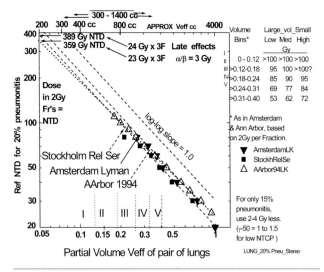

FIGURE 1.9. Extrapolating Fig. 1.8 to higher doses and smaller volumes can reach biologically equivalent doses values for late effects (αβ = 3 Gy), which are similar to those reached in clinical stereotactic body radiation therapy schedules (Table 1.2).

▶ **TABLE 1.2** **Late-reaction BED and NTD for Some SBRT Schedules, Calculated by LQ with αβ = 3 Gy. For Comparison with the Lung Tolerance Dose Versus Veff Modeling from Ann Arbor, Amsterdam, and Stockholm (Figs. 1.11 and 1.12)**

| Total dose | BED Gy3 | NTD, Gy (2-Gy Fractions) |
|---|---|---|
| **Conventional fractionation** | | |
| 70 Gy, 35 fractions | 117 | 70 |
| **SBRT** | | |
| 45 Gy, 3 fractions | 270 | 162 |
| 48 Gy, 3 fractions | 303 | 182 |
| 60 Gy, 5 fractions | 300 | 180 |
| 60 Gy, 3 fractions | 460 | 276 |
| 69 Gy, 3 fractions | 598 | 359 |

BED, biologically equivalent doses; SBRT, stereotactic body radiation therapy; NTD, normalized total dose in 2-Gy fractions.

However, the late-complication BEDs of 450 to 600 $Gy_3$ shown do correspond approximately to the total doses of 3F × 22 Gy or 3F × 23 Gy (Table 1.2) whose results are reported by Timmerman et al. to be close to tolerance doses (37), so the modeling is not impossibly wrong. More accurate clinical data are needed concerning the actual GTV and PTV volumes, together with the important mean dose to lung-minus-GTV for physical treatment plans not as concentrated as some others.

## REPOPULATION OF NON–SMALL CELL LUNG CANCER AND LENGTH OF TREATMENT SCHEDULE

Our team has pointed out that the rate of repopulation in non–small cell lung tumors (20) is about as fast as in tumors of the ear, nose and throat (38), so that the SBRT strategy of delivering the full treatment dose within 2 weeks utilizes a short enough overall time to avoid tumor repopulation (15). This is worth emphasizing when standard multifraction radiotherapy occupies 6 or 7 weeks and therefore suffers a disadvantage from repopulation of tumor cells after 3 or 4 weeks of radiotherapy (Fig. 1.2).

In 1993, the Radiation Therapy Oncology Group (RTOG) published detailed results from 397 patients treated by multiple small fractions to 69 Gy, including 70 who experienced gaps in treatment exceeding 5 days (39). The 3-year survival was 17% without delays, but 1% with delays ($p = 0.0001$). Detailed study (20) showed that the median delay was 11 days with a median actuarial loss of 19% local control at 3 years = 1.7% per day. This was equal to the loss reported from head and neck cancer patients of 1.66 % per day in recent reviews (38). It is attributed to repopulation of clonogens in the tumors during treatment as a reflection of normal tissue stimulation by depopulation, especially after 3 to 5 weeks of multiple small fractions (15–19).

There is therefore a significant advantage in shortening the overall time of radiotherapy at least to 3 or 4 weeks (15,20,21), and this is done in the SBRT protocols with only three to five fractions in 2 weeks. Previously, the shortest multifraction schedules reported were the UK Continuous Hyperfractionated Accelerated Radiation Therapy (CHART) [36 × 1.5 Gy three times daily in 11 days (40)] or a regimen of 12 fractions of 4 Gy in 2.5 weeks (41,42), both of which gave good results in NSCLC but not major gains, using standard physical dose distributions. However, until some centers explore results from 2 or 3 weeks compared with those from 3 to 5 weeks over time, we will not know with certainty whether shortening to less than 4 or 5 weeks is additionally advantageous for NSCLC from a biologic perspective, though the clinical advantage of patient convenience might be valuable. It is worth remembering that repopulation can start sooner after a high dose of 10 to 20 Gy than multiple small doses, but still after depopulation has occurred; sooner than after multiple small fractions, which generate a slower depopulation (43).

Although conveniently short, the use of a single fraction is probably the worst radiobiologic alternative, because it gives no chance for reoxygenation or any shift out of a resistant phase of cell cycle or nutritional deprivation. It would be expected to require a considerably larger total dose to be effective on tumors than even a small number of dose fractions.

## CONCLUSIONS

There is sufficient uncertainty about the continued presence of hypoxic or other radioresistant cells in tumors, especially after a short course of large dose fractions, that it would be prudent to continue to investigate the clinical effects of doses near the top of the dose ranges discussed here. For normal tissue complications, the three types of limiting doses described above—dose in the target volume, dose just outside the PTV, and mean total dose to the lungs minus GTV—all require further investigation and confirmation, but the algorithms of conventional radiobiologic modeling appear likely to be able to encompass them.

## REFERENCES

1. Timmerman R, Papiez L, McGarry R, et al. Extracranial stereotactic radioablation: results of a phase I study in medically inoperable stage I non–small cell lung cancer. *Chest* 2003;124:1946–1955.
2. Blomgren JM, Lax I, Naslund I, et al. Stereotactic high dose fraction radiation therapy of extracranial tumors using an accelerator: clinical experience of the first thirty-one patients. *Acta Oncol* 1995;34:861–870.
3. Blomgren H, Lax I, Goranson H, et al. Radiosurgery for tumors in the body: clinical experience using a new method. *J Radiosurg* 1988;1:63–74.
4. Uematsu M, Shioda A, Taharab K, et al. Focal, high dose, and fractionated modified stereotactic radiation therapy for lung carcinoma patients: a preliminary experience. *Cancer* 1988;15:82:1062–1070.
5. Uematsu M, Shioda A, Suda A, et al. Computed tomography-guided frameless stereotactic radiotherapy for stage I non–small cell lung cancer: a 5-year experience. *Int J Radiat Oncol Biol Phys* 2001;51: 666–670.
6. Nagata Y, Negoro Y, Aoki T, et al. Three-dimensional conformal radiotherapy for extracranial tumors using a stereotactic body frame [in Japanese]. *Igaku Butsuri* 2001;21;28–34.
7. Nagata Y, Negoro Y, Tetsuya A, et al. Clinical outcomes of 3D conformal hypofractionated single high-dose radiotherapy for one or two lung tumors using a stereotactic body frame. *Int J Radiat Oncol Biol Phys* 2002;52:1041–1046.
8. Wulf J, Hadinger U, Oppitz U, et al. Stereotactic radiotherapy of targets in the lung and liver. *Strahlenther Onkol* 2001;177:645–655.
9. Herfarth KK, Bebys J, Lohr F, et al. Stereotactic single-dose radiotherapy of liver tumors: results of a phase I/II trial. *J Clin Oncol* 2001;19:164–179.
10. Hara B, Itami J, Kondo T, et al. Stereotactic single high-dose irradiation of lung tumors under respiratory gating. *Radiother Oncol* 2002;63:159–163.
11. Hof H, Herfarth KK, Munter M, et al. Stereotactic single-dose radiotherapy of stage I non–small cell lung cancer. *Int J Radiat Oncol Biol Phys* 2003;56:335–341.
12. Gomi K, Koichi M, Oguchi M, et al. Clinical experience of stereotactic radiation therapy for stage IA non–small cell lung cancer. In: Proceedings of the Sixth International Stereotactic Radiosurgery Society Congress; June, 2003; Kyoto Japan. Abstract OSS X-1.
13. Fujino M, Harada T, Onimaru R, et al. Feasibility of real-time tumor-tracking radiotherapy system for lung tumors. In: Proceedings of the Sixth International Stereotactic Radiosurgery Society Congress; Month, date, 2003; Kyoto Japan. Abstract OSS X-5.
14. Martel MK, Ten Haken RK, Hazuka MB, et al. Estimation of tumor control probability model parameters from 3-D dose distributions of non–small cell lung cancer patients. *Lung Cancer* 1999;24:31–37.
15. Withers HR, Taylor JMG, Maciejewski B. The hazard of accelerated tumor clonogen repopulation during radiotherapy. *Acta Oncol* 1988;27:131–146.
16. Brenner DJ. Accelerated repopulation during radiotherapy: quantitative evidence for delayed onset. *Radiat Oncol Invest* 1993;1:167–172.
17. Roberts SA, Hendry JH. The delay before onset of accelerated tumor cell repopulation during radiotherapy: a direct-maximum likelihood analysis of a collection of worldwide tumor-control data. *Radiother Oncol* 1993;29:69–74.
18. Roberts SA, Hendry JH, Brewster AE, et al. The influence of radiotherapy treatment time on the control of laryngeal cancer: a direct analysis of data from two British Institute of Radiology trials to calculate the lag period and the time factor. *Br J Radiol* 1994;67: 790–794.
19. Robertson C, Robertson AG, Hendry JH, R, et al. Similar decreases in local control are calculated for treatment protraction and for interruptions in the radiotherapy of carcinoma of the larynx in four centres. *Int J Radiat Oncol Biol Phys* 1998;40:319–329.
20. Fowler JF, Chappell R. Non small cell lung tumors repopulate rapidly during radiation therapy [Letter]. *Int J Radiat Oncol Biol Phys* 2000;46:516–517.
21. Fowler JF. The Linear-quadratic formula and progress in fractionated radiotherapy: a review. *Brit J Radiol* 1989;62:679–694.
22. Douglas BG, Fowler JF. The effect of multiple doses of x-rays on skin reactions in the mouse and a basic interpretation. *Radiat Res* 1976;6:401–426.
23. Hall EJ. The oxygen effect and reoxygenation. In: Hall EJ, ed. Radiobiology for the Radiobiologist, 5th ed. Philadelphia, PA: Lippincott Williams & Wilkins, 2000.
24. Tomé WA, Fowler JF. On cold spots in tumor subvolumes. *Med Phys* 2002;29:1590–1598.
25. Niemierko A, Goitein M. Implementation of a model for estimating tumor control probability for an inhomogeneously irradiated tumor. *Radiother Oncol* 1993;29:140–147.

26. Niemierko A. Reporting and analyzing dose distributions: a concept of equivalent uniform dose. *Med Phys* 1997;24:103–110.
27. Goitein M, Niemierko A. Intensity modulated radiotherapy and inhomogeneous dose to the tumor: a note of caution [Editorial]. *Int J Radiat Oncol Biol Phys* 1996; 36:519–522.
28. Kwa LS, Lebesque JV, Theuws JCM, et al. Radiation pneumonitis as a function of mean lung dose: an analysis of pooled data of 540 patients. *Int J Radiat Oncol Biol Phys* 1998;42:1–9.
29. Seppenwoolde Y, Lebesque J. Partial irradiation of the lung. *Sem Radiat Oncol* 2001;11:247–258.
30. De Jaeger K, Hoogeman MS, Engelsman M, et al. Incorporating an improved dose-calculation algorithm in conformal radiotherapy of lung cancer: re-evaluation of dose in normal lung tissue. *Radiother Oncol* 2003;69:1–10.
31. Niemierko A. The "a" slopes in EUD. Invited lecture, University of Wisconsin, 1999.
32. Rancati T, Ceresoli GL, Gagliardi G, et al. Factors predicting radiation pneumonitis in lung cancer patients: a retrospective study. *Radiother Oncol* 2003;67:275–283.
33. Emami B, Lyman J, Brown A, et al. Tolerance of normal tissue to therapeutic irradiation. *Int J Radiat Oncol Biol Phys* 1991;21:109–122
34. Robertson JM, Ten Haken RK, Hazuka MB, et al. Dose escalation for non–small cell lung cancer using conformal radiation therapy. *Int J Radiat Oncol Biol Phys* 1997; 37:1079–1085.
35. Hayman JA, Martel MK, Ten Haken RK, et al. Dose escalation in non–small cell lung cancer using three-dimensional conformal radiotherapy: update of a phase I trial. *J Clin Oncol* 2001;19:127–136.
36. Gagliardi G, Bjohle J, Lax I, et al. Radiation pneumonitis after breast cancer irradiation: analysis of the complication probability using the relative seriality model. *Int J Radiat Oncol Biol Phys* 2000;46:373–381.
37. Timmerman et al, Papiez L, McGarry R et al. Extracranial stereotactic radioablation: results of a phase I study in medically inoperable stage I non–small cell lung cancer. *Chest* 2003;124:1946–1955.
38. Hendry JH, Bentzen SM, Dale RG, et al. A modelled comparison of the effects of using different ways to compensate for missed treatment days in radiotherapy. *Clin Oncol* 1996;8:297–307.
39. Cox JD, Pajak TF, Asbell S, et al. Interruptions of high-dose radiation therapy decrease long-term survival of favorable patients with unresectable non–small cell carcinoma of the lung: analysis of 1244 cases from 3 radiation therapy oncology group (RTOG. Trials:. *Int J Radiat Oncol Biol Phys* 1993;27:493–498.
40. Dische S, Saunders M, Barrett A, et al. A randomised multicentre trial of CHART versus conventional radiotherapy in head and neck cancer . *Radiother Oncol* 1997;44:123–136.
41. Slotman BJ, Antonosse IE, Njo KH, et al. Limited field irradiation in early stage (T1-2N0: non–small cell lung cancer. *Radiother Oncol* 1996;41:41–44.
42. Cheung PC, Yeung LT, Basrur V, et al. Accelerated hypofractionation for early-stage non–small cell lung cancer. *Int J Radiat Oncol Biol Phys* 2002;54:1014–1023.
43. Dörr W, Weber-Frisch M. Repopulation response of mucosal mucosa during unconventional radiotherapy protocols. *Radiother Oncol* 1995;37:230–236.

# The Cellular Signaling Response to Radiation

## Michael P. Hagan, Adly Yacoub, Steven Grant*, and Paul Dent

Stereotactic body radiation therapy (SBRT) is typically applied in a brief course of hypofractionated, high-dose radiation treatment in which the primary goal is to eradicate tumor cells within the targeted volume by destroying their reproductive capacity or inducing apoptotic cell death. However, at the same time that it exerts potentially cytotoxic effects, ionizing radiation triggers cascades of molecular signaling events. The responses that are activated can compensate for the cytotoxic effects on the tumor as a whole by promoting cellular repopulation. Likewise, individual tumor cells are partially protected as antiapoptotic and DNA repair mechanisms are turned on. Certain early reactions appear to be fully manifest after cells are exposed to very low radiation doses, while other responses increase in magnitude in a dose-dependent manner up through the range of high doses applied clinically using SBRT.

Identification of the signaling pathways activated by radiation and other cellular stresses has opened up new avenues of cancer therapy. Agents that target specific steps in these signaling pathways can abrogate their cytoprotective effects. The net result can be an enhancement of the therapeutic effect of the radiation or other treatment given. Selected radiation-induced cellular stress responses are highlighted here to foster an appreciation of the complex matrix of messages stimulated by SBRT and an understanding of potential opportunities to enhance SBRT.

## SIGNALING EVENTS AT THE CELL MEMBRANE

The ErbB family of growth factor receptors is a group of structurally and functionally related transmembrane phosphoglycoproteins. ErbB1 is more commonly known as the epidermal growth factor receptor (EGFR). ErbB2, ErbB3, and ErbB4 are also commonly referred to as

HER2, HER3, and HER4, respectively. EGFR contains a tyrosine kinase within its intracellular domain whose activity is stimulated via phosphorylation upon binding with naturally occurring autocrine ligands such as EGF or transforming growth factor alpha (TGFα). This process of phosphorylation initiates intracellular signaling pathways that promote cellular proliferation and inhibit apoptosis. EGFR is frequently overexpressed in a wide range of carcinomas and may play a major role in oncogenesis (1).

EGFR can interact (dimerize) with other ErbB family receptors, and in certain conditions, ligand binding with EGFR activates other subtypes of ErbB receptors (2). ErbB2 is similar to EGFR insofar as it contains a tyrosine kinase within its intracellular domain (3). However, because no ligand that binds to ErbB2 has yet been described, it is believed that ErbB2 primarily plays a supporting role in the activation of all ErbB family members (4–6). While ErbB3 and ErbB4 are known to bind with ligands different from those that bind to EGFR (7,8), ErbB3 does not appear to have an active tyrosine kinase domain in its intracellular component (9).

Ionizing radiation above a minimum dose of approximately 0.5 Gy activates EGFR in a manner similar to ligand-mediated activation (10,11). This threshold effect may explain, in part, why some cell types irradiated with radiation doses of 0.1 to 0.4 Gy—a dose range not expected to activate EGFR—exhibit hypersensitivity to radiation (12). Also activated downstream from EGFR are signaling pathways involving numerous distinct signaling molecules such as the proto-oncogene Raf-1, mitogen activated protein kinase (MAPK), and phosphatidyl inositol 3-kinase (PI3K) (13–15) (Fig. 2.1).

The first wave of MAPK pathway activation induced by low doses of radiation occurs within minutes and is dependent on reactive oxygen species and reactive nitrogen species generated directly by the exposure to ionizing radiation (11,16–18). A second wave of indirect MAPK pathway activation follows later and is related to radiation-induced release of TGFα (19,20). In some cell types, the

Departments of *Medicine and Radiation Oncology and Biochemistry, Virginia Commonwealth University, Richmond VA 23298

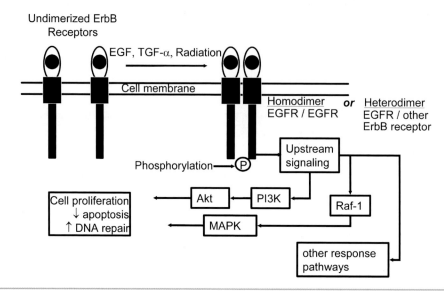

**FIGURE 2.1.** Activation of ErbB receptors by ligands or radiation. Pairs of ErbB receptors dimerize as they are phosphorylated, initiating signal transduction through numerous pathways to downstream effectors. The effect of radiation is to inhibit protein tyrosine phosphatases, shifting the equilibrium to permit enhanced tyrosine phosphorylation by the receptor's tyrosine kinase. (From Dent P, Reardon DB, Park JS, et al. Radiation-induced activations of the epidermal growth factor receptor and the mitogen activated protein kinase pathway via transforming growth factor a in autocrine-regulated carcinoma cells. *Mol Biol Cell* 1999;10:2493–2506; and Raben D, Helfrich BA, Chan D, et al. ZD1839, a selective epidermal growth factor receptor tyrosine kinase inhibitor, alone and in combination with radiation and chemotherapy as a new therapeutic strategy in non-small cell lung cancer. *Semin Oncol* 2002;29[Suppl 4]:37–46, with permission.)

released ligand has been noted to be heregulin acting through ErbB3.

Radiation causes cleavage of pro-TGFα in the plasma membrane, leading to its release into the surrounding media. Increasing the radiation dose from 2 Gy up to 10 Gy enhances the secondary activation of both EGFR and the MAPK pathway, suggesting that radiation promotes a dose-dependent increase in the cleavage of pro-TGFα that reaches a plateau at approximately 10 Gy (Fig. 2.2). Typically, SBRT fractions sizes will be at or above this level, in the range expected to cause maximum TGFα release. Interestingly, radiation can activate the other ErbB family members besides EGFR without intermediate activation of EGFR (21,22), suggesting that radiation causes an indiscriminate activation of multiple other plasma membrane receptor tyrosine kinases.

## INHIBITORS OF GROWTH FACTOR SIGNALING

Signaling by the ErbB family of receptors promotes tumor cell proliferation in most instances (23,24). Both receptor expression and autocrine growth factor levels are often increased in tumor cells compared with normal tissue, prompting efforts to inhibit signaling by these receptors. Indeed, blocking the activation and signaling of ErbB receptors has been demonstrated to retard tumor cell growth and render the cells more susceptible to various toxic stresses,

including radiation. Successful methods of inhibiting ErbB receptors include the use of inhibitory antibodies, small-molecular-weight inhibitors of receptor tyrosine kinases, dominant negative truncated receptors without a functional intracellular domain, or antisense approaches (25).

The antibody cetuximab (Erbitux), also called C225, binds to the extracellular portion of EGFR that associates with growth factor ligands such as EGF and TGFα (26), thus abolishing the ability of these ligands to activate EGFR. However, cetuximab does not block the primary activation of the receptor or MAPK by radiation, in general agreement with the ligand-independent nature of this latter process. Furthermore, it is unclear whether the antitumor effects of anti-ErbB receptor antibodies are mediated solely via receptor inhibition or are augmented by other immunologic mechanisms generated by the antibody. Small-molecule tyrosine kinase inhibitors such as ZD1839 (gefitinib; Iressa) bind to the intracellular domain of EGFR and block EGFR signaling, thereby slowing tumor cell growth and potentially enhancing the efficacy of radiotherapy (27).

## DOWNSTREAM CYTOPLASMIC SIGNALING PATHWAYS

Two examples of the multitude of downstream, primarily cytoplasmic, signaling pathways set in motion by ionizing radiation include the PI3K and aforementioned MAPK

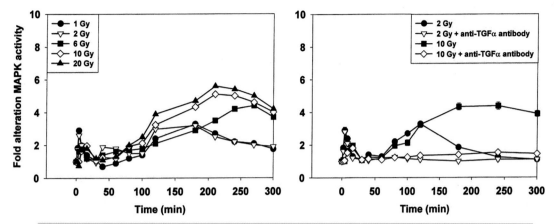

**FIGURE 2.2.** Increasing doses of radiation cause a dose-dependent increase in the secondary activation of mitogen activated protein kinase (MAPK): dependence on radiation-stimulated cleavage and release of transforming growth factor alpha (TGFα). In the experiments represented, A431 squamous carcinoma cells were treated 30 minutes before irradiation with no antibody **(A)**, control antibody, or neutralizing anti-TGFα antibody **(B)**. Cells were exposed to increasing doses of radiation (2–20 Gy). At the indicated times, media were aspirated after radiation exposure. MAPK activity was determined as fold increases relative to activity in control conditions at time = zero. Inhibition of secondary MAPK activation by anti-TGFα antibody indicates the role of TGFα in this process. (From Dent P, Reardon DB, Park JS, et al. Radiation-induced activations of the epidermal growth factor receptor and the mitogen activated protein kinase pathway via transforming growth factor a in autocrine-regulated carcinoma cells. *Mol Biol Cell* 1999;10:2493–2506, with permission.)

pathways. The PI3K pathway, which includes the key downstream target Akt kinase, inhibits apoptosis. Inhibitors of ErbB signaling have been shown to decrease the activity of the PI3K/Akt pathway in a variety of cell types and thus increase the sensitivity of cells to radiation (28). Direct inhibition of PI3K function can radiosensitize tumor cells in certain conditions (29–31).

Radiation-induced activation of the MAPK pathway can also serve to protect the tumor cell. However, there can be paradoxic radiosensitizing effects in certain cell types. An illustrative example of this dual nature of MAPK signaling is the DU145 human prostate cancer cell line. In these cells, progression through the $G_2/M$ cell cycle checkpoint is linked to MAPK signaling. If MAPK signaling is *transiently* blocked prior to irradiation, the expected temporary radiation-induced $G_2/M$ is increased and a radioprotective effect is observed, perhaps from increased DNA damage repair during the cell cycle arrest. On the other hand, *prolonged* inhibition of MAPK *following* irradiation increases the apoptotic response and reduces clonogenic survival (22,32). Therefore, the interruption of MAPK signaling can either enhance or degrade DU145 cell survival depending on its timing and duration. The key point in relation to SBRT is that when the use of agents that disrupt intracellular signaling is considered as a means of potentiating SBRT, there must be a careful evaluation of the proper sequencing and integration of these agents into the overall treatment schedule to maximize additive and synergistic therapeutic effects.

## REFERENCES

1. Khazaie K, Schirrmacher V, Lichtner RB. EGF receptor in neoplasia and metastasis. *Cancer Metastasis Rev* 1993;12:255–274.
2. Zhang K, Sun S, Liu N, et al. Transformation of NIH 3T3 cells by HER3 or HER4 receptors requires the presence of HER1 or HER2. *J Biol Chem* 1996;271:3884–3890.
3. Hsuan JJ, Panayotou G, Waterfield MD. Structural basis for epidermal growth factor receptor function. *Prog Growth Factor Res* 1989;1:23–32.
4. Huang GC, Ouyang X, Epstein RJ. Proxy activation of protein ErbB2 by heterologous ligands implies a heterotetrameric mode of receptor tyrosine kinase interaction. *Biochem J* 1998; 331:113–119.
5. Qian X, LeVea M, Freeman JK, et al. Heterodimerization of epidermal growth factor receptor and wild-type or kinase-deficient Neu: a mechanism of interreceptor kinase activation and transphosphorylation. *Proc Natl Acad Sci USA* 1994;91:1500–1504.
6. Azios NG, Romero FJ, Denton MC, et al. Expression of herstatin, an autoinhibitor of HER-2/neu, inhibits transactivation of HER-3 by HER-2 and blocks EGF activation of the EGF receptor. *Oncogene* 2001;20:5199–5209.
7. Tzahar G, Levkowitz D, Karunagaran L, et al. ErbB-3 and ErbB-4 function as the respective low and high affinity receptors of all Neu differentiation factor/heregulin isoforms. *J Biol Chem* 1994;269: 25226–25233.
8. Offterdinger M, Schneider SM, Huber H, et al. Expression of c-erbB-4/HER4 is regulated in T47D breast carcinoma cells by retinoids and vitamin D3. *Biochem Biophys Res Commun* 1990;258:559–564.
9. Yoo JY, Hamburger AW. The use of the yeast two hybrid system to evaluate ErbB-3 interactions with SH2 domain containing proteins. *Biochem Biophys Res Commun* 1998;251:903–906.
10. Schmidt-Ullrich RK, Mikkelsen RB, Dent P, et al. Radiation-induced proliferation of the human A431 squamous carcinoma cells is dependent on EGFR tyrosine phosphorylation. *Oncogene* 1997;15: 1191–1197.
11. Kavanagh BD, Dent P, Schmidt-Ullrich RK, et al. Calcium-dependent stimulation of mitogen-activated protein kinase activity in A431 cells by low doses of ionizing radiation. *Radiat Res* 1998;149: 579–587.

12. Mothersill C, Seymour CB, Joiner MC. Relationship between radiation-induced low-dose hypersensitivity and the bystander effect. *Radiat Res* 2002;157:526–532.
13. Wu J, Harrison JK, Dent P, et al. Identification and characterization of a new mammalian mitogen-activated protein kinase kinase, MKK2. *Mol Cell Biol* 1993;13:4539–4548.
14. Kyriakis J, App H, Zhang XF, et al. Raf-1 activates MAP kinase-kinase. *Nature* 1992;358:417–421.
15. Dent P, Haser W, Haystead TA, et al. Activation of mitogen-activated protein kinase kinase by v-Raf in NIH 3T3 cells and in vitro. *Science* 1992;257:1404–1407.
16. Leach JK, Van Tuyle G, Lin PS, et al. Ionizing radiation-induced, mitochondria-dependent generation of reactive oxygen/nitrogen. *Cancer Res* 2001;61:3894–3901.
17. Leach JK, Black SM, Schmidt-Ullrich RK, et al. Activation of constitutive nitric-oxide synthase activity is an early signaling event induced by ionizing radiation. *J Biol Chem* 2002;277:15400–15406.
18. Dent P, Yacoub A, Fisher PB, et al. MAPK pathways in radiation responses. *Oncogene* 2003;22:5885–5896.
19. Dent P, Reardon DB, Park JS, et al. Radiation-induced activations of the epidermal growth factor receptor and the mitogen activated protein kinase pathway via transforming growth factor a in autocrine-regulated carcinoma cells. *Mol Biol Cell* 1999;10:2493–2506.
20. Hagan M, Wang L, Hanley JR, et al. Ionizing radiation-induced mitogen-activated protein (MAP) kinase activation in DU145 prostate carcinoma cells: MAP kinase inhibition enhances radiation-induced cell killing and G2/M-phase arrest. *Radiation Res* 2000;153:371–381.
21. Bowers G, Reardon D, Hewitt T, et al. The relative role of ErbB1-4 receptor tyrosine kinases in radiation signal transduction responses of human carcinoma cells. *Oncogene* 2001;20:1388–1397.
22. Contessa JN, Hampton J, Lammering G, et al. Ionizing radiation activates Erb-B receptor dependent Akt and p70 S6 kinase signaling in carcinoma cells. *Oncogene* 2002;21:4032–4041.
23. Grant S, Qiao L, Dent P. Roles of ERBB family receptor tyrosine kinases, and downstream signaling pathways, in the control of cell growth and survival. *Front Biosci* 2002;7:376–389.
24. Schmidt-Ullrich RK, Dent P, Grant S, et al. Signal transduction and cellular radiation responses. *Radiat Res* 2000;153:245–257.
25. Dent P, Yacoub A, Contessa J, et al. Stress and radiation-induced activation of multiple intracellular signaling pathways. *Radiat Res* 2003;159:283–300.
26. Herbst RS, Langer CJ. Epidermal growth factor receptors as a target for cancer treatment: the emerging role of IMC-C225 in the treatment of lung and head and neck cancers. *Semin Oncol* 2002;29:27–36.
27. Raben D, Helfrich BA, Chan D, et al. ZD1839, a selective epidermal growth factor receptor tyrosine kinase inhibitor, alone and in combination with radiation and chemotherapy as a new therapeutic strategy in non-small cell lung cancer. *Semin Oncol* 2002;29[Suppl 4]:37–46.
28. Pianetti S, Arsura M, Romieu-Mourez R, et al. Her-2/neu overexpression induces NF-kappaB via a PI3-kinase/Akt pathway involving calpain-mediated degradation of IkappaB-alpha that can be inhibited by the tumor suppressor PTEN. *Oncogene* 2001;20:1287–1299.
29. Gupta AK, Bakanauskas VJ, Cerniglia CJ, et al. The Ras radiation resistance pathway. *Cancer Res* 2001;61:4278–4782.
30. Gupta AK, McKenna WG, Weber CN, et al. Local recurrence in head and neck cancer: relationship to radiation resistance and signal transduction. *Clin Cancer Res* 2002;8:885–892.
31. Gupta AK, Bernhard EJ, Bakanauskas VJ, et al. RAS-Mediated radiation resistance is not linked to MAP kinase activation in two bladder carcinoma cell lines. *Radiat Res* 2000;154:64–72.
32. Yacoub A, Park JS, Qiao L, et al. MAPK dependence of DNA damage repair: ionizing radiation and the induction of expression of the DNA repair genes XRCC1 and ERCC1 in DU145 human prostate carcinoma cells in a MEK1/2 dependent fashion. *Int J Radiat Biol* 2001;77:1067–1078.

# Radiation Effects and the Role of Cytokines: Mechanisms and Potential Clinical Implications

*Paul Okunieff*

Radiation consequences in normal tissue are commonly divided, temporally and biologically, into early and late effects. While this is a clinically useful distinction, the separation of effects is artificial. The immediate biologic consequences of radiation necessarily arise from the initial exposure of tissues to the irradiation per se. The progression of radiation effects over time is due to a variety of cellular, tissue, and host factors. This statement, once controversial, implies that late consequences of radiation are not inevitable since they are not an immediate consequence of the radiation injury.

The indirect consequences of radiation are moderated in large part by signal proteins called cytokines. They are a diverse group of proteins that induce necrosis, apoptosis, inflammation, proliferation, and stem cell differentiation. Cytokines are produced within the irradiated field and released by irradiated tissues; they stimulate other cells to produce a biologic response by binding to receptors on cells within the same tissues (paracrine response) and by entering the circulation to stimulate cells that are distant from the field of irradiation (endocrine response). They can cause proliferation and also increase cell cycle arrest, and they can promote or inhibit inflammation. Examples of radiation-induced cytokines include tumor necrosis factor (TNF), interleukin-1 (IL-1), and stem cell factor (1,2).

Fibrosis is a late sequela of radiation therapy that occurs in many normal tissues within the field of irradiation. The tissues in which fibrosis has been noted to produce the greatest degree of pathology include the lung, liver, and skin. While the mechanism of fibrosis is not completely understood, it is believed to be mediated by the cascade of cytokines released as part of the inflammatory response. Ultimately, chronic elevation of TGFβ precipitates fibrosis (3,4).

In this chapter, we will review the basic mechanisms of radiation response, presenting our current understanding of the process by which radiation effects progress over time during the hours, days, weeks, and years following exposure. We will emphasize the role that cytokines appear to play in the early and late processes after irradiation of normal and, to a lesser extent, tumor tissue. We will divide these mechanisms into three major categories: (a) biologic basis of radiation toxicity and direct, radiation-induced damage; (b) apoptotic and growth factor–related signaling processes important in the production of tumor and normal tissue responses; (c) cytokine-mediated inflammatory processes that begin during the early phase of toxicity and persist chronically. All three mechanisms interact and must be understood in the context in which they are expressed: Tissues that have specific intercellular interactions and specific physiologic responsibilities toward the health of the host.

## BIOLOGIC BASIS OF RADIATION-INDUCED TOXICITY

Ionizing radiation interacts with $H_2O$, and, to a lesser extent, with lipids, proteins, or DNA within cells to generate reactive oxygen species (ROS)—often more correctly termed "reactive radical intermediates" since many of the reactive pathways include nonoxygen-related steps (5). The incremental increase in concentration of ROS induced by radiation compared with that already present is small. Thus, it is assumed that radiation-induced ROS are produced in microregions within the cell that are expediently protected from chemical exposure by antioxidant scavenging. The nucleus, or perhaps just the DNA itself, is likely one of those "microregions."

Department of Radiation Oncology, University of Rochester School of Medicine and Dentistry, Rochester, NY 14642

## Contrasting Mechanisms of Cell Inactivation: Reproductive Sterilization versus Apoptosis

DNA damage from radiation is quantitatively predictable: a 1-Gy dose of radiation delivers 1 J of ionization to 1 kg of irradiated mass. For diploid DNA and low, linear energy transfer (LET) radiation, this amount of ionization results in approximately 20 to 40 DNA double-strand breaks per cell and a 100- to 500-fold higher level of single-strand breaks. Classical experiments have demonstrated that most cell "deaths" observed after radiation are due to double-strand DNA damage (6–8). In these studies, death is measured by clonogenic survival rather than metabolic dysfunction. This effect is called sterilization and can occur without metabolic cell death.

Another effect commonly initiated by DNA damage is apoptosis, which is an active process of cell deletion requiring complex cell signaling. Most cells do not undergo apoptosis even after very high radiation doses, and thus, cells and tissues that are not prone to divide, and those that do not undergo substantial apoptosis in response to irradiation are presumed to be protected from significant radiation toxicity (Fig. 3.1). It is critical to keep the relative impact of apoptosis and reproductive sterilization in mind when thinking about developing therapies with differential effects on tumor and normal tissue. Of note, cytokines have a powerful effect on apoptosis and can thus be manipulated to alter tumor and normal tissue toxicity at early and late time points following irradiation (9,10).

## Role of Stem Cells

Loss of stem and progenitor cells also contributes to the temporal progression of radiation effects in tumor and normal tissue. In this context, we define stem cells as being pleuripotent, whereas progenitor cells are committed cells that proliferate. Tumor cells might be considered in the second category. Phenotypic expression of toxicity in these cell populations is delayed until the cells are called upon to proliferate, perhaps after surgery or chemotherapy. Thus, the delay observed in "late-reacting" tissues is due, in part, to the natural loss of progenitor cells that occurs over the lifetime of the host, though more rapidly in irradiated tissue.

Maintaining stem cells can be accomplished by altering the cytokine exposure of cells. Furthermore, replacement of progenitor cells, when possible, results in improved radiation tolerance. The obvious example for this is bone marrow transplantation, wherein lethal toxicity is easily prevented by infusion of bone marrow stem cells. It is reasonable to assume that, eventually, mucosal, cutaneous, endothelial, astrocytic, and mesenchymal progenitor cells might be identified and similarly reimplanted in irradiated patients. Growing these progenitors for ulti-

mate transplantation should be possible with appropriate cytokine stimulation (11–13).

Reproductive damage and cellular depopulation of reproducing cells account in part for the observation of a "volume effect" seen in patients treated with radiation. The severity of cell loss is mitigated by shrinking the field size exposed to radiation, thereby allowing the functional reproducing cells and tissues that surround the damaged volume to help with repopulation. While shrinking field size does not, dose for dose, decrease the damage to the individual irradiated cells (hence the tumor is still controlled), it does affect the tissue's ability to repair itself, and it significantly affects the organ's ability to maintain function. Improved delivery techniques and better tumor localization continue to make some of the greatest modern improvements we have seen in preventing normal tissue toxicity.

## APOPTOTIC AND GROWTH FACTOR–RELATED SIGNALING PROCESSES IMPORTANT IN THE PRODUCTION OF TUMOR AND NORMAL TISSUE RESPONSES

While DNA is the major target responsible for reproductive inactivation of cells, there are also a number of other signals that occur following irradiation that can affect tumor and normal tissue response to irradiation. Many components of postradiation tissue damage are mediated through ROS-induced signal responses. In particular, ROS can react with cellular lipids, which are the main components of the membrane of the nucleus, cytoplasm, and intracellular organelles. The interaction of ROS with fatty acids within the cell membrane leads to oxidization, and the oxidized lipids are then hydrolyzed by a number of enzymes within the cell membrane (14,15). These enzymes generate products termed "second messengers" that activate a cascade of enzymes within the cytoplasm. The cascade of enzymes typically includes kinases that phosphorylate, as well as other proteins such as transcription factors or inhibitors of transcription factors. Transcription factors are proteins that can either up- or down-regulate gene expression.

As mentioned previously, ROS can induce factors that precipitate apoptosis, the active process of programmed cell death that occurs in many tissues. Apoptosis appears to account for only a minority of cell death in most adult solid tumors following radiation; however, the excellent responses of some pediatric, hematopoietic, and germ cell tumors are often ascribed to this phenomenon (16). Therefore, promoting apoptosis in irradiated tumors has been an area of active research.

As discussed in the previous sections, however, apoptosis definitely contributes to worsening normal tissue toxicity. Indeed, modification of apoptosis may not im-

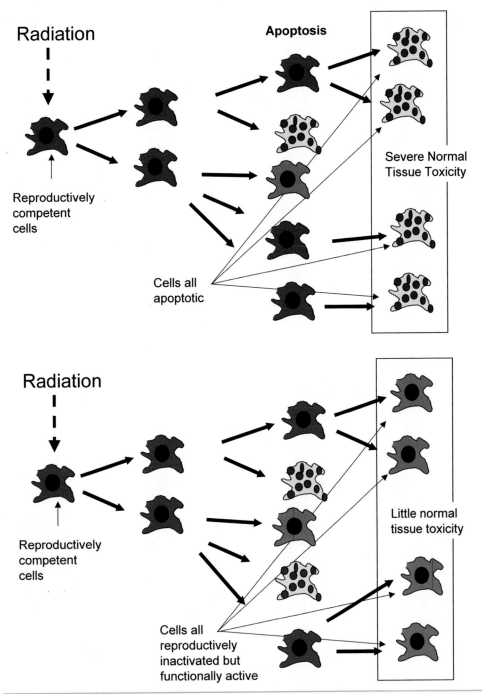

**FIGURE 3.1.** Following irradiation, reproductively competent cells can undergo several cell divisions before progeny undergo a metabolic death. Divisions can be very aberrant, including trifurcations. The aberrant segregation of DNA at each division, however, ultimately results in progeny not receiving a full complement of DNA. Thus, at any given division one or more progeny might not survive. In the case of tumor, the goal is to achieve this reproductive sterilization in all reproductively competent cells. For successful treatment, it is sufficient for cells to undergo only reproductive sterilization and not apoptosis. If tumor cells undergo apoptosis, there can be a complete or partial response. Complete and partial responses are desirable but are not always sufficient for permanent tumor control. If apoptosis occurs in normal tissues, there can be sudden loss of organ function (e.g. mucosal disruption) leading to clinical toxicity (*top*). In the case of normal tissues, therefore, reproductive sterilization alone can lead to less toxicity than apoptosis since cellular metabolic function is preserved. Conveniently, contrary to intuition, most normal tissues have regulation of their apoptosis. Thus, chemotherapy can be given safely without massive apoptosis of the brain, lung, heart, liver, but commonly with impressive apoptosis of tumor cells.

prove therapeutic gain (the ratio of tumor response to normal tissue toxicity) because tumor cells that are already reproductively inactivated due to DNA damage cannot be "killed" a second time by apoptosis. Rather, only their mode of death can be altered. In contrast, nonproliferating normal tissue cells could continue to perform their functions indefinitely unless they are forced to undergo apoptosis.

In the category of treatments aimed at improving apoptosis of tumor following irradiation, the commonly mutated tumor suppressor protein p53 has been a major target. Drugs that correct the p53 signal pathway, block the cell-cycle inhibitor p21, or more directly affect potentially cytoprotective tyrosine kinase activity have been evaluated in clinical trials. Tumors that have transformed from a low grade to a higher grade, for example, frequently have abnormal p53 function. Likewise, in tumors that recur following irradiation, p53 mutations may be more common; however, it has been very difficult to evaluate the degree to which p53 affects radiation response. In genetically defined *in vitro* tumor models, p53 can decrease and increase intrinsic radiation response (9,17,18). Restoring normal p53 function should signal tumors with abnormal DNA to spontaneously undergo apoptosis.

The role of apoptotic induction as a component of combined-modality therapeutic strategies has been contested. Clinical data to date that have featured apoptosis-modifying drugs in combination with radiation are mostly negative, and, in some cases, toxicity has been seen [e.g., interferon (19,20), and tyrosine kinase inhibitors (21)]. We await the findings of current studies on promising new agents (22).

A few drugs that have been very successful in the clinic appear to work by blocking cytokines and therefore predisposing cells to apoptosis. The most important of these is trastuzumab (Herceptin). For women with breast cancer that expresses her-2, a growth factor receptor in the epidermal growth factor (EGF) family, suppression of the receptor by this blocking antibody can precipitate apoptosis. It remains unclear whether radiation acts synergistically with growth factor blocking agents. Both animal and clinical studies are very encouraging; for example, Kunala and Macklis (23) found that CD20 antibodies can produce dramatic tumor responses (24). As treatments move forward with antibodies and drugs that block growth factors or induce apoptosis, it is expected that concurrent or sequential radiotherapy will play a large role.

## Radiation-induced Effects on Blood Vessels

All tissues are dependent on blood flow for nutrition and maintenance of homeostasis. The effects of radiation on blood vessels, therefore, are important moderators of all normal tissue radiation responses. Studies have indicated that vascular radiation response begins with oxidative

damage of the endothelium (15). The endothelium responds with endothelial cell loss and the induction of compensatory mechanisms to maintain homeostasis. Indeed, apoptosis of capillary endothelial cells appears to occur very soon after irradiation in many organs, including the bowel and lung (25,26). Some investigators have proposed that the apoptosis of endothelium triggers apoptosis of the parenchymal cells in these organs (27). The homeostatic mechanisms reducing the impact of vascular toxicity focus on preserving the barrier function in blood vessels (28,29). The mechanism by which radiation activates these homeostatic responses is, in part, through the expression of cell adhesion molecules and the induction of a procoagulative state. Radiation also leads to the expression of a host of other signaling proteins, whose downstream effects include a long-lasting suppression of angiogenesis in irradiated tissue (30–34).

The long-term homeostatic cost of irradiating normal vasculature includes persistent vascular dysfunction and/or a chronic proinflammatory condition (Fig. 3.2). This subclinical damage can precipitate early atherosclerotic disease, telangiectasia, or thromboembolic disease. All of these progressive effects are controlled by cytokines. Thus, endothelial damage, inflammation, fibroblast pro-

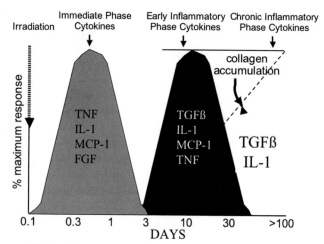

NORMAL TISSUE EFFECTS OF HIGH DOSE RADIATION

**FIGURE 3.2.** Cytokines are important modulators of radiation toxicity. The balance of cytokines produced during the various periods after irradiation determines the severity of radiation toxicity. Immediately after irradiation, a number of cytokines are produced and maintained for a period of hours. Some of these cytokines are probably produced to offset the toxic effects of radiation. Some can recruit mononuclear cells into the irradiated volume. Some can signal stem cells to proliferate or mature. The early inflammatory phase of radiation toxicity begins a few days after irradiation and continues for approximately a month. The chronic progression of radiation damage over time is also augmented by inflammatory responses controlled by cytokines. Ultimately, collagen accumulation and fibrovascular accumulation are common. The latter are probably under the control of TGFβ.

liferation, thrombosis, and so forth can be managed by adjusting expression or responsiveness to various signaling molecules.

## GROWTH FACTORS

Growth factors are a class of cytokines that cause proliferation. Growth factors often only affect specific classes of cells that express the appropriate receptors. They control proliferation and manage differentiation of progeny cells.

### Acidic and Basic Fibroblast Growth Factors

The first angiogenic factors discovered were acidic and basic fibroblast growth factors (aFGF, bFGF, respectively), now designated FGF1 and FGF2. There are at least 14 members of the fibroblast growth factor family. Angiogenic factors are proving to be critically important modifiers of radiation response. They can inhibit radiation-induced apoptosis and improve radiation-induced DNA repair. Perhaps more important, they can prevent radiation-induced bone marrow death following whole-body irradiation (35) and gastrointestinal death (36,37). The most powerful angiogenic cytokines implicated in the radioprotective process come from the FGF family, and the most efficacious for the protection of normal tissues and inhibition of radiation-induced apoptosis appears to be basic fibroblast growth factor (FGF2) (25). Acidic fibroblast growth factor (FGF1) and keratinocyte growth factors appear to be important as well. In addition to the prevention of acute toxicities of radiation, they also appear to be able to downregulate late complications of radiation such as bone growth retardation (38). The mechanism for radiation protection by angiogenic cytokines is unclear, but it is tempting to suggest that they interfere with the apoptotic processes. FGFs protect normal tissues when given before radiation and still provide benefit when given after radiation. While there is substantial concern that these factors can also promote tumor growth, tumor resistance to therapy, and tumor metastases, low dose and brief exposure might be sufficient to protect normal tissues and not affect tumors (39).

### Keratinocyte Growth Factors

The keratinocyte growth factors (KGF1, KGF2) are in the FGF family and are designated FGF7 and FGF10, respectively. They are distinguished from other members of the family in that their receptors are on epithelial cells rather than mesenchymal cells. Moreover, numerous studies (36,37) have failed to demonstrate that KGFs protect tumor from the effects of radiation *in vivo* or *in vitro*. Furthermore, KGF1 and KGF2 have both been shown to pro-

tect bowel from radiation effects (37). The mechanism is multifactorial and includes mucosal thickening and hypertrophy. It also includes suppression of apoptosis of crypt cells and perhaps an expansion of the stem cells of the small bowel. KGFs also have a small radioprotective effect against bone marrow as determined by whole body LD50/30 studies. KGFs work additively with other growth factors, suggesting that cytokine combinations might be an optimal clinical approach to cytokine therapy.

### Vascular Endothelial Growth Factor

Vascular endothelial growth factor (VEGF) is a growth factor that increases in response to hypoxia and causes relatively specific proliferation of endothelial cells. VEGF has some other effects, including induction of vascular leakage (40). It is a component, perhaps a major component, of vasogenic edema in the brain after irradiation (40). Like the FGFs, it has some protective effects against crypt loss in the small bowel, and it increases the whole-body LD50/7. Its radioprotective effects, however, are less pronounced than those of the FGFs. Many aggressive tumors produce VEGF, and tumors can be made less chemotherapy-responsive by transfection with VEGF (41). The new drugs being developed to suppress VEGF signaling might prove most intriguing for combination with radiation for brain tumors.

### Erythropoietin

Erythropoietin (Epo) stimulates bone marrow to produce erythroblasts. It has anti-apoptotic effects on irradiated blood vessels. Epo is commonly given to patients with anemia and cancer. The increase in hemoglobin parallels an improvement of energy and decrease in fatigue. Epo alters neither the radiation response of skin, nor the LD50/30 (42, Okunieff P, unpublished data, May, 1995). Recently there has been concerning evidence that Epo increases metastases formation (43). Early results of randomized clinical trials involving the combination of radiation and Epo for solid tumors have suggested a possible adverse interaction, and a role for Epo given in combination with radiotherapy has not been established.

### Granulocyte Growth Factors

Granulocyte growth factors [granulocyte colony-stimulating factor (GCSF) and granulocyte-macrophage colony-stimulating factor (GMCSF)] are used clinically to improve recovery after chemotherapy. While *in vitro* they can stimulate growth of tumor cells (44), there is little if any evidence that clinically they affect rates of recurrence of hematopoietic tumors in humans. Their effects on radiation response are more modest. There is probably some improvement in LD50/30, but the benefit is most evident when this drug is given in combination with other growth factors (45). These drugs, although weak, are among the very few treatments available for either radiation sickness or other radiation-induced toxicity (46).

## Epidermal Growth Factor

EGF was discussed in Chapter 2. It is probably involved in the accelerated repopulation of tumor that can occur after insufficient or prolonged course-radiation. There is evidence in a number of models that blocking EGF improves tumor response to irradiation (47,48). There is little evidence of an increase in toxicity, thus agents that block EGF signaling may ultimately be beneficial.

## INFLAMMATORY FACTORS

Inflammatory factors mediate a wide range of effects in normal and malignant tissue (Fig. 3.3). Several important examples are discussed here.

## Tumor Necrosis Factor

TNF, also termed "cachexin," is a cytokine that is released by leukocytes and tumor cells following exposure to ionizing radiation (1,14). The role of TNF is complex. It probably improves tumor response to irradiation and is therefore the subject of some experimental gene therapies (22). It probably also worsens normal tissue toxicity; however,

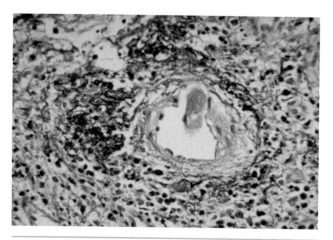

**FIGURE 3.3.** Pulmonary artery in a lobectomy specimen removed 3 months after 60 Gy. A macrophage stain (*black*) and collagen stain (*red*) are shown. A platelet clot is seen attached to the exposed arterial basement membrane. The endothelial cells are atypical and hypertrophic. The picture is one of proliferation rather than cell depopulation. The proliferating inflammatory cells were therefore recruited to the irradiated volume by cell signaling phenomena in the tissues that were damaged by the irradiation. The entire process is governed by a cascade of cytokines.

its effects have yet to be fully elucidated. TNF binds to its receptor on leukocytes and endothelial cells to activate the inflammatory response (49). TNF causes tumor cells, normal epithelial cells, and endothelial cells to undergo apoptosis, and that effect is at least additive to apoptosis caused by radiation alone. TNF also plays a role in the paraneoplastic anorexia and weight loss that occurs in patients with cancer (50). TNF has been proposed to play a role in radiation-induced pneumonitis and subsequent pulmonary fibrosis (3,51).

## Interleukin-1

The radiation-induced expression of IL-1 has been demonstrated in a number of studies (2). This was the first cytokine studied in combination with radiation, in the pioneering work by Neta et al. (45). IL-1 may be the most important cytokine governing toxicity after irradiation. There are two main isoforms of IL-1: the α form appears to be most important for late effects in the lung, while the β isoform is important as an initial response of most nonhematopoietic cells to irradiation including lung, brain, and skin. There are two main IL-1 receptors. Receptor IL-1R1 is active, while the IL-1R2 receptor has no kinase activity and is therefore a decoy. There is also an important natural competitive receptor blocker termed "IL-1Ra" that binds IL-1R1 but not IL-1R2. IL-1Ra does not cause kinase activity by IL-1R1.

The positive and negative balance of IL-1 signal pathways probably influences the severity of both early and late reactions to irradiation in a number of tissues. The *in vivo* expression of the IL-1β gene is dependent on the dose and timing of radiation. Expression of IL-1 corresponds to the level of fibrosis seen months after mouse irradiation. Chen et al. (52) have shown that IL-1 levels in the blood of patients undergoing chest irradiation is a powerful predictor of patients at risk for subsequent pneumonitis. Thus, the predisposition to develop some inflammatory toxicities after irradiation may be predicted by IL-1 levels, and blockage of IL-1 using drugs like IL-1Ra may prevent toxicities. IL-1 may or may not alter tumor response; this question has not yet been sufficiently studied (53).

## Transforming Growth Factor Beta

One of the well-characterized mechanisms of fibrosis is through the induction of the gene encoding transforming growth factor beta (TGFβ). TGFβ is a proliferative cytokine associated with radiation-mediated injury to the lung and liver (54–56). TGFβ biology is exceptionally complex; there are many isoforms, with the β1 form being the most heavily studied. TGFβ can suppress growth of several epithelial cancers including breast cancers. Interestingly, it can also suppress inflammation even though it promotes fibrosis. It causes maturation of fibroblasts but also proliferation of fibroblasts.

The actions of TGFβ are mediated by intracellular factors called SMADs. Several SMADs (e.g., SMAD6 and SMAD7) inhibit TGFβ signals and others are critical for TGFβ signaling (SMAD3). TGFβ is secreted and accumulates in the extracellular matrix in an inactive form. Activation occurs when the latent peptide is removed by oxidation of the disulphide bond connecting it to the active protein. TGFβ levels in platelets are orders of magnitude higher than what is found in blood and help platelets to coagulate. Thus, serum TGFβ levels are much higher than plasma levels.

In laboratory animals, levels of TGFβ were found to be elevated after lung irradiation (3). Similar changes in TGFβ are seen in the skin after irradiation. Inhibitors of TGFβ are being developed in part because inhibition of its fibrotic properties might prevent over-exuberant scarring following trauma and surgery, and not just after irradiation.

## CONCLUSION

A number of cytokines and growth factors have been demonstrated to participate in radiation-induced toxicity (Table 3.1). IL-1, TGFβ, and TNF are important examples. Growth factors are radiation-inducible, as are apoptotic factors. Single-dose radiation causes a different sequence of factor production than does fractionated radiation. Host effects prominently alter cytokine responses in unpredictable ways. Markers from serum and tumor and of host genetic origin are being identified. Ultimately, using simple combinations of cytokine-modifying drugs, we should be able to improve tumor response and prevent many severe late treatment sequelae.

▶ **TABLE 3.1** Cytokines.

| Cytokines Generally Considered To: | |
|---|---|
| *Benefit Normal Tissue Radiation Response* | *Increase Normal Tissue Toxicity* |
| GCSF, FGFs, KGFs, Epo, SCF, ?VEGF | TGFβ, IL-1, IL-2, TNF, IFN, ?VEGF |
| *Increase Tumor Radiation Sensitivity* | *Increase Tumor Growth or Metastasis* |
| IL-2, TNF, IFN | EGF, FGFs, VEGF, IL-1?, GCSF?, Epo? |

GCSF, granulocyte colony-stimulating factor; FGF, fibroblast growth factor; VEGF, vascular endothelial growth factor; IL-1, interleukin-1; KGF, keratinocyte growth factor; SCF, stem cell factor; TNF, tumor necrosis factor; TGF, transforming growth factor; Epo, erythropoietin; IFN, interferon.
This table is a general summary of data from cell culture, *in vivo* animal models, and clinical studies. Our understanding of the role that cytokines play is constantly evolving. Likewise, the effects of various cytokines vary between tumor histologies, normal organs, and animal strains. As can be seen in the table, many cytokines have both beneficial and deleterious effects. For more information on the various cytokines, the reader may refer to articles in the reference list.

## REFERENCES
### Introduction

1. Hallahan DE, Spriggs DR, Beckett MA, et al. Increased tumor necrosis factor alpha mRNA after cellular exposure to ionizing radiation. *Proc Natl Acad Sci USA* 1989;86(24):10104–10107.
2. Linard C, Marquette C, Mathieu J, et al. Acute induction of inflammatory cytokine expression after gamma-irradiation in the rat: effect of an NF-kappaB inhibitor. *Int J Radiat Oncol Biol Phys* 2004;58:427–434.
3. Rubin P, Johnston CJ, Williams JP, et al. A perpetual cascade of cytokines postirradiation leads to pulmonary fibrosis. *Int J Radiat Oncol Biol Phys* 1995;33:99–109.
4. Anscher MS, Kong FM, Murase T, et al. Short communication: normal tissue injury after cancer therapy is a local response exacerbated by an endocrine effect of TGF beta. *Br J Radiol* 1995;68:331–333.

### Biologic Basis of Radiation-induced Toxicity

5. Hill RP. Cellular basis for radiotherapy. In: Tannock IF, and Hill RP, eds. *The basic science of oncology.* New York: Pergammon Press, 1987:237–255.

### Contrasting Mechanisms of Cell Inactivation: Reproductive Sterilization Versus Apoptosis

6. Painter RB. Chemical changes induced by DNA by ionizing radiation and the relationship of their repair to survival of mammalian cells. In: Nygaard OF, Adler EF, Sinclair WK, eds. *Proceedings of the Fifth International Congress of Radiation Research. Seattle, July 14–20 1974.* New York: Academic Press, 1975:735–739.
7. Painter RB. The role of DNA damage and repair in cell killing induced by ionizing radiation. In: Meyn RE, Withers HR, eds. *Radiation biology in cancer research.* New York: Raven Press, 1980: 59–70.
8. Munro TR. The relative radiosensitivity of the nucleus and cytoplasm of Chinese hamster fibroblasts. *Radiat Res* 1970;42: 451–470.
9. Belka C, Jendrossek V, Pruschy M, et al. Apoptosis-modulating agents in combination with radiotherapy: current status and outlook. *Int J Radiat Oncol Biol Phys* 2004;58:542–554.
10. Younes A, Kadin ME. Emerging applications of the tumor necrosis factor family of ligands and receptors in cancer therapy. *J Clin Oncol* 2003;21:3526–3534.

### The Role of Stem Cells

11. Noble M, Dietrich J. Intersections between neurobiology and oncology: tumor origin, treatment and repair of treatment-associated damage. *Trends Neurosci* 2002;25:103–107.
12. Noble M. Can neural stem cells be used to track down and destroy migratory brain tumor cells while also providing a means of repairing tumor-associated damage? *Proc Natl Acad Sci USA* 2000;97: 12393–12395.
13. Quesenberry PJ, Stewart FM, Becker P, et al. Stem cell engraftment strategies. *Ann N Y Acad Sci* 2001;938:54–61.

### Apoptotic and Growth Factor Related Signaling Processes Important in the Production of Tumor and Normal Tissue Responses

14. Hallahan DE, Virudachalam S, Kuchibhotla J, et al. Membrane-derived second messenger regulates x-ray-mediated tumor necrosis factor alpha gene induction. *Proc Natl Acad Sci USA* 1994;91: 4897–4901.
15. Haimovitz-Friedman A, Kan CC, Ehleiter D, et al. Ionizing radiation acts on cellular membranes to generate ceramide and initiate apoptosis. *J Exp Med* 1994;180:525–535.

16. Rosen EM, Fan S, Rockwell S, et al. The molecular and cellular basis of radiosensitivity: implications for understanding how normal tissues and tumors respond to therapeutic radiation. *Cancer Invest* 1999;17910:56–72.
17. Scott SL, Earle JD, Gumerlock PH. Functional p53 increases prostate cancer cell survival after exposure to fractionated doses of ionizing radiation. *Cancer Res* 2003;63:7190–7196.
18. El Deiry WS. The role of p53 in chemosensitivity and radiosensitivity. *Oncogene* 2003;22:7486–7495.
19. McDonald S, Chang AY, Rubin P, et al. Combined Betaseron R (recombinant human interferon beta) and radiation for inoperable non-small cell lung cancer. *Int J Radiat Oncol Biol Phys* 1993; 27:613–619.
20. Bradley JD, Scott CB, Paris KJ, et al. A phase III comparison of radiation therapy with or without recombinant beta-interferon for poor-risk patients with locally advanced non-small-cell lung cancer (RTOG 93-04). *Int J Radiat Oncol Biol Phys* 2002;52:1173–1179.
21. Giaccone G, Herbst RS, Manegold C, et al. Gefitinib in combination with gemcitabine and cisplatin in advanced non-small-cell lung cancer: a phase III trial—INTACT 1. *J Clin Oncol* 2004;22:777–784.
22. Hallahan DE, Qu S, Geng L, et al. Radiation-mediated control of drug delivery. *Am J Clin Oncol* 2001;24:473–480.
23. Kunala S, Macklis RM. Ionizing radiation induces CD20 surface expression on human B cells. *Int J Cancer* 2001;96:178–181.
24. Friedberg JW, Fisher RI. Iodine-131 tositumomab (Bexxar): radioimmunoconjugate therapy for indolent and transformed B-cell non-Hodgkin's lymphoma. *Exp Rev Anticancer Ther* 2004;4:18–26.

### Radiation-induced Effects on Blood Vessels

25. Fuks Z, Persaud RS, Alfieri A, et al. Basic fibroblast growth factor protects endothelial cells against radiation-induced programmed cell death *in vitro* and *in vivo*. *Cancer Res* 1994;54:2582–2590.
26. Maj JG, Paris F, Haimovitz-Friedman A, et al. Microvascular function regulates interstitial crypt response to radiation. *Cancer Res* 2003;63:4338–4341.
27. Garcia-Barros M, Paris F, Cordon-Cardo C, et al. Tumor response to radiotherapy regulated by endothelial cell apoptosis. *Science* 2003;300:1155–1159.
28. Li YQ, Chen P, Jain V, et al. Early radiation-induced endothelial cell loss and blood-spinal cord barrier breakdown in the rat spinal cord. *Radiat Res* 2004;161:143–152.
29. Tan J, Hallahan DE. Growth factor-independent activation of protein kinase B contributes to the inherent resistance of vascular endothelium to radiation-induced apoptotic response. *Cancer Res* 2003;63:7663–7667.
30. Terry NH, Ang KK, Hunter NR, et al. Tissue repair and repopulation in the tumor bed effect. *Radiat Res* 1988;114:621–626.
31. Milas T, Hunter N, Peters LJ. Tumor bed effect-induced reduction of tumor radiocurability through the increase in hypoxic cell fraction. *Int J Radiat Oncol Biol Phys* 1989;16:139–142.
32. Okunieff P, Dols S, Lee J, et al. Angiogenesis determines blood flow, metabolism, growth rate, and ATPase kinetics of tumors growing in an irradiated bed: 31P and 2H nuclear magnetic resonance studies. *Cancer Res* 1991;51:3289–3295.
33. Okunieff P, Urano M, Kallinowski F, et al. Tumors growing in irradiated tissue: oxygenation, metabolic state, and pH. *Int J Radiat Oncol Biol Phys* 1991;21:667–673.
34. Rubin P, Williams JP, Riggs PN, et al. Cellular and molecular mechanisms of radiation inhibition of restenosis, I: role of the macrophage and platelet-derived growth factor. *Int J Radiat Oncol Biol Phys* 1998;40:929–941.

### Acidic and Basic Fibroblast Growth Factors

35. Neta R, Okunieff P. Cytokine-induced radiation protection and sensitization. *Semin Radiat Oncol* 1996;6:306–320.
36. Ning S, Shui C, Khan WB, et al. Effects of keratinocyte growth factor on the proliferation and radiation survival of human squamous cell carcinoma cell lines *in vitro* and *in vivo*. *Int J Radiat Oncol Biol Phys* 1998;40:177–187.

37. Okunieff P, Li M, Liu W, et al. Keratinocyte growth factors radioprotect bowel and bone marrow but not KHT sarcoma. *Am J Clin Oncol* 2001;24:491–495.
38. Wang X, Ding I, Wu T, et al. Hyperbaric oxygen and basic fibroblast growth factor promote growth of irradiated bone. *Int J Radiat Oncol Biol Phys* 1998;40:189–196.
39. Okunieff P, Abraham EH, Moini M, et al. Basic fibroblast growth factor radioprotects bone marrow and not RIF1 tumor. *Acta Oncol* 1995;34:435–438.

### Vascular Endothelial Growth Factor

40. Li YQ, Ballinger JR, Nordal RA, et al. Hypoxia in radiation-induced blood-spinal cord barrier breakdown. *Cancer Res* 2001;61:3348–3354.
41. Kern FG, Lippman ME. The role of angiogenic growth factors in breast cancer progression. *Cancer Metastasis Rev* 1996;15:213–219.

### Erythropoietin

42. Glaspy JA. Hematopoietic management in oncology practice. *Oncology (Huntingt)* 2003;17:1724–1730.
43. Henke M, Laszig R, Rube C, et al. Erythropoietin to treat head and neck cancer patients with anaemia undergoing radiotherapy: randomized, double-blind, placebo-controlled trial. *Lancet* 2003;362: 1255–1260.

### Granulocyte Growth Factors

44. Natori T, Sata M, Washida M, et al. G-CSF stimulates angiogenesis and promotes tumor growth: potential contribution of bone marrow-derived endothelial progenitor cells. *Biochem Biophys Res Commun* 2002;297:1058–1061.
45. Neta R, Oppenheim JJ, Douches SD. Interdependence of the radioprotective effects of human recombinant IL-1, TNF, G-CSF, and murine recombinant G-CSF. *J Immunol* 1988;140:108–111.
46. Tejedor M, Valerdi JJ, Arias F, et al. Hyperfractionated radiotherapy concomitant with cisplatin and granulocyte colony-stimulating factor (filgrastim) for laryngeal carcinoma. *Cytokines Cell Mol Ther* 2000;6:35–39.

### Epidermal Growth Factor

47. Raben D, Bianco C, Helfrich B, et al. Interference with EGFR signaling: paradigm for improving radiation response in cancer treatment. *Exp Rev Anticancer Ther* 2002;2:461–471.
48. Ochs JS. Rationale and clinical basis for combining gefitinib (IRESSA, ZD1839) with radiation therapy for solid tumors. *Int J Radiat Oncol Biol Phys* 2004;58:941–949.

### Tumor Necrosis Factor

49. Zhang K, Gharaee-Kermani M, McGarry B, et al. TNF-α-mediated lung cytokine networking and eosinophil recruitment in pulmonary fibrosis. *J Immunol* 1997;158:954–959.
50. Pitsiou G, Kyriazis G, Hatzizisi O, et al. Tumor necrosis factor-alpha serum levels, weight loss and tissue oxygenation in chronic obstructive pulmonary disease. *Resp Med* 2002;96:594–598.
51. Rubin P, Finkelstein J, Shapiro D. Molecular biology mechanisms in the radiation induction of pulmonary injury syndromes: interrelationship between the alveolar macrophage and the septal fibroblast. *Int J Radiat Oncol Biol Phys* 1992;24:93–101.

### Interleukin-1

52. Chen Y, Williams JP, Ding I, et al. Radiation pneumonitis and early circulatory cytokine markers. *Semin Radiat Oncol* 2002;12: 26–33.

53. Bubenik J, Indrova M, Holas V. Anti-tumor efficacy of IL-1 and IL-2. *Folia Biol (Praha)*1988;34:42–47.

## *Transforming Growth Factor Beta*

54. Anscher MS, Crocker IR, Jirtle RL. Transforming growth factor-beta 1 expression in irradiated liver. *Radiat Res* 1990;122:77–85.

55. Anscher MS, Peters WP, Reisenbichler H, et al. Transforming growth factor beta as a predictor of liver and lung fibrosis after autologous bone marrow transplantation for advanced breast cancer. *N Engl J Med* 1993;328:1592–1598.

56. Anscher MS, Murase T, Prescott DM, et al. Changes in plasma TGF beta levels during pulmonary radiotherapy as a predictor of the risk of developing radiation pneumonitis. *Int J Radiat Oncol Biol Phys* 1994;30:671–676.

# Normal Tissue Dose Constraints Applied in Lung Stereotactic Body Radiation Therapy

*Robert D. Timmerman and *Frank Lohr*

## ANATOMIC, ARCHITECTURAL, AND FUNCTIONAL ASPECTS RELATING TO RADIATION INJURY

Respiration is the process of drawing oxygen-enriched air into the lungs where it can be exchanged for carbon dioxide, a waste product of metabolism. The mechanics of respiration require that a negative pressure gradient (vacuum) be generated between the terminal air sacs in the lung (alveoli) and the atmosphere via forces generated by the musculature of the chest wall and diaphragm. These forces are transmitted through to the alveoli by the lung parenchyma itself, which normally maintains a pliable and elastic character. Oxygen-enriched air is pulled into the lungs via a series of branching tubes and tubules (pharynx, trachea, bronchi, bronchioles), which must remain patent and of sufficient caliber to channel air to the alveoli. Within the alveoli, the oxygen must diffuse across the alveolar membranes, across any interstitial tissues, and ultimately across the endothelial membranes of the adjacent capillaries in order to find its way into the bloodstream and attach to hemoglobin. The same structures must be traversed by carbon dioxide coming from the blood stream, but in reverse order, toward the alveoli. The air in the alveoli, now rich in carbon dioxide, is expelled back into the atmosphere mostly by the recoil elasticity of the lung tissue and chest wall. This respiratory process is repeated nearly 30,000 times per day in the healthy adult.

The lung is a large organ and most people have a great deal more respiratory capacity than is actually required constituting a reserve. Diseases and conditions that damage pulmonary tissue (hence, respiratory processes)

Department of Radiation Oncology, University of Texas Southwestern Medical Center, Dallas, TX 75390; and *Department of Radiation Oncology, Mannheim Medical Center, University of Heidelberg, Mannheim, Germany

eventually may reduce this reserve to a threshold below which symptomatic disease becomes apparent. As noted in Table 4.1, radiation-related normal tissue injury may affect several of the essential respiratory processes simultaneously. This radiation toxicity is a consequence of damage to any of the various anatomic structures of the lung to a variable degree (e.g., bronchi, bronchioles, alveoli, interstitial tissues, chest wall, and vasculature) depending on *dose, volume, and inherent predisposition (radiosensitivity).* In conventionally fractionated radiation (CFR), the predominant dose-limiting toxicity has been radiation pneumonitis. Radiation pneumonitis is predominantly an inflammation of end bronchioles and alveoli characterized by fluffy infiltrates on chest radiograph and symptoms of fever, cough, shortness of breath, and chest pain. The symptoms of radiation pneumonitis after CFR present clinically in an acute to subacute timeframe (weeks to months). Radiation pneumonitis affects the ability of lung tissue to draw air into the alveoli (i.e., obstruction) and to exchange oxygen for carbon dioxide, effectively decreasing the patient's pulmonary reserve. Often, perhaps always, radiation pneumonitis will be followed by the formation of scar tissue called radiation fibrosis as a late effect. Dense radiation fibrosis disrupts the recoil elasticity of the lung and blocks oxygen exchange via interstitial thickening around terminal airways and small blood vessels.

Formal analysis of dose-limiting toxicity of CFR for lung cancer would indicate that radiation pneumonitis is both dose- and volume-dependent. Radiation pneumonitis is commonly graded by the Common Terminology Criteria for Adverse Events Version 3.0 (1) shown in Table 4.2. Armstrong and colleagues (2) determined that the volume of total lung getting 25 Gy or more ($V_{25}$) correlated significantly with grade 3 or higher toxicity If this volume was kept below 30% of total lung volume, symptomatic radiation pneumonitis was only 4%. Marks and colleagues (3) saw a

▶ **TABLE 4.1** **Functional and Structural Aspects of Respiratory Tissue with Relationship to Disease Conditions.**

| Essential Respiratory Function | Structure Performing Respiratory Function | Associated Dysfunctional Conditions |
|---|---|---|
| Generate negative pressure gradients in relation to the atmosphere | Diaphragm and chest wall musculature | Neuromuscular disorders (including paraneoplastic disorders)<br>Phrenic nerve palsy<br>Chest wall injury (including previous surgery)<br>Generalized weakness<br>Lack of respiratory drive (central nervous system dysfunction) |
| Transmit negative pressure gradients to alveoli | Elastic parenchyma of lung tissue | Lung fibrosis (caused by occupational exposure, radiation therapy, chemotherapy, etc.)<br>Pneumo- and hydrothorax |
| Pull oxygen-rich air into alveoli | Branching tubular airway structures (pharynx, trachea, bronchi, bronchioles) | Obstructive diseases (including chronic bronchitis, asthma, pneumonia, radiation pneumonitis, etc.)<br>Foreign body<br>Mucous plugging<br>Bronchial stenosis |
| Exchange oxygen for carbon dioxide with bloodstream | Alveolar walls, interstitial tissues, endothelial walls | Interstitial lung disease, emphysema (absence of alveoli)<br>Lung fibrosis<br>Vascular disorders |
| Discharge carbon dioxide–rich air back to atmosphere | Recoil elasticity of lung and chest wall via tubular airways | "Air trapping" disorders (including emphysema, asthma, and obstructive diseases)<br>Lung fibrosis<br>Chest wall injury |

similar toxicity correlation in a subgroup of patients with greater than 40% predicted pretreatment spirometry ("good" pulmonary function test [PFT] group) using total lung getting 30 Gy or more ($V_{30}$) as the cutoff. This same variable correlated well in this group with posttreatment diffusing capacity. Graham and colleagues (4) found significant correlation between the volume of lung getting 20 Gy or more ($V_{20}$) and development of grade 2 or higher pneumonitis. That group concluded that measures should be taken to try to improve plans with $V_{20}$ greater than 25% to avoid pneumonitis. Finally, an extensive analysis of two

▶ **TABLE 4.2** **Common Terminology Criteria for Adverse Events Version 3.0 for Radiation Pneumonitis.**

| Grade | Clinical Description |
|---|---|
| 0 | No pneumonitis |
| 1 | Asymptomatic; radiographic findings only |
| 2 | Symptomatic; not interfering with activities of daily living (ADLs); steroids indicated |
| 3 | Symptomatic; interfering with ADLs; supplemental oxygen indicated |
| 4 | Life threatening; ventilatory support indicated |
| 5 | Death |

large center's experience by Seppenwoolde and colleagues (5) indicated that mean lung dose (MLD) correlated best with grade 2 or higher pneumonitis. However, greater than 50% pneumonitis is observed with MLD of just 30 Gy for their model. Furthermore, they found that at a threshold dose of only 13 Gy ($V_{13}$), a strong correlation with pneumonitis was observed. Altogether, these data would indicate that radiation pneumonitis occurs at a relatively low dose (13–30 Gy) after CFR, and its clinically symptomatic form is highly volume dependent.

In most of these series, the spatial character of the dose distribution is very similar for all dose levels. This is highlighted by the fact that all dose–volume parameters such as $V_{20}$, $V_{30}$, MLD, and so forth, are correlated. If the spatial character of the dose distribution differs from the pattern that forms the basis of these studies, it is not clear if the predictive models are still valid. Indeed, a dosimetrist could construct three-dimensional (3D) dose plans with a wide variety of beam numbers, entrance/exit trajectories, and beam weights that may have a variety of clinical toxicity implications and yet have identical $V_{20}$ or MLD. A more recent series tried to formulate dose–volume statistics templates that may serve as better guidelines for evaluating plans with unconventional dose distributions (6). None of these models rigorously account for the dramatic changes in dose per fraction utilized in SBRT. Altogether, an encompassing description of relevant dose–volume statistical parameters as related to toxicity is still evolving.

Another issue that mandates reevaluation of all the parameters discussed in the preceding paragraph relates to tissue heterogeneity modeling. Most of the lung treatment data was collected using no heterogeneity correction. Current-generation dose calculation engines used for modeling heterogeneities are often inaccurate or inconsistent in determining dose at air–tissue interfaces, potentially overestimating minimum tumor dose (especially in the peripheral region of smaller tumors) and underestimating dose in normal lung (7). Improved dose calculation engines based on collapsed-cone or Monte-Carlo algorithms will provide more accurate data for future analysis. As discussed in other chapters of this text, such considerations may be of even greater importance for the estimates of lung tolerance for SBRT than for CFR.

In SBRT, due to various immobilization methods, tumor mobility is better accounted for than in historic reports using CFR. As a result, adequate tumor treatment is accomplished with overall less normal tissue irradiation to the prescription dose levels. For SBRT, dosimetry is constructed such that high-dose volumes are reduced in exchange for larger low-dose volumes. Furthermore, moderate-dose volumes are compacted around the target itself, making this tissue's volume and location within the lung critical. Finally, the use of large dose per fraction changes the biologic response characteristics dramatically, especially in tissue near the target. As such, the shell of tissue immediately around the target receives the very high target dose, the shells several centimeters around the target receive a rapidly declining high to moderate dose, and a large volume of tissue beyond this region receives a low dose all delivered over a few fractions. This is in strong contrast to CFR where essentially a large volume gets a homogeneously large dose but via small daily dose fractions. From SBRT dose–volume characteristics for the typical 60 Gy in three fraction treatments given at Indiana University, $V_{13}$ through $V_{30}$ are generally less than 10% of total lung volume and MLD values are only 4 to 7 Gy. As such, the predicted pneumonitis rates based on models established for CFR would be less than 5%. Aoki and colleagues (8) described radiographic changes after SBRT to a dose of 48 Gy in four fractions for primary lung cancer. They found radiographic changes correlated well to $V_{20}$; however, they did not have enough clinical toxicity events to assess this parameter with clinical outcome. Whether dose–volume limits appreciated for CFR lung tolerance will apply to SBRT remains to be seen. Whatever the case, data derived from SBRT series will certainly expand the knowledge about dose–volume relationships in the lung, just as it was the case for the liver with the tolerance data for high-dose treatments of small volumes (9).

As noted in the previous paragraph, the location of the targeted lesions is of paramount concern for SBRT. In

SBRT giving high daily dose treatments, there is a clear component of bronchial injury in addition to the more typical pneumonitis seen with conventional radiotherapy (Fig. 4.1). Along with this bronchial injury is the appearance of atelectasis of "downstream" lung tissue even into areas receiving very little dose as shown in Fig. 4.2. Interestingly, in this regard, SBRT may be similar to surgery where "downstream" lung tissue is removed beyond any transected bronchus and vascular pedicle in the vicinity of the tumor. Whether this pattern of injury is related to bronchial damage with airway obstruction or vascular pedicle injury with starvation of downstream tissues (or perhaps both) remains to be determined. However, the observation of "wedgelike" imaging changes starting at the location of tumor treatment and extending outward toward the pleural surface is a common finding related to higher dose SBRT.

## LESSONS FROM RADIOBIOLOGIC MODELING OF LUNG INJURY

Wolbarst and colleagues (10) described a model where tissue is broken down into relatively small *functional subunits* (FSUs) useful for describing normal tissue changes after therapeutic radiation. These FSUs are composed of an organized population of differentiated cells and a smaller population of clonogenic (stem) cells capable of replenishing the differentiated cells. Wolbarst et al. divided FSUs into two general groups: (a) *structurally defined units* with discrete anatomic structure limiting stem cell migration, and (b) *structurally undefined units* where stem cell migration was not bounded by anatomic barriers. The alveoli–capillary complex is an example of a tissue with structurally defined functional subunits. In this model, if all clonogenic cells within a single alveolus are damaged, all functional capability of that alveolus will be lost. This is in contrast to a structurally undefined FSU, like the mucosa of the esophagus, where clonogens are free to migrate long distances to rescue damaged epithelium as demonstrated in Fig. 4.3. As such, structurally defined subunits have a much lower radiation tolerance per FSU.

Again, considering the Wolbarst model, one can identify a threshold dose beyond which all clonogens within a particular structurally defined FSU are incapable of rescue and the FSU will become totally dysfunctional. Moreover, delivering additional dose beyond the threshold dose within a particular volume containing a defined number of FSUs will not increase the dysfunction since all function is already lost at the threshold dose. Based on the radiation pneumonitis data presented above, this threshold dose is probably quite low, in the range of 13 to 30 Gy given in 2-Gy fractions. The fact that large volumes of lung can be irradiated to these doses without untoward

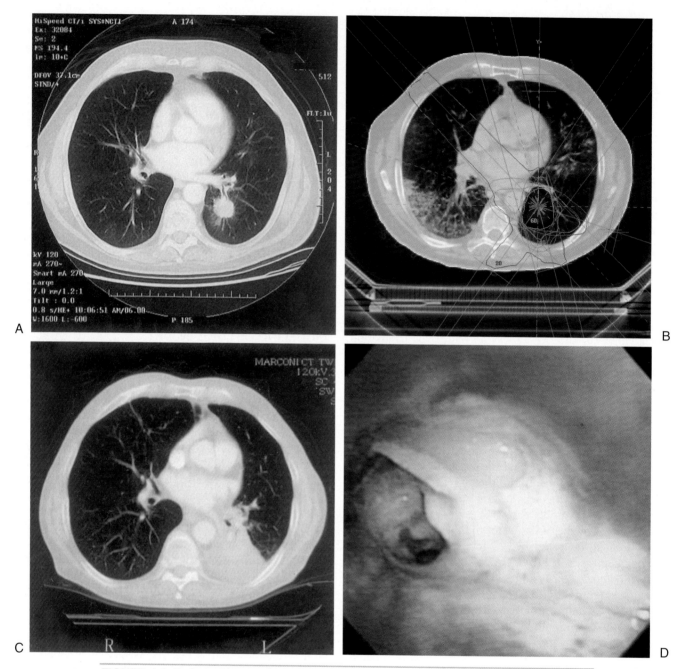

**FIGURE 4.1.** Patient with T1, N0, M0 non–small cell lung cancer treated with 60 Gy to the edge of the planning target volume (PTV) in three fractions using stereotactic body radiation therapy (SBRT). **A:** Pretreatment diagnostic scan. **B:** Treatment planning scan with superimposed isodose curves (magenta color corresponds to prescription dose). **C:** One year after treatment showing segmental collapse and consolidation. Repeated bronchial brushings, transbronchial biopsy, and positron emission tomography (PET) scanning all negative for cancer. **D:** Appearance of segmental bronchus on bronchoscopy shows mucosal damage with loss of airway patency.

consequences attests to the large functional reserve inherent to the lung.

Tissues that are made up predominantly of structurally defined FSUs are called *parallel functioning tissues* (including peripheral lung, peripheral kidney, peripheral liver, etc.) and occur within organs that are characterized by redundancy of function and large inherent reserves. In contrast, tissues that are made up of predominantly structurally undefined FSUs are called *serially functioning tissues* [including the gastrointestinal (GI) tract, large airways, large vascular trunks, spinal cord, etc.] and occur within organs that involve a "chain"

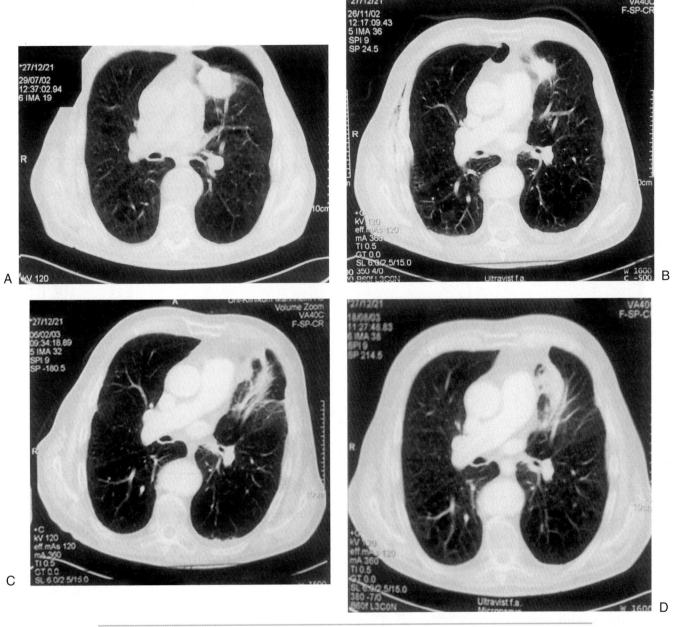

**FIGURE 4.2.** Evolution of radiographic changes on computed tomography after stereotactic body radiation therapy (SBRT) to a early-stage lung cancer using 50 Gy in five fractions. Images include pretreatment diagnostic scan **(A),** 2 months after therapy **(B),** 5 months after therapy **(C),** and 11 months after therapy **(D).** Irregular-shaped patchy opacities are situated in close proximity to the treated tumor within the region of high dose, making assessment of local tumor shrinkage difficult to quantify.

of function. In treating a lung cancer in the peripheral lung, a parallel functioning tissue, high tumor doses are required to control the clonogenic capability inherent to most lung cancers. Adjacent lung tissue will be exposed to relatively the same dose as the tumor. According to the "Critical Volume Model" proposed by Yeas and Kalend (11), any dose beyond the threshold dose defined above will not add additional toxicity to a given volume. Therefore, according to this model, organ dysfunction is not avoided by limiting the magnitude of *dose* beyond the threshold but rather by limiting the *volume* exposed to any dose beyond the threshold. Again, the similarities between surgery and SBRT are apparent. Surgeons contemplating a lung resection first try to quantify the amount of reserve in a given patient by measuring surrogate markers (e.g., pulmonary function tests). The surgeon then determines if following removal of a certain fraction of lung whether the patient will be left with

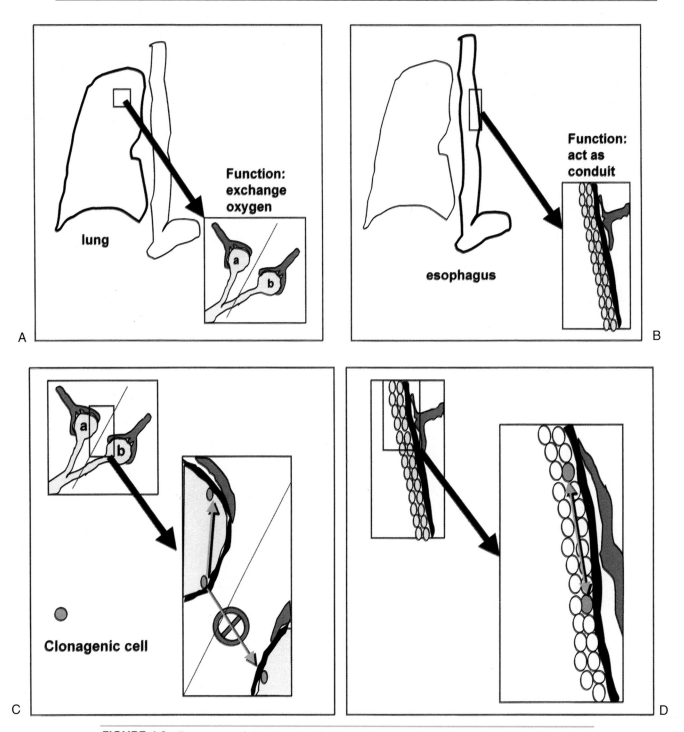

**FIGURE 4.3.** Illustrations of the concepts of structurally defined (peripheral lung tissue) and structurally undefined (esophagus) normal tissue architecture. **A:** Structurally defined relationship between functional subunits (separate alveolus–capillary complexes). **B:** Structurally undefined relationship of functional subunits (esophageal mucosa). **C:** Inherent limitation of migration of clonogens within structurally defined functional subunits. **D:** Relative freedom of migration of clonogens within structurally undefined functional subunits.

enough respiratory function to carry on daily activities. Overall, these considerations account for the inherent function of the lung (respiration), the organizational structure of the lung (branching airways leading to ter- minal alveoli), the redundancy of lung function (e.g., the left lung carries out the same activity as the right lung), and appreciation and quantification of the additional ca- pability (reserve) inherent to the lung. These same considerations are paramount to understanding normal tissue and host responses after SBRT of the lung.

The biggest shortcoming of the models of Wolbarst et al. and Yeas and Kalend relates to the fact that an organ such as the lung is composed of both parallel and serial tissue entwined in proximity to each other. The actual organization of the lung is similar to a tree or bush with a very large trunk (trachea) branching into large main branches (mainstem bronchi), branching further into smaller branches and twigs (lobar bronchi and bronchioles), and finally into terminal buds or leaves (alveoli–capillary complexes). All of the airways described above are serially functioning tissues since air is being directed along a single path as a chain of function and the clonogens within the airways are situated in the epithelium without anatomic boundaries. The vascular pedicles to the lobes and segments follow a relatively similar course to the airways and are serially functioning as well. In contrast, the alveoli–capillary complexes are parallel functioning tissues with basement membranes and septa separating one alveolus from another, limiting clonogen migration.

The type of anatomic arrangement seen in the lung may be referred to as a *branching tubular structure* and is in contrast to organs of the GI tract in which the lumen follows a single straight path known as a *linear tubular structure* as demonstrated in Fig. 4.4. An important consideration in relation to SBRT between these structures follows because if the dose is intense enough to totally disrupt the function of the serial-functioning component (e.g., the bronchus, vascular pedicles, or esophagus), all downstream functioning tissue will be lost as well (even if they were not irradiated) via collapse of the lumen or inadequate blood supply. In a branching tubular structure, such damage will result in a collapse of the particular branch affected, not the entire organ. The same damage to a linear tubular structure will obstruct all downstream function of the organ (e.g., complete bowel obstruction), a more catastrophic problem for the patient. In striking contrast to conventionally fractionated treatment, with potent doses of SBRT delivered to a bronchus, bronchiole, or vascular pedicle, distal atelectasis or pulmonary injury will occur, which may be permanent. As long as the volume lost is less than the organ reserve for the particular individual, no significant symptomatic toxicity will result. If the lost volume is larger than the patient's reserve, the patient will have symptomatic respiratory decline. As such, with potent treatment doses to serially functioning pulmonary tissues (e.g., ablative doses), the loss of functional lung tissue may be larger than the actual volume ir-

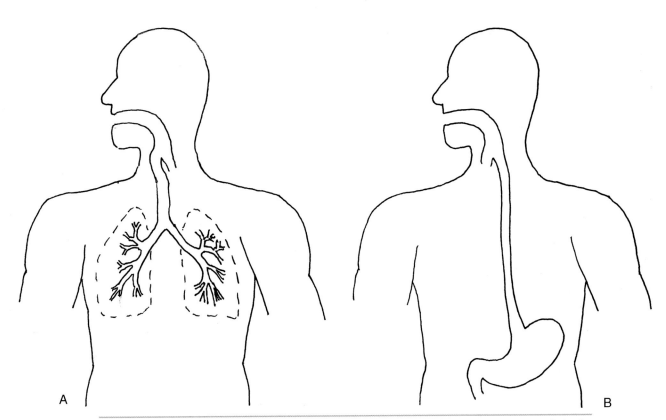

**FIGURE 4.4.** Architectural arrangements of intrathoracic serially functioning tissues include the *branching tubular* arrangement of the lung airways shown in **A**, and the *linear tubular* arrangement of the esophagus shown in **B**.

radiated beyond the threshold dose for parallel functioning tissues. It may still be reasonable to use such a strategy in order to control tumor proliferation; however, the treating physician must be aware of these two components of lung dysfunction, serial and parallel tissue injury, when formulating the treatment plan. In this regard, high-dose SBRT is different from conventionally fractionated radiation where long-term toxicity is predominantly just to the parallel functioning pulmonary tissues.

## RADIATION TOLERANCE OF PULMONARY TISSUES

Within the lung itself, there are a variety of tissues that possess unique radiation tolerance characteristics, namely, the airways (both large and small functioning as serial structures), vascular trunks and pedicles following similar routes as the bronchial tree (functioning as serial structures), and the alveoli–capillary complexes (functioning as parallel structures). In addition, the thoracic cavity includes the serially functioning esophagus, serially functioning nerve tissue (e.g., phrenic nerves, brachial plexus, etc.), heart, pericardium, and pleura (all difficult to categorize as parallel or serial), and the bones and musculature of the chest wall. All of these structures will have a unique mechanism of injury and tolerance after SBRT.

Conventional radiotherapy commonly causes large serially functioning airway irritation, such as cough, but rarely causes dose-limiting toxicity. In contrast, high-dose SBRT schemes may cause significant large airway damage by both mucosal injury and ultimate collapse of the airway. Along the routes of bronchial airways, a similar injury is experienced by blood vessels following a similar route. Altogether, this collective radiation injury appears to mostly affect oxygenation parameters including diffusing capacity for carbon monoxide (DLCO), arterial oxygen tension (pressure) on room air [partial pressure of oxygen ($Po_2$)], and supplemental oxygen requirements [fraction of inspired oxygen ($FiO_2$)] (12). Decline in spirometry indices, including forced expiratory volume ($FEV_1$) and forced vital capacity (FVC), are less commonly observed. Because the degree of this airway injury toxicity is related to the proximity of the target to proximal trunks of the branching tubular lung structure, great care should be taken when considering treatment to tumors near the hilum or central chest. More protracted fractionation schedules for central tumors may facilitate treatments in these locations at the expense of potentially less effective tumor control.

Unexpected toxicity may also occur when treating central chest targets relating to toxicity to mediastinal structures, including esophagus and heart. While acute and sometimes severe esophageal toxicity is commonly seen after conventionally fractionated radiation for lung cancer,

most of the injury is self-limiting and resolves after treatment. After high-dose SBRT, esophageal strictures may form as a late effect. Another more unique toxicity from SBRT relates to pericardial injury. In the Indiana University phase 1 study, several patients with tumors adjacent to the heart had asymptomatic pericardial effusions, while one patient treated at the highest dose level had a large and symptomatic pericardial effusion that required a surgical intervention to resolve (unpublished data, Timmerman R, 2004). Probably by a similar mechanism, pleural effusions commonly develop after SBRT treatment of tumors treated adjacent to the chest wall. Usually these fluid collections will reabsorb without intervention after several months of follow-up. Rarely, such fluid collections will need to be drained via thoracentesis in patients symptomatic with shortness of breath, pleurisy, or hypoxia.

Most reports of SBRT do not include long-term follow-up data. As such, there may be unexpected toxicities that need to be recognized, monitored, and evaluated. Particularly with large doses per fraction, there may be unexpected injury related to nerve tissue and vascular tissue. Ideally, dose to brachial plexus, spinal cord, phrenic nerves, and intercostal nerves will be kept low via prudent treatment planning. Furthermore, avoiding large blood vessels in the central chest would be reasonable as well. In the Indiana University collective phase 1 and 2 experience prospectively treating early-stage lung cancer, a single patient of approximately 100 patients studied died of massive hemoptysis 1 year from completion of therapy (unpublished data). Although not a mainstem bronchus lesion, this patient's tumor target was located just 1 cm inferior to the right mainstem bronchus and received three treatments of 20 Gy each (60 Gy total). Incidentally and possibly related, this patient was one of a small minority of patients in the study who continued to smoke cigarettes heavily after treatment. At any rate, neurovascular calamities including aneurysms, fistulas with bleeding, or neuropathies (including phrenic or vagal nerve palsies) have rarely been reported but may only manifest after many years of follow-up.

With a paucity of long-term data relating tissue effects after large-dose-per-fraction radiation, it is difficult and somewhat dangerous to identify specific normal tissue tolerances. Nonetheless, for thoughtful investigation to proceed, a starting point must be established. The Radiation Therapy Oncology Group (RTOG) in the United States has developed a protocol for using stereotactic radiation to treat early-stage lung cancer. The prescription dose to the margin of the planning target volume (PTV) for this protocol that treats tumors up to 5 cm in dimension is 60 Gy total over three fractions (20 Gy per fraction). A committee of experienced radiation oncologists, physicists, and biologists has established organ dose limits for this protocol on the basis of limited institutional follow-up and linear-quadratic conversions (13) of known dose tolerance parameters from conventional radiation

▶ **TABLE 4.3** Radiation Therapy Oncology Group–Proposed Radiation Tolerances of Thoracic Normal Tissue with Tumor Prescription of 60 Gy Total in Three Fractions.

| Organ | Volume | Dose (cGy) |
|---|---|---|
| Spinal cord | Any point | 18 Gy (6 Gy per fraction) |
| Esophagus | Any point | 27 Gy (9 Gy per fraction) |
| Ipsilateral brachial plexus | Any point | 24 Gy (8 Gy per fraction) |
| Heart | Any point | 30 Gy (10 Gy per fraction) |
| Trachea and ipsilateral bronchus | Any point | 30 Gy (10 Gy per fraction) |

fractionation schemes. The tolerances for this protocol are shown in Table 4.3 for several critical organs. These are absolute limits relating to a point rather than a volume. Obviously, a goal of radiation dosimetry for planning stereotactic lung radiation therapy should be to minimize the volume of normal tissue even getting lower doses than those listed in Table 4.3. It must be emphasized that these tolerance figures have *not* been validated with long-term follow-up.

A proposed tolerance of the lung itself is not identified in Table 4.3. Lung toxicity is correlated to target volume. Toxicity related to serially functioning tissues is more predominant in the central chest. The RTOG study only allows high-dose SBRT treatment for tumors more than 2 cm distal to the central bronchi and large pulmonary vessels. Ideally, SBRT should demonstrate a high degree of conformality between the prescription dose and the PTV. At least 95% of the PTV should be covered by the prescription dose without spilling prescription dose into the surrounding normal lung. Lung within the PTV exceeds tolerance and is no longer functional after high-dose SBRT. A dose fall-off region exists outside of the PTV, the volume of which depends on the size of the PTV, the location of the PTV within the chest, the quality of the radiation dosimetry (e.g., number of beams, beam arrangements, radiation energy, etc.), and the type of radiation (e.g., photon vs. proton, etc.). This dose fall-off region, also called the gradient region, constitutes unintended radiation exposure and should be kept as small as possible. Rates of symptomatic pneumonitis should be acceptable if the $V_{13}$ is kept at or below 10% and mean lung dose at or below 7 to 8 Gy. It should be possible to keep these parameters relating to normal lung considerably less for smaller targeted lesions.

## SUMMARY

Lung injury after SBRT is derived from damage to both parallel and serial functioning tissues. Unlike CFR where significant damage to serially functioning tissue has mostly been limited to the esophagus, SBRT may cause significant subacute and late toxicity to serially functioning bronchi, bronchioles, and vascular pedicles. Knowledge of the branching tubular architecture of the lung and experience from prudent dosimetry construction is essential for safe treatment. Early recognition of toxicity and effective management strategies may still allow adequate dose to be delivered. SBRT constitutes a great opportunity to deliver large dose per fraction and biologically potent total dose for tumors historically poorly controlled by CFR. Ongoing dose–volume data collection and reporting with correlation to imaging changes and clinical toxicity effects will be required for effective utilization of SBRT.

## REFERENCES

1. Cancer Therapy Evaluation Program. Common Terminology Criteria for Adverse Events. Version 3.0, DCTD, NCI, HIH, DHHS, March 31, 2003.
2. Armstrong J, Raben A, Zelefsky M, et al. Promising survival with three-dimensional conformal radiation therapy for non-small cell lung cancer. *Radiother Oncol* 1997;44:17–22.
3. Marks LB, Munley MT, Bentel GC, et al. Physical and biological predictors of changes in whole-lung function following thoracic irradiation. *Int J Radiat Oncol Biol Phys* 1997;39:563–570.
4. Graham MV, Purdy JA, Emami B, et al. Clinical dose-volume histogram analysis for pneumonitis, after 3D treatment for non-small cell lung cancer. *Int J Radiat Oncol Biol Phys* 1999;45:323–329.
5. Seppenwoolde Y, Lebesque JV, De Jaeger K, et al. Comparing different NTCP models that predict the incidence of radiation pneumonitis. *Int J Radiat Oncol Biol Phys* 2003;55:724–735.
6. Willner J, Jost A, Baier K, et al. A little to a lot or lot to a little? An analysis of pneumonitis risk from dose-volume histogram parameters of the lung in patients with lung cancer created with 3-D conformal radiotherapy. *Strahlenther Onkol* 2003;179:548–556.
7. De Jaeger K, Hoogeman MS, Engelsman M, et al. Incorporating an improved dose-calculation algorithm in conformal radiotherapy of lung cancer: re-evaluation of dose in normal tissue. *Radiother Oncol* 2003;69:1–10.
8. Aoki T, Nagata Y, Negoro Y, et al. Evaluation of lung injury after three-dimensional conformal stereotactic radiation therapy for solitary lung tumors: CT appearance. *Radiology* 2004;230:101–108.
9. Dawson LA, Normalle D, Balter JM, et al. Analysis of radiation-induced liver disease using the Lyman NTCP model. *Int J Radiat Oncol Biol Phys* 2002;53:810–821.
10. Wolbarst AB, Chin LM, Svensson GK. Optimization of radiation therapy: integral-response of a model biological system. *Int J Radiat Oncol Biol Phys* 1982;8:1761–1769.
11. Yeas RJ, Kalend A. Local stem cell depletion model for radiation myelitis. *Int J Radiat Oncol Biol Phys* 1988;14:1247–1259.
12. Timmerman R, Papiez L, McGarry R, et al. Extracranial stereotactic radioablation: results of a phase I study in medically inoperable stage I non-small cell lung cancer patients. *Chest* 2003;124:1946–1955.
13. Douglas BG, Fowler JF. The effects of multiple small doses of x-rays on skin reactions in the mouse and a basic interpretation. *Radiat Res* 1976;66:401–426.

## Chapter 5

# Normal Tissue Dose Constraints in Stereotactic Body Radiation Therapy for Liver Tumors

*Jörn Wulf and *Klaus K. Herfarth*

## INTRODUCTION

In the management of liver tumors, stereotactic body radiation therapy (SBRT) has the advantage of being entirely noninvasive when compared with surgical resection or thermoablative approaches. Additionally, SBRT is also feasible for tumors adjacent to larger intrahepatic vessels and the inferior vena cava, regions where surgical resection often is impossible and the success of thermoablation is limited by a cooling effect due to the blood flow.

The goal of treatment is to induce tumor cell death within the volume irradiated. With the high doses needed to provide a good chance of controlling tumors present, there is a risk of injury to the adjacent normal tissue surrounding the tumor. The risk of serious toxicity in organs at risk can be minimized by precisely defining the target and reproducing the patient setup with a high level of accuracy, allowing for a reduction in the planning target volume (PTV). Treatment plans that provide a sharp dose gradient in surrounding areas are also highly advantageous.

The reaction of functional normal liver tissue is an important issue for liver SBRT. Many patients, especially with hepatocellular carcinoma (HCC), have underlying liver cirrhosis causing borderline liver function. Patients with limited metastatic disease in the liver might have decreased liver volume because of prior surgical resection. Numerous questions arise: How much liver tissue will be affected by SBRT? Is there a dose–effect relation to predict the reaction? What is the equivalent dose to compare normal liver tissue reaction from SBRT compared with conventionally fractionated radiotherapy? How can follow-up radiographic images after SBRT be interpreted to differentiate treatment-related changes from tumor recurrence?

## RADIATION-INDUCED LIVER DISEASE

### Histopathologic Features

In 1965, Ingold and colleagues (1) applied the term "radiation hepatitis" to describe a clinicopathologic condition characterized by a rise in liver enzymes, hepatomegaly, and ascites occurring 2 to 6 weeks after whole-liver irradiation. More commonly now called radiation-induced liver disease (RILD), the syndrome was observed after irradiation of the whole liver with doses ranging from 30 Gy to 51 Gy in 13 of 40 patients. Clinically, the syndrome ranged from asymptomatic presentation with reversibility of enzyme levels within months to chronic liver damage and death in three of 13 patients. Histopathologically, changes in the centrolobular region were noted within 60 days after irradiation: severe sinusoidal congestion, hyperemia, or hemorrhage, some atrophy of the central hepatic cells; and a mild dilatation of the central veins with erythrocytes but without thrombi. The general liver architecture was intact, the portal spaces and periportal liver cells were normal as were the bile ducts, periportal arteries, and veins. The authors concluded from their findings that the maximum safe dose to the entire liver is in the range of 30 to 35 Gy in 3 to 4 weeks.

Reed and Cox (2) recognized radiation injury of the liver to be a form of "veno-occlusive disease" (VOD), and the potential pathologic mechanism has been described by Fajardo and Colby (3). Radiation-induced endothelial cell damage of the central veins, not injury to hepatocytes themselves, is believed to be the principal causative factor. Endothelial cell injury leads to the adhesion of fibrin with

Department of Radiotherapy, University of Würzburg, D-97080 Würzburg, Germany; and *Department of Radiation Oncology, University of Heidelberg, D-69120 Heidelberg, Germany

consecutive partial or complete obliteration. Erythrocytes are captured in these plaques. Later, the fibrin is organized by invading fibroblasts producing collagen. Hepatocytes are absent around many of the involved central veins; the atrophy is likely due to increased pressure at the sinusoids of the congested liver (4). Stimulation of fibroblasts by transforming growth factor beta (TGFβ) is also implicated in the pathophysiologic mechanism. Additionally, the fibrinolytic activity is reduced in the irradiated liver volume (3). A detailed review distinguishing radiation-induced VOD from combined modality–induced liver disease, observed most commonly in the setting of high-dose chemotherapy and total body irradiation prior to allogeneic bone marrow transplantation, is provided by Lawrence et al. (5).

## Clinical Presentation and Patient Workup

Fortunately, with careful attention to technique and volume of liver irradiated, RILD after SBRT is very uncommon. In the unusual severe case, obliteration of the central veins induces severe congestion that can result in liver engorement and an increase of the portal venous pressure. The patient complains of rapid weight gain, fatigue, increased abdominal volume, and occasionally discomfort in the right upper abdominal quadrant. Jaundice is rare. The typical onset is 4 to 8 weeks after irradiation with occasionally early onset after 2 weeks or late onset after 7 months.

Physical examination reveals hepatomegaly and ascites. Laboratory findings can include moderate elevation of liver transaminases on the order of a 2-fold increase above the normal level and a substantial rise of alkaline phosphatase to the 3- to 10-fold above normal (5). Bilirubin is rarely elevated. Viral hepatitis should be excluded by serologic testing. To rule out progression of malignant disease, paracentesis with diagnostic workup of ascites and a computed tomography (CT) scan of the liver and abdomen are recommended. In the case of VOD, the ascites contains no malignant cells. CT scan will reveal a hypodensity in the liver in the portal venous contrast phase, which becomes a hyperdense area minutes after contrast agent administration (6–8).

## Patient Management

The clinical syndrome of RILD ranges from incidental asymptomatic laboratory test abnormality to life-threatening condition. Therefore, management decisions have to be adjusted to the potential individual risk. The amount of liver exposed to radiotherapy and the volume of unirradiated functional liver tissue should be considered. A uniform consensus regarding optimal therapy is not established. Anticoagulants and thrombocyte aggregation inhibitors have been tried, as have diuretics to treat ascites and steroids to reduce swelling and edema of the congested liver tissue. Most patients recover with this or similar conservative therapy within 1 to 2 months (5). In an extremely severe case with marked increase of the portal venous pressure, a transjugular intrahepatic portosystemic shunt can be used to reduce the gradient of pressure (9,10).

## DOSE–VOLUME EFFECTS IN RADIATION-INDUCED LIVER DISEASE

### Radiobiologic Modeling

Fisher and Hendry (11,12) studied the clonogenic survival of hepatocytes using the quantitative transplantation assay. They varied the fraction dose from 1 Gy to 8 Gy and calculated an α/β value of less than 2 Gy for hepatocytes for fractionated radiotherapy and a $D_0$ (dose that cause one natural log of cell kill, or survival $1/e$) of 2.4 Gy with an extrapolation number of 1.6 for single-dose irradiation. Similar results had previously been achieved by Jirtle et al. (13), who evaluated the clonogenic potential of irradiated rabbit liver, also noting a $D_0$ of 2.4Gy. However, because hepatocytes are not generally thought to be the primary target cells in the pathophysiologic process of RILD, analyses of *in vivo* tissue effects are more informative.

There is not a well-established animal model of RILD from which translatable radiobiologic knowledge may be reliably gained. Most animals do not develop liver injury in response to radiation alone (5,14,15). However, Brase et al. (16) irradiated rabbit liver with single doses ranging from 5 to 30 Gy and found modest changes after 10 Gy, persistent vascular changes after 12 Gy, and lethal damage after 16 Gy. Geraci et al. (17) irradiated parts of rat liver with doses between 17 and 30 Gy followed by resection of two thirds of the entire liver. They observed steeply escalating mortality with increasing dose and determined the dose for 50% lethality ($LD_{50}$) to be 24 Gy.

Using the clinical data of Ingold et al. (1), Trott and colleagues (14) estimated a dose–effect curve for whole-liver irradiation whereby the incidence of RILD is expected to be 0% at 25 Gy and 100% at 45 Gy. The fractionation schedule might influence these predictions. Early observations of Delclos et al. (18), Wharton et al. (19), and Perez et al. (20) evaluating the hepatic toxicity of moving-strip irradiation of the whole abdomen showed no hepatotoxicity with 8 × 2.25 Gy but severe toxicity in eight of 25 patients irradiated with 8 × 3.5 Gy.

### Clinical Experience with Whole-liver Irradiation

The most extensive experience in whole-liver irradiation was obtained in a series of Radiation Therapy and Oncology Group (RTOG) studies. In the first study, different dose-fractionation schedules were evaluated in 109 patients: Patients with solitary lesions received 30.4 Gy in 1.6 Gy fractions or 30 Gy in 2 Gy fractions with an optional boost of 10 × 2 Gy to residual disease. Patients with multiple lesions or extrahepatic disease received 15 × 2 Gy, 16 × 1.6 Gy, 10 × 2 Gy, or 7 × 3 Gy. No cases of RILD were observed. Because there was no difference in palliative effect, the 7 × 3 Gy approach was established as a "standard" (21).

The next study evaluated the potentially beneficial effect of misonidazole as a radiosensitizer in combination with 7 × 3 Gy whole-liver irradiation. Again, no RILD was observed in 187 evaluable patients (22). In the following study, the potential for radiation dose escalation was analyzed: A total of 173 patients were treated by hyperfractionated whole-liver irradiation of two daily fractions of 1.5 Gy with at least 4 hours in between to increasing total doses from 27 Gy to 33 Gy. While none of the 122 patients at the 27 or 30 Gy level showed clinical or biochemical evidence of RILD, severe (grade 3) RILD was observed in five of 51 patients at the 33 Gy level (23). The results indicate that hyperfractionation did not appear to raise the maximum safe whole-liver radiation dose above 30 Gy.

## Effects of Chemotherapy on Risk of Radiation-induced Liver Disease

Patients receiving SBRT for liver tumors have frequently received one or more chemotherapeutic agents in the past. The effect, if any, upon susceptibility to RILD likely depends on the amount and type of prior chemotherapy, although data specifically addressing this issue are limited. VOD is a common problem with an incidence of up to 25% in patients undergoing conditioning for bone-marrow transplantation by chemotherapy and whole-body irradiation with single doses of up to 10 Gy (3,24–27). Other authors reported increased liver toxicity due to doxorubicin (Adriamycin®) or actinomycin D (28–30). However, 5-fluorouracil (5-FU) does not appear to increase the risk of RILD; Rotman et al. (31,32) observed no cases of RILD among 23 patients treated with 27.5 Gy (±5 Gy) in fractions of 1.5 to 2 Gy, who received continuous-infusion 5-FU during portions of the treatment.

Similarly, no evidence of significant RILD was observed despite concomitant 5-FU in a large, prospective, randomized study evaluating the role of 21-Gy prophylactic liver irradiation for patients with colon cancer. Komaki et al. (34) reported on 16 patients treated for pancreatic cancer with doses up to 61 Gy including prophylactic liver irradiation (23.4 Gy/1.8 Gy fractions) with concomitant intravenous 5-FU. Although they do not report specifically on increased liver toxicity, in ten patients transient elevation of serum levels of liver enzymes were observed, indicating at least mild VOD.

## Partial Liver Irradiation and Radiation-induced Liver Disease

While assessment of liver toxicity due to whole-liver irradiation is important to assess radiotolerance of the complete organ, the analysis of data on partial liver irradiation gives more insight on the effects of dose escalation as it is intended in SBRT. Partial liver irradiation is mainly aimed on nonsurgical treatment of HCC, cholangiocarcinoma (CCC), and liver metastases.

Because HCC is frequently associated with liver cirrhosis and impaired baseline liver function, minimizing the risk of additional RILD is a very important goal. One of the first analyses was reported by Austin-Seymour et al. (35), who irradiated 11 patients with pancreas or bile duct carcinomas with heavy charged particles. One patient developed RILD. They concluded from dose–volume histogram (DVH) analysis that partial liver doses exceeding 30 to 35 Gy should be limited to a maximum of 30% of the total organ volume if the whole liver receives 18 Gy in 2-Gy fractions.

The most extensive experience of partial liver irradiation together with or without whole-liver irradiation and intraarterial chemotherapy has been achieved at the University of Michigan (36–39). From 1987 to 1999, 203 inoperable patients with normal liver function were irradiated for HCC ($n = 58$), CCC ($n = 47$), or liver metastases ($n = 98$). Forty-one patients were treated with whole-liver irradiation (24–36 Gy), 20 patients were treated with whole-liver irradiation followed by a boost to a partial liver volume (to 45–66 Gy), and 142 patients were treated with partial liver irradiation alone (48–90 Gy) in 11 fractions per week of 1.5 to 1.65 Gy (4–6 hours between fractions). The median dose was 52.5 Gy (range, 24–90 Gy), with a 2-week break in radiotherapy after 2 weeks. Simultaneously, intraarterial chemotherapy with 5-FU ($n = 69$) or bromodeoxyuridine (BrdU) ($n = 34$) was administered. Treatment plans and total dose were adjusted to an expected level of normal liver toxicity of 10% using a modified Lyman–normal tissue complication probability (NTCP) model (37,39).

Consistent with the investigators' predictions, in 19 patients (9%) RILD of RTOG grade 3 or higher (treatment required) was observed. Six cases occurred after whole-liver irradiation alone, six occurred after whole-liver irradiation plus boost, and seven occurred after partial liver irradiation alone. The strongest parameter predicting liver toxicity was the mean liver dose, with no cases of RILD below 31 Gy. In patients with hepatic toxicity, the mean liver dose was 37 Gy (NTCP 0.17) compared to 31 Gy in patients without RILD (NTCP 0.04), which is in agreement with prior estimations (40). The fact that the mean dose was an important predictor of RILD is consistent with an understanding of the liver as an organ containing a parallel structure of functional subunits (41). It is predicted from these data that small portions of the liver could tolerate very high doses of radiation as long as the mean dose to the entire organ was kept at a safe level.

The effect of partial liver irradiation with transarterial chemoembolization (TACE) in patients with HCC (*n* = 12) and liver cirrhosis (*n* = 11) was evaluated by Ohara et al. (42), again using the NTCP model. Partial liver volumes were irradiated with conventionally fractionated doses ranging from 50 to 77.4 Gy. Similar to the experience, the probability of RILD was overestimated by the original Lyman parameters. In patients with impaired liver function, the complication risk correlated well with the unirradiated liver volume, which was evaluated in accordance to surgical prediction scores for assessment of resectability of liver tumors (43,44). For that purpose, the authors related the effectively resected volume to the irradiation volume receiving 30 Gy or more. The authors concluded that the preserved functional capacity, the volume receiving less than 30 Gy, predicted radiation tolerance better than parameters concerned with the volume receiving a higher dose.

Seong et al. (45,46) combined focal liver irradiation with transarterial chemoembolization (TACE) in 158 patients with HCC. The irradiation was performed either with TACE (*n* = 107) or after progression following previous TACE (*n* = 51). The total dose given was titrated according to the percent of the nontumor liver volume receiving more than half of the prescribed total dose. If more than 75% of nontumor tissue received more than 50% of the prescription dose, no treatment was given. If 50% to 75% of nontumor tissue received more than 50% of the prescription dose, 30.6 to 41.4 Gy was given. If 25% to 50% of nontumor tissue received more than 50% of the prescription dose, 45 to 54 Gy was given. If less than 25% of nontumor tissue received more than 50% of the prescription dose, 59.4 Gy was given.

The mean tumor size was 9.0 ± 3.0 cm. Ninety percent of patients had underlying liver cirrhosis (Child A, 74%; Child B, 26%); patients with advanced liver cirrhosis Child C were excluded. The mean prescription radiation dose was 48.2 Gy (range, 25.2–60 Gy). Eleven patients developed RILD. The risk of RILD was not analyzed from the viewpoint of nontumor volume dose but rather with reference to the prescription dose. RILD was observed in 4.2% (*n* = 1) of patients who received a prescription dose less than 40 Gy, 5.9% (*n* = 3) of those who received 40 to 50 Gy, and 8.4% of those who received prescription doses above 50Gy (*n* = 7). RILD was slightly more common in patients with a worse baseline level of liver cirrhosis (Child B), but the number of cases overall was too low to establish a statistically significant relationship. Nevertheless, the evaluation demonstrates that partial liver irradiation can be performed in considerable large volumes even in patients with substantial baseline impairment of liver function.

## Summary of Clinical Data

The presented data suggest that the incidence of RILD is strongly correlated to the volume of liver irradiated. The tolerance dose to the whole liver is approximately 30 Gy in fractions of 1.5 to 2.0 Gy. Higher doses may be safely administered to parts of the liver if the mean dose to uninvolved liver is held to a safe level. Even patients with significant baseline impairment of liver function can tolerate high-dose irradiation to parts of the liver as long as an adequate functional reserve of tissue is preserved.

## RADIOGRAPHIC CHANGES AFTER STEREOTACTIC BODY RADIATION THERAPY FOR LIVER TUMORS

The incidence of clinical RILD after SBRT is extremely low and is discussed additionally elsewhere in the book. However, characteristic changes are routinely observed on follow-up radiographic imaging. A focal radiation reaction in the tumor and surrounding normal liver tissue in the follow-up CT scans is common.

The Heidelberg group (47) has evaluated the radiologic appearance of the focal reaction in detail. Follow-up CT images for 36 patients treated with a single fraction of SBRT were analyzed. The median dose was 22 Gy (range, 16–24 Gy) at the isocenter. The PTV was encompassed by the 80% isodose line. The median PTV was 93 cc (range 9–295). Typically, the reaction volume was sharply demarcated from the surrounding liver tissue.

Tumor and radiation reaction could be well differentiated in the portal-venous contrast-enhanced CT scans. Liver vessels running through the liver reaction were not displaced, as would be expected in the setting of expanding tumor. The area of radiation reaction was hypodense in most nonenhanced CT scans. Three different types of appearance of the reaction could be defined on the basis of the liver density in the portal-venous and the late phase after contrast agent administration:

- *Type 1 reaction:* Hypodensity in portal-venous contrast phase, isodensity in the late contrast phase (Fig. 5.1)
- *Type 2 reaction:* Hypodensity in portal-venous contrast phase, hyperdensity in the late contrast phase (Fig. 5.2)
- *Type 3 reaction:* Isodensity / hyperdensity in portal-venous contrast phase, hyperdensity in the late contrast phase (not shown)

The median time of onset for reactions observed was 1.8 months. While the type 1 or type 2 reactions usually showed up earlier, type 3 reactions appeared later than the other types. It was also noted for individual cases that there was a progression of the appearance during follow-

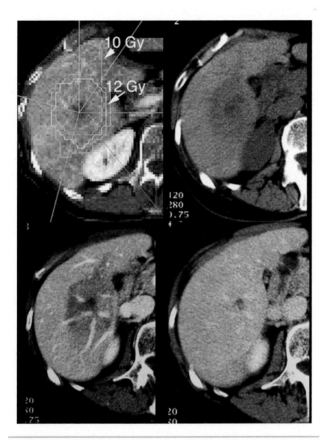

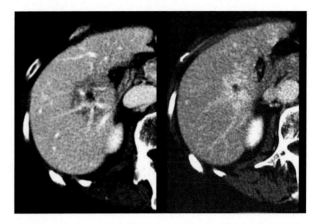

**FIGURE 5.2.** Radiation reaction 6 months after therapy (same patient as shown in Fig. 5.1). The reaction stills shows a hypodense appearance in the portal-venous phase (*left*). It is hyperdense in the later contrast phase (*right*) (type 2 reaction). The volume of the reaction is decreased compared with that seen in Fig. 5.1.

**FIGURE 5.1.** Dose distribution of a liver metastasis treated with stereotactic body radiation therapy (*upper left*) and the focal radiation reaction 6 weeks after therapy on a nonenhanced image (*upper right*) and during the portal-venous contrast phase (*lower left*). The sharply demarcated area corresponds to a dose between 10 and 12 Gy. The radiation reaction is not visible in the late contrast phase (*lower right*) at this time (type 1 reaction).

up toward type 3 appearances. Furthermore, the volume of the radiation reaction decreased with longer follow-up time (Fig. 5.2). The most dramatic shrinkage was observed during the first months after appearance. This led to the speculation that the reaction goes through different radiographic stages as it is schematically illustrated in Fig. 5.3. The histologic basis of these stages was not determined because no biopsies were taken. However, others have reported a type 2 appearance after single-dose radiation therapy and it was histologically confirmed veno-occlusive disease (48).

What is the threshold single dose that causes a radiographic indication of focal VOD? Based on reconstruction of the dose-volume histograms, the mean threshold dose was 13.7 Gy with a wide range between 8.9 and 19.2 Gy given in a single fraction. One reason for this large variance might be the fact that the reaction volume decreases steadily over time. Unless patients were scanned frequently soon after treatment, the examination might have not detected large initial reaction volumes; consequently,

the calculated threshold doses might have been overestimated. Supporting this hypothesis was the significant correlation between the threshold dose and the time of detection (correlation coefficient $r = 0.709$). Apart of the time factor, other factors, which might influence the individual radiation sensitivity (e.g., additional toxic liver agents like alcohol), might have been another reason of the variance. There is no evidence that other therapies after SBRT influenced the radiographic findings. More data are needed to strengthen the estimation of threshold doses. However, currently, we estimate the volume of potential VOD as the volume that receives a dose of more than 11 Gy when we perform a radiosurgical (single dose) form of SBRT. The radiation reaction after hypofractionated SBRT to the liver treatment has not been as thoroughly characterized.

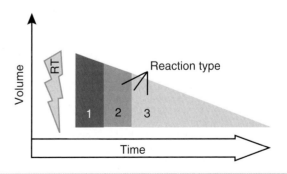

**FIGURE 5.3.** Schematic plot of the time course of a focal radiographic liver reaction to stereotactic body radiation therapy. A radiation reaction appears with its maximal volume at a definite time after radiotherapy. At this time, the reaction shows an appearance of a type 1 reaction. With follow-up time, the volume of the reaction shrinks and the appearance turns to a type 2 and type 3 reaction.

## SUMMARY

The incidence of clinical RILD is closely correlated to the volume of normal liver irradiated. High-dose tumor treatment using well-focused, stereotactic technique should be feasible as long as the uninvolved liver receives a mean dose expected to yield a low risk of RILD.

In view of the available information concerning liver tolerance to radiation, the German multicenter randomized trial of SBRT comparing a hypofractionated (three fraction) regimen with a single fraction (radiosurgery-like) schedule for liver metastases specifies the following normal tissue constraints:

- For hypofractionation (three fractions) arm: 50% of the liver ($L_{50}$) should not receive more than 5 Gy per fraction (total, 15 Gy), and 30% of the liver ($L_{30}$) should not receive more than 7 Gy per fraction (total, 21 Gy).
- For the single-fraction, radiosurgical arm: $L_{50}$ and $L_{30}$ are 7 Gy and 12 Gy, respectively.

The University of Colorado–Indiana University multi-institutional phase I/II dose escalation study of SBRT for liver metastases and phase I/II dose escalation study of SBRT for hepatocellular carcinoma each stipulate the following:

- At least 700 mL of normal liver (entire liver minus cumulative gross tumor volume) receives a total cumulative dose of less than 15 Gy over the course of the three fractions administered.

## REFERENCES

1. Ingold JA, Reed GB, Kaplan HS, et al. Radiation hepatitis. *Am J Roentgenol* 1965;93:200–208.
2. Reed GB, Cox AJ Jr. The human liver after radiation injury: a form of veno-occlusive disease. *Am J Pathol* 1966;48: 597–611.
3. Fajardo L, Colby T. Pathogenesis of veno-occlusive disease after radiation. *Arch Pathol Lab Med* 1980;104:584–588.
4. Djakova AM, Stefani NV, Zagrebin VM, et al. Postradiogene Effekte im Lebergewebe von Patienten mit Magenkarzinomen nach Radiosensibilisation mit Mitronidazol. *Radiobiol Radiother (Berl)* 1985;26:343–350.
5. Lawrence TS, Robertson JM, Anscher MS, et al. Hepatic toxicity resulting from cancer treatment. *Int J Radiat Oncol Biol Phys* 1995;31:1237–1248.
6. Jeffrey RB, Jr., Moss AA, Quivey JM, et al. CT of radiation-induced hepatic injury. *Am J Roentgenol* 1980;135:445–448.
7. Unger EC, Lee JK, Weyman PJ. CT and MR imaging of radiation hepatitis. *J Comput Assist Tomogr* 1987;11:264–268
8. Kolbenstvedt A, Kjøseth I, Klepp O, et al. Postirradiation changes of the liver by computed tomography. *Radiology* 1980;135:391.
9. Bischof M, Zierhut D, Gutwein S, et al. Die Venenverschluβkrankheit der Leber nach infradiaphragmaler total lymphatischer Bestrahlung. *Strahlenther Onkol* 2001;177:296–301.
10. Shen-Gunther J, Walker JL, Johnson GA, et al. Hepatic venoocclusive disease as a complication of whole abdominopelvic irradiation and treatment with the transjuglar intrahepatic portosystemic shunt: case report and literature review. *Gynecol Oncol* 1996;61:282–286.
11. Fisher DR, Hendry JH. Dose fractionation and hepatocyte clonogens: alpha/beta congruent to 1-2 Gy, and beta decreases with increasing delay before assay. *Radiat Res* 1988;113:51–57.
12. Fisher DR, Hendry JH, Scott D. Long-term repair in vivo of colony-forming ability and chromosomal injury in X-irradiated mouse hepatocytes. *Radiat Res* 1988;113:40–50.
13. Jirtle RL, Michalopoulos G, McLain JR, et al. Transplantation system for determining the clonogenic survival of parenchymal hepatocytes exposed to ionizing radiation. *Cancer Res* 1981;41:3512–3518.
14. Trott KR, Herrmann T. Radiation effects on abdominal organs. In: Scherer, E, Streffer C, Trott KR, eds. *Radiopathology of organs and tissues.* New York: Springer, 1991:329–338.
15. Fajardo LFC. Liver. In: Fajardo LFC, ed. *Pathology of radiation injury.* New York, Paris, Barcelona: Masson Publications, 1982:88–96.
16. Brase A, Bockslaff H, Emminger E. Angiographische Untersuchungen der portalen Lebergefäβe bei Kaninchen nach Strahleninsult. *Strahlenther Onkol* 1974;147: 278–289.
17. Geraci JP, Jackson KL, Mariano MS, et al. Hepatic injury after whole-liver irradiation in rats. *Rad Res* 1985;101:508–518.
18. Delclos L, Braun EJ, Herrera JR Jr., et al. Whole abdominal irradiation by cobalt-60 moving-strip technique. *Radiology* 1963;81:632–641.
19. Wharton T, Delclos L, Gallager S, et al. Radiation hepatitis induced by abdominal irradiation with the cobalt 60 strip technique. *Am J Roentgenol Radium Ther Nucl Med* 1973;117:73–80.
20. Perez CA, Korba A, Zivnuska F, et al. 60Co moving strip technique in the management of carcinoma of the ovary: analysis of tumor control and morbidity. *Int J Radiat Oncol Biol Phys* 1978;4:379–388.
21. Borgelt BB, Gelber R, Brady LW, et al. The palliation of hepatic metastases: results of the radiation therapy oncology pilot study. *Int J Radiat Oncol Biol Phys* 1981;7:587–591.
22. Leibel SA, Pajak TF, Massullo V, et al. A comparison of misonidazole sensitized radiation therapy to radiation therapy alone for the palliation of hepatic metastases: results of a radiation oncology group randomized prospective trial. *Int J Radiat Oncol Biol Phys* 1987;13:1057–1064.
23. Russell AH, Clyde C, Wasserman TH, et al. Accelerated hyperfractionated hepatic irradiation in the management of patients with liver metastases: results of the RTOG dose escalating protocol. *Int J Radiat Oncol Biol Phys* 1993;27:117–123.
24. McDonald GB, Sharma P, Matthews DE, et al. Venocclusive disease of the liver after bone marrow transplantation: diagnosis, incidence, and predisposing factors. *Hepatology* 1984;4:116–122.
25. Girinsky T, Benhamou E, Bourhis JH, et al. Prospective randomized comparison of single-dose versus hyperfractionated total-body irradiation in patients with hematologic malignancies. *J Clin Oncol* 2000;18:981–986.
26. Lee JL, Gooley T, Bensinger W, et al. Veno-occlusive disease of the liver after busulfan, melphalan, and thiotepa conditioning therapy: incidence, risk factors, and outcome. *Biol Blood Marrow Transplant* 1999;5:306–315.
27. Bradley J, Reft C, Goldman S, et al. High-energy total body irradiation as preparation for bone marrow transplantation in leukemia patients: treatment technique and related complications. *Int J Radiat Oncol Biol Phys* 1998;40:391–396.
28. Tefft M, Mitus A, Jaffe N. Irradiation of the liver in children: acute effects enhanced by concomitant chemotherapeutic administration? *Am J Roentgenol Radium Ther Nucl Med* 1971;111:165–173.
29. Kun LE, Camitta BM. Hepatopathy following irradiation and adriamycin. *Cancer* 1978;42:81–84.
30. Flentje M, Weirich A, Potter R, et al. Hepatotoxicity in irradiated nephroblastoma patients during postoperative treatment according to SIOP9/GPOH. *Radiother Oncol* 1994;31:222–228.
31. Rotman M, Kuruvilla AM, Choi K, et al. Response of colo-rectal hepatic metastases to concomitant radiotherapy and intravenous infusion 5 fluorouracil. *Int J Radiat Oncol Biol Phys* 1986;12: 2179–2187.
32. Rotman MZ. Chemoirradiation: a new initiative in cancer treatment: 1991 RSNA annual oration in radiation oncology. *Radiology* 1992;184:319–327.
33. GI_Tumor_Study_Group. Adjuvant therapy with hepatic irradiation plus fluorouracil in colon carcinoma: the Gastrointestinal Tumor Study Group. *Int J Radiat Oncol Biol Phys* 1991;21:1151–1156.
34. Komaki R, Hansen R, Cox JD, et al. Phase I-II study of prophylactic hepatic irradiation with local irradiation and systemic chemotherapy for adenocarcinoma of the pancreas. *Int J Radiat Oncol Biol Phys* 1988;15:1447–1452.

35. Austin-Seymour MM, Chen GT, Castro JR, et al. Dose volume histogram analysis of liver radiation tolerance. *Int J Radiat Oncol Biol Phys* 1986;12:31–35.
36. McGinn CJ, Ten Haken RK, Ensminger MD, et al. Treatment of intrahepatic cancers with radiation doses based on a normal tissue complication probability model. *J Clin Oncol* 1998;16:2246–2252.
37. Lawrence TS, Ten Haken RK, Kessler ML, et al. The use of 3-D dose volume analysis to predict radiation hepatitis. *Int J Radiat Oncol Biol Phys* 1992;23:781–788.
38. Dawson LA, McGinn CJ, Normolle D, et al. Escalated focal liver radiation and concurrent hepatic artery fluorodeoxyuridine for unresectable intrahepatic malignancies. *J Clin Oncol* 2000;18:2210–2218.
39. Dawson LA, Normolle D, Balter JM, et al. Analysis of radiation-induced liver disease using the lyman NTCP model. *Int J Radiat Oncol Biol Phys* 2002;53:810–821.
40. Emami B, Lyman J, Brown A, et al. Tolerance of normal tissue to therapeutic irradiation. *Int J Radiat Oncol Biol Phys* 1991;21:109–122.
41. Jackson A, Ten Haken RK, Robertson JM, et al. Analysis of clinical complication data for radiation hepatitis using a parallel architecture model. *Int J Radiat Oncol Biol Phys* 1995;31:883–891.
42. Ohara K, Tsuji H, Tatsuzaki H, et al. Radiation tolerance of the liver in relation to the preserved functional capacity. *Acta Oncol* 1994;33:819–823.
43. Yamanaka N, Okamoto E, Kuwata K, et al. A multiple regression equation for prediction of posthepatectomy liver failure. *Ann Surg* 1984;200:658–663.
44. Yamanaka N, Okamoto E, Oriyama T, et al. A prediction scoring system to select the surgical treatment of liver cancer: further refinement based on 10 years of use. *Ann Surg* 1994;219:342–346.
45. Seong J, Park HC, Han KH, et al. Clinical results and prognostic factors in radiotherapy for unresectable hepatocellular carcinoma: a retrospective study of 158 patients. *Int J Radiat Oncol Biol Phys* 2003;55:329–336.
46. Park HC, Seong J, Han KH, et al. Dose-response relationship in local radiotherapy for hepatocellular carcinoma. *Int J Radiat Oncol Biol Phys* 2002;54:150–155.
47. Herfarth KK, Hof H, Bahner ML, et al. Assessment of the focal liver reaction after stereotactic single dose radiation therapy of liver tumors by multiphasic CT. *Int J Radiat Oncol Biol Phys* 2003;57:444–451.
48. Willemart S, Nicaise N, Struyven J, et al. Acute radiation-induced hepatic injury: evaluation by triphasic contrast enhanced helical CT. *Br J Radiol* 2000;73:544–546.

## Chapter 6

# Special Problems in Stereotactic Body Radiation Therapy: Dose Rate Effect, Dose Inhomogeneity, and Target Margin Selection

*Brian D. Kavanagh and \*Robert M. Cardinale*

## INTRODUCTION

Special problems at the interface of radiobiology and medical physics emerge during stereotactic body radiation therapy (SBRT). Several important examples are addressed here.

## The Dose Rate Problem

Routinely ignored in conventionally fractionated radiotherapy administration, the rate at which tumor cells are exposed to radiation within a single treatment can have a profound impact on the expected cytotoxicity of the radiation. The problem is relevant to cranial radiosurgery, high dose rate brachytherapy, and intensity-modulated radiotherapy (IMRT). Given that SBRT typically involves technically complex patient setups and multiple treatment fields, with individual treatments lasting considerably longer than conventional radiation treatments, it is expected that the dose rate problem is a potential concern for SBRT, also.

The potential detrimental effect of lengthy treatment times in linear accelerator–based cranial radiosurgery was well demonstrated experimentally by Benedict and colleagues (1). U-87MG human glioma cells were irradiated with 6 mV x-rays to doses ranging from 6 to 18 Gy over a range of total irradiation times representing the range of what is sometimes required for multiple-isocenter, multiple-arc treatment delivery. The cell survival increased with increasing total irradiation time, pre-

Department of Radiation Oncology, University of Colorado Comprehensive Cancer Center, Aurora, Colorado 80010; and \*Princeton Radiology Associates, Kendall Park, New Jersey 08824.

sumably a consequence of induced cellular repair mechanisms that can compromise the efficacy of treatment if the duration of an individual fraction is excessively prolonged (Fig. 6.1).

Arnfield and colleagues (2) evaluated a situation that can occur commonly during a high-dose-rate (HDR) brachytherapy treatment. Because the distance between a point within a tumor and the radioactive source can vary considerably as the source moves through the planned sequence of dwell positions, the dose rate at that point may vary by a factor of 100 or more. It was hypothesized that the sequence of dose delivery might affect the radiobiologic effect. Tumor cell survival was assayed in two conditions of dose rate sequence: initial exposure at a true, HDR-caliber, high exposure rate (240 Gy per hour) prior to exposure at an intermediate dose rate (3.5 Gy per hour), or vice versa. The results indicted that when the intermediate-dose-rate component was given before the HDR component, there was increased tumor cell survival even if the same nominal total dose was given. This effect was suspected to result from induced radioresistance or sublethal damage repair. Welsh and colleagues (3) calculated the average dose rates for IMRT. They observed that since the average time required to treat patients using IMRT was prolonged to a range of dose rates much lower than those of conventional treatment rates, raising concern about possible adverse effect on the treatment efficacy due to intrafraction repair.

In summary, SBRT is unavoidably more complex and time-consuming than conventional radiation treatments, and there can be extra delays during treatment in the early stages of an SBRT program as quality assurance issues are addressed with extra caution. However, as the treatment team (physician, therapist, physicist, and other

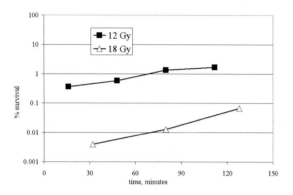

**FIGURE 6.1.** Time to deliver exposures of 12 or 18 Gy (*x-axis*) versus percent survival of U-87MG cells (*y-axis*). Note that for the 18-Gy dose level, increasing the length of treatment from approximately ½ hour to 2 hours corresponds to an order of magnitude decrement in cytotoxicity. (From Benedict SH, Lin PS, Zwicker RD, et al. The biological effectiveness of intermittent irradiation as a function of overall treatment time: development of correction factors for linac-based stereotactic radiotherapy. *Int J Radiat Oncol Biol Phys* 1997;37:765–769, with permission.)

support staff) becomes more comfortable with patient setup and treatment delivery techniques, it appears advantageous to make every effort to administer each individual SBRT treatment within as short a time as possible to avoid the problem of intrafraction cellular radiation repair responses.

## The Dose Inhomogeneity Problem

There is a common misconception that radioresistant hypoxic cells are preferentially located within the geographic center of a solid tumor, suggesting that it might be beneficial during SBRT to create dose "hotspots" centrally within a tumor to address that particular problem. While it is true that some tumors develop frankly necrotic, fluid-filled cavities centrally, it is not true that the outer edges of a tumor would necessarily contain less hypoxia than any other subvolume. Ljungkvist and colleagues (4) described several patterns of hypoxia with a variety of squamous cell cancers, all of which contained regions of marked variability in oxygen pressure occurring within distances well below 1 mm. These findings are consistent with conceptual approaches to understanding and solving the problem of tumor hypoxia (5).

While intentionally placing high-dose regions within the geographic center of a tumor does not necessarily resolve the problem of hypoxic cells, there is certainly no particular disadvantage to the dose inhomogeneity. Indeed, significant dose inhomogeneity within the tumor is unavoidable and probably desirable, because the SBRT treatment plans often involve multiple static fields or arcing beams designed in an effort to sharpen the dose gradient between the surface of the planning target volume

and adjacent normal tissue (see below). Furthermore, a higher dose of radiation administered anywhere within the tumor will enhance the composite cytotoxic effect of treatment and increase the tumor control probability (TCP).

A problem might arise, however, in the interinstitutional comparison of SBRT dose prescriptions. Variations in SBRT delivery techniques between institutions and interpatient variability within institutions can cause significant differences in the true biologic effect of the same nominal prescription dose, depending on the extent of dose inhomogeneity present within the dose distribution. We have attempted to address this issue by comparing the relative merits of two commonly used indices that describe the composite biologic effectiveness of a complex dose distribution: equivalent uniform dose (EUD) and TCP (6). The EUD (7) was calculated as follows:

$$EUD = 2Gy \frac{\ln\left[\frac{1}{V} \sum_{i=1}^{N} V_i(SF_2)^{\frac{D_i}{2Gy}}\right]}{\ln(SF_2)}$$

where $V$ is total volume, $V_i$ is the volume of the $i$th subvolume within the dose-volume histogram (DVH), $D_i$ is the dose to the $i$th subvolume, and $SF_2$ is the surviving fraction after 2 Gy. TCP was calculated according to the following formulas:

$$TCP = \Pi \, BCP_j$$
$$BCP = \exp(-N \times SF)$$

where $BCP$ is the bin control probability of a subpopulation of cells, $N$ is the number of cells in the bin, $SF$ is the surviving fraction after the dose given, and $BCPj$ is the $j$th bin.

By analyzing differences in representative SBRT DVHs from several institutions, it was concluded that EUD is more robust for the prospective description of SBRT because it is less sensitive to estimates of SF and number of tumor clonogens. TCP remains more valuable for a post hoc estimation of radiosensitivity parameters. Of note, the presence of hypoxic cells does, indeed, have a profound effect on TCP. For a small volume tumor of approximately 5 cc total volume, a three-fraction SBRT regimen of nominal dose 15 Gy that yields a TCP of 75% is predicted to give a TCP of only around 25% if 5% of the cells are effectively hypoxic.

## The Target Margin Problem

In one of their first reports of SBRT methodology, Lax and colleagues (8) describe the use of so-called negative block margin, whereby the beam aperture is smaller than the target when considered from a "beam's eye view" perspective. They propose that this method can achieve a higher dose centrally within the tumor with only modest increases in the dose within the volume of normal tissue just outside the tumor.

In a quantitative assessment of the potential biologic impact of margin selection upon both tumor and normal tissue dose, we previously analyzed the impact of varying the margin around the planning target volume (PTV) for a lung and liver SBRT case (9). For each of the two targets, plans were generated with block margins of −2.5 to 10 mm around the PTV. All plans were normalized such that 99% of the PTV was covered by the prescription isodose volume. The following indices were calculated for each plan: (a) maximum dose divided by prescription dose (MDPD); (b) the volume of the prescription isodose surface divided by the PTV volume (PITV); (c) the volume of non-PTV tissue contained in the 100%, 90%, 80%, 50%, and 25% of prescription isodose volumes; and (d) the normal tissue complication probabilities (NTCPs) based on the Lyman model parameters.

As it would have been expected, with increasing margin the MDPD decreases while the PITV increases. There were notable differences, however, in the volume of non-PTV normal tissue covered as margin varied. Although we also analyzed NTCP predictions, it can be argued that for parallel organs such as liver and lung, mean dose would be a better prediction of functional compromise.

Let us consider, then, a simplified example case of a spherical 2.5 cm liver mass. For the purpose of this analysis, we can define a therapeutic ratio, TR, that represents the quotient of the effective dose to the tumor divided by the mean dose to the surround normal liver tissue:

$$TR = \frac{EUD}{Dm}$$

where EUD to the tumor is defined as above (estimating $SF_2 = 0.5$) and $Dm$ is the mean dose to the surrounding normal tissue, in this case the entire liver volume minus the gross tumor volume (GTV). From the 2.5-cm GTV, a PTV was constructed by adding 5-mm margins radially and 7-mm margins in the superior–inferior direction. Given this PTV, a single-plane, dynamic conformal arc plan was normalized so that the minimum dose to 99% of the PTV was 16 Gy (Fig. 6.2). Treatment planning was performed using the Novalis system (BrainLAB, Inc., Westchester, IL).

The block margin specified around the PTV was varied, and the EUD, Dm, and TR were calculated for the case in which at least 99% of the PTV received 16 Gy per fraction for each of three fractions. Results are shown in Fig. 6.3. For this particular setup and this particular PTV, the EUD was highest with the furthest negative margin evaluated

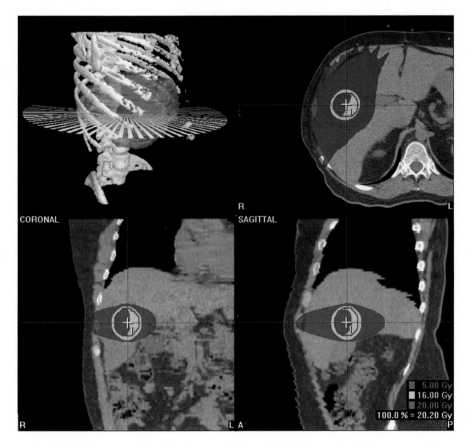

FIGURE 6.2. Example case used for planning target volume (PTV) margin versus therapeutic ratio (TR) determination (see Target Margin Problem section). Three-dimensional rendering of bony anatomy, liver (*orange*), path of dynamic conformal arc (*yellow coplanar rays*), and PTV (*maroon structure inside liver*) **(upper left)**. Axial, coronal, and sagittal reconstruction of planning CT scan with isodose volumes in color wash as per legend in lower right corner **(upper right, lower left, and lower right panels)**. The doses indicated (*blue*, 5 Gy; *green*, 16 Gy; *red*, 20 Gy) represent the stereotactic body radiation therapy dose per fraction. The distribution shown represents the case of adding 2 mm of block margin around the PTV.

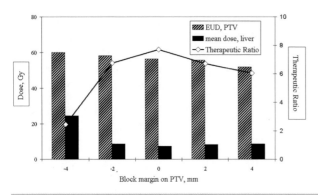

**FIGURE 6.3.** Block margin versus equivalent uniform dose (EUD), mean dose to normal liver, and therapeutic ratio (TR) for the sample case described in the Target Margin Problem section on page 49. EUD and mean dose to liver are represented by the left y-axis; TR is represented by the right y-axis (see text for definitions).

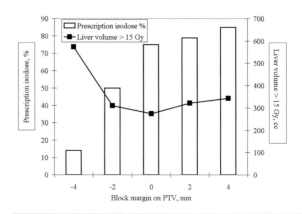

**FIGURE 6.4.** For the case analyzed in Fig. 6.3, the block margin (on the x-axis) is plotted against the normal liver volume less than 15 Gy (right y-axis) and the prescription isodoses required to satisfy the requirement that 99% of the PTV receive the specified minimum dose (left y-axis).

(−4 mm). However, the TR was highest with a 0-mm block margin around the PTV.

In this particular case, the liver is rather large, and the mean dose is therefore relatively low. Another relevant index to consider would be the absolute volume of liver receiving more than 15 Gy. It is noted in Chapter 5 that in the University of Colorado–Indiana University Phase 1 studies of liver SBRT, there is a requirement that at least 700 mL of normal liver receives less than 15 Gy in three fractions. In Fig. 6.4 the relationship between block margin and normal liver volume less than 15 Gy is illustrated, along with the effective prescription isodoses (relative to maximum point dose equal to 100%) required in each case to satisfy the requirement that 99% of the PTV receive the specified minimum dose. For this specific example case, the liver volume more than 15 Gy was lowest with a block margin of 0 mm.

The optimum block margin for the example PTV and specific plan tested were derived using an iterative method rather than analytic solution, and the results shown in Fig. 6.3 and Fig. 6.4 should not be viewed as universally applicable. Furthermore, the choice of coplanar arc versus noncoplanar static beam arrangement is open to debate—a strong argument is made for noncoplanar arrangements in Chapter 8. Nevertheless, it is useful to recognize that in planning SBRT at any given institution, it might be helpful to consider unconventional block margins around the PTV, specifically either 0-mm margins or even a negative margin.

Each commercially available system of treatment planning and delivery is likely to vary somewhat. As the

dosimetrists and physicists at a particular institution experiment with nonstandard beam arrangements and block margins to gain experience with SBRT, they will gain insight into the particular features of their own system and develop consistent approaches for optimizing the therapeutic ratio in cases treated.

## REFERENCES

1. Benedict SH, Lin PS, Zwicker RD, et al. The biological effectiveness of intermittent irradiation as a function of overall treatment time: development of correction factors for linac-based stereotactic radiotherapy. *Int J Radiat Oncol Biol Phys* 1997;37:765–769.
2. Arnfield MR, Lin PS, Manning MA, et al. The effect of high-dose-rate brachytherapy dwell sequence on cell survival. *Int J Radiat Oncol Biol Phys* 2002;52:850–857.
3. Welsh JS, Howard SP, Fowler JF. Dose rate in external beam radiotherapy for prostate cancer: an overlooked confounding variable? *Urology* 2003;62:204–206.
4. Ljungkvist AS, Bussink J, Rijken PF, et al. Vascular architecture, hypoxia, and proliferation in first-generation xenografts of human head-and-neck squamous cell carcinomas. *Int J Radiat Oncol Biol Phys* 2002;54:215–228.
5. Kavanagh BD, Secomb TW, Hsu R, et al. A theoretical model for the effects of reduced hemoglobin-oxygen affinity on tumor oxygenation. *Int J Radiat Oncol Biol Phys* 2002;53:172–179.
6. Kavanagh BD, Timmerman RD, Benedict SH, et al. How should we describe the radiobiologic effect of extracranial stereotactic radiosurgery: equivalent uniform dose or tumor control probability? *Med Phys* 2003;30:321–324.
7. Niemierko A. Reporting and analyzing dose distributions: a concept of equivalent uniform dose. *Med Phys* 1997;24:103–110.
8. Lax I, Blomgren H, Naslund I, et al. Stereotactic radiotherapy of malignancies of the abdomen. *Acta Oncol* 1994;6:677–683.
9. Cardinale RM, Wu Q, Benedict SH, et al. Determining the optimal block margin on the planning target volume for extracranial stereotactic radiotherapy. *Int J Radiat Oncol Biol Phys* 1999;45:515–520.

# The Physics and Dosimetry of Stereotactic Body Radiation Therapy

## Chapter 7

### Immobilization, Localization, and Repositioning Methods in Stereotactic Body Radiation Therapy

*Stanley H. Benedict*

## INTRODUCTION

Our current three-dimensional (3D) conformal radiotherapy and intensity-modulated radiotherapy techniques can deliver radiation beams shaped tightly to the target volume, particularly with the micro-multileaf collimator (mlc) technology now available. However, the

Department of Radiation Oncology, Medical College of Virginia Hospitals, Virginia Commonwealth University, Richmond, VA 23298

standard approach for patient setup introduces uncertainties that can directly impair delivery of the planned treatment, especially for extracranial tumors. An accurate system that accounts for patient positioning and motion compensation is especially important for the successful delivery of stereotactic body radiation therapy (SBRT).

In general, the basic prerequisite for high-dose-per-fraction radiotherapy is a high level of confidence in targeting and delivery. An accurate patient positioning, motion detection, and compensation system is essential. With conventional radiation therapy techniques, patient positioning is accomplished by using laser alignment to skin marks. Inherent difficulties include any operator-related laser misalignment and patient-related skin mark movements, given the fact that the skin is mobile. This method is at best within 2.0 to 2.5 mm for a perfectly immobilized phantom, and inadequate immobilization adds approximately 1 to 4 mm of additional error, depending on the site treated (1). Nonimmobilized patients with thoracic lesions are reported to have treatment-to-treatment and simulation-to-treatment target position variations on the order of 4 to 6 mm (2). It has been argued that an acceptable standard deviation for the systematic and random setup errors in routine clinical practice for lung cancer would be around 3.5 mm (3).

Many methods have been used to achieve spatial accuracy when treating patients with SBRT. In this chapter we review reported techniques with which patients were treated with hypofractionated, high dose radiation and multiple beams.

## OVERVIEW OF IMMOBILIZATION AND REPOSITIONING FOR STEREOTACTIC BODY RADIATION THERAPY

### Clinical Procedures

The sequence of clinical procedures for patients undergoing SBRT include (a) computed tomography (CT) simulation, (b) immobilization, (c) treatment planning, (d) repositioning of the patient in the simulated immobilization device, (e) relocalization of the target and isocenter within the patient, and (f) treatment delivery.

The CT simulation is used to assess tumor size, location, and range of motion. The range of motion in particular provides necessary data for required planning target volume (PTV) margin and can influence the decision of whether respiratory gating should be incorporated in the treatment delivery. At the time of CT simulation, immobilization is achieved by constructing some form of custom-fitting device to minimize motion and breathing effects and to provide a reproducible setup during treatment. It is important to provide comfortable immobilization, since the CT simulation and treatment procedures can be lengthy.

Treatment planning for SBRT includes numerous special considerations and is discussed in more detail in Chapter 8. *Repositioning* addresses the accurate setup of the patient in the planned position, whereas *relocalization* addresses the specific identification of the tumor and planned isocenter in the treatment field. Finally, treatment delivery is performed using any of a wide array of high-precision beam delivery techniques.

### Initial Reports for Patient Immobilization, Positioning, and Relocalization for Stereotactic Body Radiation Therapy

The first "frame" established for body stereotactic was reported by Lax and colleagues (4) and designed as a body cast in a box frame with scales and fiducial markers for imaging data acquisition. The patient was placed in a vacuum pillow in a frame equipped with indicators on the inner walls that are visible on CT and magnetic resonance imaging (MRI). The scales mounted on the frame, corresponding to fiducials, were used to set up isocenter coordinates in the treatment room. Diaphragmatic motion was minimized by applying pressure to the abdomen. The topic of target position uncertainty is addressed in more detail in Chapter 9.

Whereas the Lax system was designed to treat soft-tissue tumors, Hamilton et al. (5) described a system for stereotactic spinal cord irradiation using a screw fixation technique. The Hamilton system was based on the principles of rigid skeletal fixation. A rigid box is used for the patient to lie prone, and a clamp is fixated on the exposed spinous process above and below the target areas. Once the coordinates of the target have been acquired from the

CT images, the box is transferred to the linear accelerator (linac) treatment couch and aligned using conventional lasers. The reported repositioning accuracy with this frame is on the order of 2 mm.

Tokuuye et al. (6) included CT evaluations to determine the effect of respiration in the treatment of hepatocellular carcinoma. Patients were treated in the ventral position without a belt or body cast, and the patient's jaw and arms were strapped in place. Three reference points were marked on the skin. With an abdominal pressure belt, the motion was reduced to approximately 1 cm. Repeated CT examinations by Tokuuye et al. revealed targeting error to be less than 5 mm.

Sato and colleagues (7) described a frameless stereotactic technique for metastatic liver cancer in which 14 patients were instructed to keep shallow respiration with an oxygen mask and abdominal belt on the treatment table. All patients received transarterial chemoembolization (TACE) with iodized poppy seed oil (Lipiodol), which played a role as a high contrast marker for x-ray simulation and CT monitoring. The craniocaudal motion of the liver tumor was generally within 1.5 cm on x-ray simulation monitoring.

## BODY FIXATION AND IMMOBILIZATION SYSTEMS AND ACCESSORIES

There are several commercially available frame-based body stereotactic immobilization systems. The Elekta Stereotactic Body Frame (Norcross, GA), the Leibinger frame (Stryker, Kalamazoo, Michigan), and the Medical Intelligence BodyFIX (Schwabmünchen, Germany) all have features suitable for use during SBRT.

### Elekta Stereotactic Body Frame

The Elekta stereotactic body frame (Fig. 7.1) was developed in cooperation with Radiumhemmet at Karolinska Hospital, Stockholm, and Elekta. As the name implies, the Elekta Stereotactic Body Frame is a reference system that is external to the patient's body. Using this external stereotactic reference system, the coordinates of an internal target can be reproducibly localized during diagnostic examination and treatment.

The frame has built-in reference indicators for CT or MRI determination of target coordinates. A diaphragm control attached to the frame can be used to minimize respiratory movements. Horizontal positioning of the frame, in the scanner or on the treatment couch, is achieved using an adjustable base on the frame. Marker devices are used for reproducible positioning after fixation of the patient in a vacuum pillow. A chest marker device, attached to the arc-ruler on the frame, is used for alignment of the patient. This is based on two skin marks over the patient's sternum. Longitudinal alignment is con-

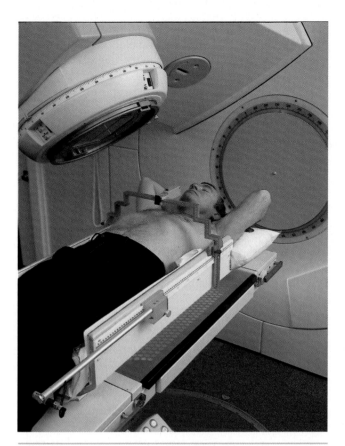

FIGURE 7.1. Elekta stereotactic body frame. (Photo courtesy of Elekta, Norcross, GA).

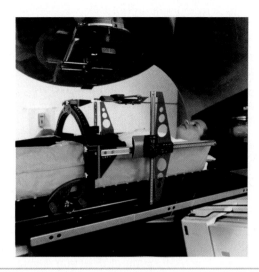

FIGURE 7.2. Leibinger stereotactic body fixation system. (Courtesy of Stryker, Kalamazoo, MI).

trolled by skin marks over the tibia using a frame-mounted laser. The coordinates used for patient positioning can be easily read on the arc-ruler and on the longitudinal ruler, along which the arc-ruler can be moved.

The stereotactic body frame fits the most commonly used CT and MRI scanners. The frame is specifically designed to avoid artifacts on the scanner images with copper or copper sulphate solution reference indicators on the frame to produce fiducials on the CT or MRI images. The fiducials permit x-, y-, and z-coordinate determination for localization of the target.

## Leibinger Stereotactic Body Frame

The Leibinger stereotactic body frame was developed at the German Cancer Research Center, Heidelberg, and manufactured by Leibinger (Freiburg, Germany). It consists of a carbon fiber–compound base plate that covers the full patient length. A metal arch is rigidly mounted to this base plate. Three V-shaped indicators (lateral and anterior) that are visible on CT are attached to this metal arch, and a fourth posterior indicator is mounted on the base plate. The indicators can be moved in defined steps along the longitudinal axis of the base plate to adequately define a stereotactic system around the region of interest (Fig. 7.2).

In the treatment room, the frame can be leveled using a mechanism that is part of the treatment couch. For setup of isocenter coordinates, metric scales are used that are mounted on the frame and correspond to the CT indicators. Fixation of the patient within the frame can be obtained with a vacuum pillow, or, as shown in the figure, with a Scotchcast (Orthopedic Products, 3M, St. Paul, MN) body cast. A body cast such as this one is made out of thermoplast or fiberglass/polyurethane resin that becomes rigid after contact with water. The cast may provide both small intratreatment patient movement and stability for several weeks, can be more rigidly attached to a stereotactic body frame than vacuum pillows, and can provide an adequate surface for reliably marking isocenter and portals.

## Medical Intelligence BodyFIX

The Medical Intelligence BodyFIX patient immobilization system (Medical Intelligence, Schwabmuenchen, Germany) (Fig. 7.3) uses two vacuums, one of which is affixed to a large full body length Vac-Lok pillow (Med-Tec, Or-

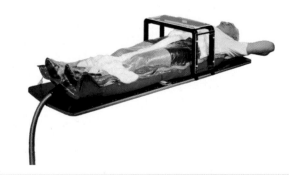

FIGURE 7.3. Medical Intelligence BodyFIX system. (Courtesy of Medical Intelligence, Schwabmuenchen, Germany).

ange City, IA) under the patient and another that provides a vacuum seal over the top of the patient. In this setup, the patient's respiration is minimized and a high degree of conformality can be achieved. The system includes a CT localizer for simulation and a laser localizer for positioning the isocenter within the treatment room.

## OPTICAL TRACKING AND PHOTOGRAMMETRY FOR PATIENT REPOSITIONING AND SETUP

Optical tracking is a means of determining in real-time the position of an object by tracking the positions of either active or passive infrared markers attached to the object. The position of the point of reflection is determined using a camera system. Optical guidance can be incorporated for frameless stereotaxis and can provide high-precision SBRT setup and positioning using either passive (reflective) markers or active (emitting) markers and fixed camera detection systems in the treatment delivery room.

Photogrammetry-based patient positioning systems have infrared charged-coupled device (CCD) cameras. The 3D positions of the markers are calculated by well-established conventional photogrammetry methods and provide reference information to determine the treatment plan isocenter location. It can be used to actively position the target at the isocenter of the treatment linear accelerator. Several authors have used this type of system and reported high precision and accuracy when applied to patients with head immobilization devices (8–10).

Such a system has also been used to measure the accuracy of conventional laser centering techniques for patient repositioning. The ExacTrac (BrainLAB, Heimstetten, Germany) is a commercially available photogrammetry-based patient positioning system developed for extracranial relocalization. Soete et al. (11) evaluated this system in 17 patients receiving conformal radiotherapy for prostate cancer. The standard deviation of measured setup errors along anterior to posterior, lateral and longitudinal axes were 2 mm, 1.6 mm, and 3.5 mm, respectively. At the Medical College of Virginia, we have observed an averaged reproducibility of around 3.5 mm for lung SBRT. It appears advantageous to use a pattern of surface marker placement that is relatively small and asymmetric.

## IMPLANTABLE MARKERS FOR IMPROVED VISUALIZATION AND RELOCALIZATION

Harada et al. (12) have reported on the performance of real-time tumor tracking radiation therapy (RTRT) using implanted gold seeds. In their studies, a 1.5- to 2.0-mm gold marker was safely inserted in or near peripheral-type lung tumors through bronchofiberscopy and used efficiently in the fluoroscopic RTRT system. Since that re-

port, a variety of implantable seeds has been developed that include novel shapes for radiolucent identification and minimization of motion. Radiofrequency (RF) emitting markers (Calypso, Seattle, WA) can identify and triangulate tumor and target position at up to 10 Hz (10 positions per second).

The system known as pReference (Med-Tec) is the original frameless system for fractionated stereotactic radiotherapy and single-dose radiosurgery. The pReference means "point reference" implanted fiducial technology for verified-accuracy stereotaxis. pReference is available in several planning configurations. In cranial cases, three markers are implanted in the skull; in SBRT cases, one to three markers are implanted directly at the target site. The bone markers are pure gold spheres. They are placed during a 20-minute outpatient procedure under local anesthesia. Tools to facilitate marker placement include drill bits, guides, and a tool for holding the marker during implantation. The soft-tissue P-ref marker surface is specially treated to prevent migration after implantation. The markers are implanted under ultrasound (US) or CT guidance with special needles. Also available from Med-Tec is the ISOLOC localization software featuring localization, image-guided setup, electronic portal image or film compatibility, marker tracking, concise couch translation output, and rotational information.

Several other manufacturers have developed markers for implanting into targets for improved visualization, and these markers have been demonstrated to be quite useful. VISICOIL linear fiducial markers (Fig. 7.4) are visible by US, radiography, CT, MRI, and high-energy photons (portal images), allowing the physician to implant the markers under one mode and later visualize them by another technique for treatment planning. These markers can be inserted by a fine needle, from 22- to 18-gauge, resulting in a less traumatic procedure to the patient. Actual needle gauge is dependent on the diameter of the marker to be implanted. Typically, a 17-gauge or larger needle has been used to introduce the 1.2-mm marker shown. The coiled-wire design of VISICOIL provides flexibility and allows the marker to conform to highly mobile soft tissue.

## ULTRASOUND VERIFICATION OF TARGET AND ORGAN POSITIONING

US identification of organ positioning is another methodology that has been applied in verification of tumor positioning prior to radiotherapy. Currently there are several vendors marketing US products for assistance with SBRT: SonArray (Zmed, Ashland, MA), ExacTrac Ultrasound Localization (BrainLAB, Heimstetten, Germany), and the BAT® (B-mode Acquisition and Targeting) ultrasound system (Nomos, Sewickley, PA). The SonArray is described and illustrated in Chapter 16, and the others are presented here.

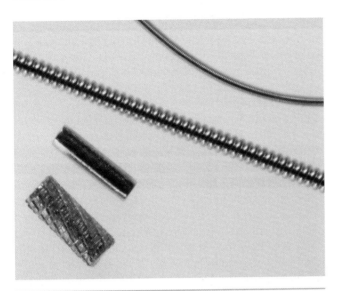

**FIGURE 7.4.** Implantable markers: Comparison of a 0.75-mm VISICOIL **(top)**, 0.35-mm VISICOIL **(center)**, and solid 1.2-mm "seed" markers. (Courtesy of RadioMed, Tyngsboro, MA).

The ExacTrac Ultrasound Localization allows a daily verification of the position of an internal reference structure (e.g. the liver) with live US images. The system can automatically compensate for internal organ shift, thereby aiding relocalization throughout the entire course of SBRT. For US scanning a reflective marker array is attached to an US probe, which is calibrated with respect to the reflective markers attached to the patient's body. The patient on the treatment couch is roughly positioned at isocenter, and an US image is then acquired in one position relative to the patient and saved with the target volume in the field of view. The software automatically reconstructs a CT image based on the previously acquired CT data scaled to represent the same position as the US image.

This procedure allows comparison of the current target volume, as seen in the US, with its position at the time of CT scanning. To compensate for any positional shift, the target volume originally contoured in the CT data set is superimposed on the US screen. Using the mouse or touch screen, these superimposed contours may be positioned interactively in the US image to the location of the target as seen in the US image. The software calculates the target volume shift in the vertical, lateral, and longitudinal coordinates and translates that information into the automatic couch movement necessary to reposition the target volume appropriately for treatment. Figure 7.5 depicts the BrainLAB ExacTrac system integrated with US and a sample output from the system indicating the required movements necessary to accurately position the isocenter.

The BAT system is another US-based stereotactic tumor localization device. It has been used at many centers for relocalization during conventionally fractionated radiotherapy for prostate cancer, and the technology is adaptable to SBRT. The operator technique is similar to the BrainLAB US system insofar as an US image of the tumor is obtained to allow a reconstruction of the target location based on previously obtained CT images, from which the necessary relocalization parameters are generated.

## SYSTEMS TO ACCOUNT FOR RESPIRATORY MOTION DURING STEREOTACTIC BODY RADIATION THERAPY

Respiration affects the instantaneous position of almost all thoracic and abdominal structures (lung, liver, pancreas, etc.), posing significant problems in the SBRT of tumors located at these sites by obliging typically an extra 2 cm or more PTV margin to account for the expected range of tumor motion during diaphragmatic excursion. It is highly desirable to reduce this standard practice of including an

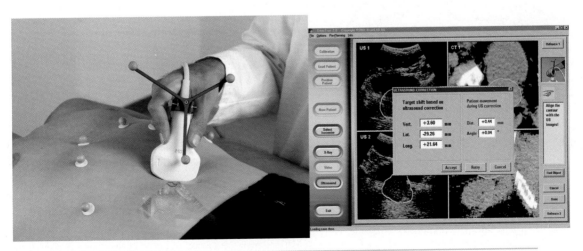

**FIGURE 7.5.** BrainLAB US ExacTrac System reflective markers and ultrasound probe **(left)**; typical screen view of relocalization parameters **(right)**. (Courtesy of BrainLAB, Munich, Germany).

additional margin in an effort to minimize the volume of normal tissue that receives radiation during SBRT.

Currently, there are two major methods to reduce the uncertainty of lung tumor location caused by respiratory motion. One includes some form of breathing regulation in which patients either hold their breath at a certain respiratory level during the irradiation or are otherwise restricted in their motion during respiration. The other method is the respiration-gated intermittent irradiation system, by which the movements of the skin surface or other physiologic parameters are monitored to coordinate the "beam-on" time with a specific portion of the respiratory cycle.

The abdominal compression method for limiting respiratory motion has been mentioned in several other chapters and generally involves placing a plate or other restrictive device above or around the torso, sometimes in combination with supplemental oxygen, in an effort to minimize diaphragmatic motion during treatment. Alternatively, patients may be instructed to hold their breath intermittently: Planning CT images are then obtained in segments of a few slices at a time while the tumor is moving less. Treatment is then administered at times of breath-hold as the beam is turned on and off intermittently.

A device call the Active Breathing Coordinator (Elekta) is designed specifically for the purpose of standardizing such a breath-hold technique for planning and treatment during SBRT or other radiotherapy (Fig. 7.6). Patients are coached to hold their breath at a certain consistent depth of inspiration, and beam-on time is coordinated with breath holding. At the moment of fixed inspiration, a valve device engages to prevent additional inspiration or expiration; patients always have access to a safety button to release the valve in the event of discomfort or anxiety. Patients with poor baseline pulmonary function will sometimes be unable to comply with breath-holding techniques.

*Respiratory-gated* radiotherapy is distinguished from *respiration-synchronized* radiotherapy as a method of accounting for respiratory motion. Respiratory-gated radiotherapy involves turning the beam on only during selected portions of the respiratory cycle, and this method has been successfully implemented in some centers. Respiration-synchronized treatment, in which the beam aperture or position is adjusted in concert with respiration, is currently under investigation at several institutions.

Varian's Real-time Position Management (RPM) Respiratory Gating System (Palo Alto, CA) uses a video monitor to characterize the patient's breathing pattern, and the pattern is obtained by tracking the motion of a reflective marker placed on the patient. Through video image analysis and signal processing, the system identifies both the full range of chest wall motion during respiration and the normal pattern of that motion. By correlating these data with the motion of the tumor in simulation, the treatment plan is designed whereby the treatment beam is on only when the tumor falls within the planned beam aperture.

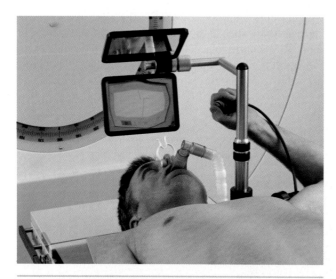

**FIGURE 7.6.** Elekta Active Breathing Coordinator. During treatment, the patient watches a monitor displaying the pattern of breathing and the signal indicating the period of breath-holding. The green button must be pressed for the respiration-control valve to engage, and patients may discontinue usage at any time in the event of discomfort or anxiety. (Courtesy of Elekta, Norcross, GA).

## REFERENCES

1. Verhey LJ. Immobilizing and positioning patients for radiotherapy. *Semin Radiat Oncol* 1995;5:100–114.
2. Rabinowitz I, Garelik-Wyler R. Accuracy of radiation field alignment in clinical practice. *Int J Radiat Oncol Biol Phys* 1985;11:1857–1867.
3. Hurkmans CW, Remeijer P, Lebesque JV, et al. Setup verification using portal imaging: review of current clinical practice. *Radiother Oncol* 2001;58:105–120.
4. Lax I, Blomgren H, Naslund I, et al. Stereotactic radiotherapy of malignancies in the abdomen: methodological aspects. *Acta Oncol* 1994;33:677–683.
5. Hamilton AJ, Lulu BA, Fosmire H, et al. Preliminary clinical experience with linear accelerator-based spinal stereotactic radiosurgery technique and application. *Neurosurgery* 1995;36:311–319.
6. Tokuuye K, Sumi M, Ikeda H, et al. Technical considerations for fractionated stereotactic radiotherapy of hepatocellular carcinoma. *Japan J Clin Oncol* 1997;27:170–173.
7. Sato M, Uematsu M, Yamamoto F, et al. Feasibility of frameless stereotactic high-dose radiation therapy for primary or metastatic liver cancer. *J Radiosurg* 1998;1:233–238.
8. Rogus RD, Stern RL, Kubo HD. Accuracy of a photogrammetry-based patient positioning and monitoring system for radiation therapy. *Med Phys* 1999;26:721–728.
9. Bova J, Buatti JM, Friedman WA, et al. The university of Florida frameless high-precision stereotactic radiotherapy system. *Int J Radiat Oncol Biol Phys* 1997;38:875–882.
10. Menke M, Hirschfeld F, Mack T, et al. Stereotactically guided fractionated radiotherapy: technical aspects. *Int J Radiat Oncol Biol Phys* 1994;29:1147–1155.
11. Soete G, Van de Steene J, Verellen D, et al. Initial clinical experience with infrared-reflecting skin markers in the positioning of patients treated by conformal radiotherapy for prostate cancer. *Int J Radiat Oncol Biol Phys* 2002;52:694–698.
12. Harada T, Shirato H, Ogura S, et al. Real-time tumor-tracking radiation therapy for lung carcinoma by the aid of insertion of a gold marker using bronchofiberscopy. *Cancer* 2002;95:1720–1727.

# Dosimetry of Stereotactic Body Radiation Therapy

Lech Papiez, Vadim Moskvin, and *Robert D. Timmerman

## INTRODUCTION

Stereotactic body radiation therapy (SBRT) (1–40) reproduces physical and biologic aspects of the intracranial stereotactic radiosurgery (SRS) experience. In particular, the SRS feature of high dose per fraction prescription applied for SBRT treatments requires minimization of volume of tissue exposed to avoid late normal tissue toxicity (1–3,25,31,32,41–43). In turn, this objective can be best achieved by imitating SRS techniques for stereotactic radiation delivery in SBRT.

One essential feature of SRS of the brain is the ability to rigidly secure an immobilization device, which serves also as frame of reference for stereotaxy to the skull. Securing the skull fastens the brain tissue in the system of coordinates defined by stereotactic frame. In contrast, extracranial targets inherently move (6–8,22,44–53), and thus cannot be absolutely held in reference to the isocenter of the radiation delivery machine. As such, stereotactic treatments in the body are inherently imprecise unless adequate immobilization or compensation for the target and organ motions, both inter- and intrafractional is achieved. Thus even though the precise stereotactic targeting is as important in SBRT as it is for intracranial radiosurgery, dosimetric benefits of this targeting are essentially tied to the appropriate utilization of immobilization devices (1–4,9–13,17,18,20,25,31,32,38,40) and/or to precise organ motion compensation techniques (6–8,22, 33–35,37,43,45,47–51,53,54).

In this chapter, we assume that devices and techniques for suitable simulation, planning, and delivery of SBRT treatments exist and are properly used in precise targeting of tumor volumes and organs. We concentrate our attention on dose distribution parameters that should be achieved in SBRT for clinically advantageous treatments.

Department of Radiation Oncology, Indiana University School of Medicine, Indianapolis, IN 46202; and *Department of Radiation Oncology, University of Texas Southwestern Medical Center, Dallas, TX 75390

## METHODS

### General Dosimetric Considerations and Measures of Quality of Dose Distributions for Stereotactic Body Radiation Therapy

The proper conduct of high-dose-per-fraction SBRT requires both precise targeting and isotropic and rapid dose falloff to normal surrounding tissues (1,2,15,25,31,32). This type of "imitation" of Gamma Knife (Elekta, Stockholm, Sweden) treatments by a linear accelerator–based delivery is achievable though generally not practiced in radiation therapy (23). In practical terms, the imitation of properties of Gamma Knife treatments in SBRT will take place if the following conditions of delivery are satisfied (25):

i. The shape of the isosurface defined by the dose prescribed conforms to the outline of the target and highest doses delivered outside of the tumor are confined to regions that spread uniformly on the outer boundary of the targeted volume.

ii. Rapid falloff of dose from the tumor volume to healthy tissue isotropically in all directions.

iii. Nonuniform dose distribution throughout the volume of the tumor, with the highest dose delivered to the central portion of the tumor where hypoxic cells potentially reside.

iv. Delivery of high dose per fraction to the tumor volume (on the order of 10 to 20 Gy).

v. A small number of fractions per course of treatment (e.g., one to five).

Conditions (i) and (ii) require that a relatively large number of preferably noncoplanar beams be used for SBRT treatments. Conditions (i), (ii), and (iii) are achieved for SBRT treatments in a somewhat deferent manner than for Gamma Knife therapy. Instead of combining multiple shots with various weighting factors, these distributions can be realized by appropriate shaping of intensities of a limited number of noncoplanar beams.

These two approaches lead to equivalent dose distributions (23). In particular, formulas that relate beam intensities of modulated linear accelerator therapy with weighting factors of equivalent Gamma Knife therapy can be uniquely defined (23). Conditions (iv) and (v), together with their justification and clinical validation, have been discussed in other publications (1,2,31,32) and will not be elaborated on in this presentation.

The assessment of the dose shaping in SBRT is important for the evaluation of the quality of the applied treatment. This evaluation should provide information about the target coverage by the prescription dose, the proximity of the dose cloud wrapping around the target, and the uniformity of the gradient of dose decrease away from the target. Some traditional parameters, or functions, that are used in radiation therapy for measuring quality of dose distributions are useful but not quite adequate for our purposes. Some previously used measures include radiation conformality index (59,60), ratios of organ volumes exposed below given value of the dose [e.g. $V_{20}$- portion of the organ exposed to 20 Gy or more per course of treatment (61,62)] and other parameters derived from dose–volume histograms (DVHs). None of these indexes, however, properly characterizes the critical aspects of SBRT dosimetry discussed in this section. For example, the radiation conformality index may indicate that the volume of the PTV is the same as the volume of tissue exposed to given level of dose; however, it

does not specify how much of both volumes overlap each other. $V_{20}$ may tell us how big portion of the lung (liver, rectum, etc.) is protected from a threshold level dose exposure but it will not tell us if the portion of the lung exposed to large dose is close to the tumor where such spillage dose may actually be beneficial for treating microscopic disease. Finally, the DVH functions give us detailed information of how large portions of organ have been exposed to different levels of dose but again it will not show where in the organ these volumes exposed to different levels of dose are located.

As SBRT is an emerging field, there is still no firm consensus on the ultimate clinical appropriateness of various methods for dosimetry evaluation. At Indiana University (IU) we are carefully following a large group of patients treated on prospective trials for both tumor control and toxicity. On the basis of our observations and the observations described at other centers, we have formulated criteria and constraints for treatment planning. These constraints have been adopted for the first Radiation Therapy Oncology Group (RTOG) trial using SBRT (Protocol number L-0236) for dosimetry evaluation. These constraints will be discussed below and are listed in Table 8.1. These constraints are used in clinical practice at the time of publication of this text, but the reader is cautioned to appreciate that these constraints have changed over the years at our own center and may change in the relatively near future as well. Practitioners of SBRT must

▶ **TABLE 8.1 RTOG Criteria for Dosimetry Evaluation of SBRT of Early-stage Lung Cancer.**

| PTV Volume (cc) | Ratio of Prescription Isodose Volume to the PTV | | Ratio of 50% Prescription Isodose Volume to the PTV, $R_{50\%}$ | | Maximum Dose 2 cm from PTV in any Direction, $D_{2cm}$ (Gy) | | Percent of Lung receiving 20 Gy total or more, $V_{20}$ (%) | |
|---|---|---|---|---|---|---|---|---|
| | Deviation | | Deviation | | Deviation | | Deviation | |
| | none | minor | none | minor | none | minor | none | minor |
| 1.8 | <1.2 | 1.2-1.4 | <3.9 | 3.9-4.1 | <28.1 | 28.1-30.1 | <10 | 10-15 |
| 3.8 | <1.2 | 1.2-1.4 | <3.9 | 3.9-4.1 | <28.1 | 28.1-30.1 | <10 | 10-15 |
| 7.4 | <1.2 | 1.2-1.4 | <3.9 | 3.9-4.1 | <28.1 | 28.1-30.1 | <10 | 10-15 |
| 13.2 | <1.2 | 1.2-1.4 | <3.9 | 3.9-4.1 | <28.1 | 28.1-30.1 | <10 | 10-15 |
| 21.9 | <1.2 | 1.2-1.4 | <3.8 | 3.8-4.0 | <30.4 | 30.4-32.4 | <10 | 10-15 |
| 33.8 | <1.2 | 1.2-1.4 | <3.7 | 3.7-3.9 | <32.7 | 32.7-34.7 | <10 | 10-15 |
| 49.6 | <1.2 | 1.2-1.4 | <3.6 | 3.6-3.8 | <35.1 | 35.1-37.1 | <10 | 10-15 |
| 69.9 | <1.2 | 1.2-1.4 | <3.5 | 3.5-3.7 | <37.4 | 37.4-41.7 | <10 | 10-15 |
| 95.1 | <1.2 | 1.2-1.4 | <3.3 | 3.3-3.5 | <39.7 | 39.7-41.7 | <10 | 10-15 |
| 125.8 | <1.2 | 1.2-1.4 | <3.1 | 3.1-3.3 | <42.0 | 42.0-44.0 | <10 | 10-15 |
| 162.6 | <1.2 | 1.2-1.4 | <2.9 | 2.9-3.1 | <44.3 | 44.3-46.3 | <10 | 10-15 |

RTOG, Radiation Therapy Oncology Group; PTV, planning target volume; SBRT, stereotactic body radiation therapy.
RTOG dosimetry evaluation criteria for early-stage lung cancer for low and high-dose "spillage." Optimally, the criteria would fit within the "none" deviation category. These criteria coupled with information in the section 2 (see text) and respect of normal tissue dose and volume tolerance are used to evaluate specific stereotactic body radiation therapy treatment plans. The criteria were written on the basis of a protocol giving 60 Gy total in three fractions to the margin of the PTV. Absolute doses in Gy listed in this table should be scaled for different dose fractionation schedules. These criteria may also be applied to abdominal and pelvic tumor sites.

keep abreast of new developments in the field since both the benefits of and harm caused by SBRT are potentially extreme.

Evaluation of SBRT dosimetry at IU includes scrutiny of three categories: (a) target coverage, (b) high-dose "spillage," and (c) low-dose "spillage." In regard to target coverage, it is our practice to normalize the dose (i.e., set to 100%) to the center of mass of the planning target volume (PTV), which for our equipment is the isocenter. With such normalization, the edge of the PTV is usually encompassed by around the 80% isodose curve. The prescription dose is given to the isodose line encompassing at least 95% of the PTV volume. Furthermore, it is required that 99% of the PTV volume get at least 90% of the prescription dose. Since we prescribe to the 80% line for most cases, there is considerable target heterogeneity, which is manipulated to occur within the gross tumor volume (GTV). High-dose "spillage" into normal tissue is evaluated by location and volume. In regard to location, any dose greater than 105% of the prescription dose (not the overall maximum dose) should occur primarily within the PTV. Therefore, the cumulative volume of any tissue outside of the PTV receiving a dose greater than 105% of prescription dose should be no more than 15% of the PTV volume (preferably less than 10% of the PTV volume). In regard to high-dose "spillage" volume, we require that the conformality ratio defined as the volume of the prescription isodose coverage over the PTV volume be less than 1.2. As with high-dose "spillage," low-dose "spillage" is critiqued by criteria relating to location and volume. Low-dose "spillage" location requires that the dose to any point 2 cm away from the PTV surface ($D_{2 cm}$) be below a limit that is a function of PTV volume as shown in Table 8.1. Finally, the volume of low-dose "spillage" is required to fit within a low-dose conformality ratio defined as the ratio of the 50% isodose coverage to the PTV. This parameter, called $R_{50\%}$, is also a function of the PTV volume as shown in Table 8.1. These evaluations, coupled with a respect for normal tissue dose–volume absolute limits, must be satisfied in most circumstances for a plan to be used in treating a patient with SBRT at IU.

## Minimization of Volume of Tissue Exposed by Minimizing Field Margins

As we described in the prior sections, the most important factor for SBRT dose shaping is the minimization of volume of tissue exposed. At our center, we generally only treat tumor targets where it is reasonable to assume GTV equals CTV (CTV is the clinical target volume that includes margin for microscopic tumor infiltration) based on anatomic, histologic, and imaging characteristics. At any rate, it is important to keep beam security margins as small as possible when transforming GTV (or CTV) into PTV (1,2,31,32). Nevertheless, these margins have to ac-

count for all motions of targeted tissue plus uncertainties inherent in patient positioning, error in the target recognition, treatment planning etc. Linear margins for SBRT planning (i.e., lengths of intervals connecting GTV and PTV surfaces along particular lines) are most commonly chosen (on the basis of validation of immobilization equipment) to be equal to 0.5 cm along any radius pointing away from target center in any direction in transverse planes and equal to 1.0 cm along all parallel lines perpendicular to the axial plane (1,2,9,16). These margins may need to be increased in the cases where equipment has not been critically evaluated or in particular patients whose target motion is difficult to control. These margins may also be decreased. However, care should be taken to insure that confidence in setup justifies smaller margins based on the immobilization and motion accounting equipment employed.

The final assessment of adequacy of target margins for SBRT treatments is appreciated in tumor control probabilities confirmed by clinical results (1–3,5,9–12,17,18,38–40). However, it is clear from a straightforward analysis of a cumulative error arising from all steps of the SBRT delivery that typically used margins are not large enough to ensure that the prescribed dose will be delivered to the entire GTV with a probability of 1. It may be noticed that if the isotropic gradient of dose in all directions away from PTV is present for SBRT treatments, the target volume is immersed in the shell of high-dose region (70% to 90% of prescribed dose) of thickness of approximately 1 cm. Thus, highly potent dose levels are delivered to the target volume in SBRT treatments even if the PTV region is few millimeters outside of the isosurface of prescribed dose.

Minimization of volume of tissue exposed to potentially toxic levels of dose may seem more difficult to achieve when simultaneously increasing dose gradients within the target volumes. The rationale for requiring these gradients of increased dose toward the center of the PTV region is based on the assumption that in SBRT treatments defined targets should contain little normal tissue (31,32). In fact, as long as an acceptable minimum dose is delivered to all parts of the target, higher target doses (hot spots) may be desirable if they can be manipulated with intensity modulation to occur within the central core of the tumor target where hypoxic, radioresistant cells may be more prevalent. Furthermore, this increase in the gradient of dose toward the center of the PTV does not generally contribute to enlargement of tissue volumes exposed to high dose outside of the PTV as discussed earlier in the prologue.

## Dose Conformity in Stereotactic Body Radiation Therapy

The angular allocation of directions of multiple non-coplanar beams in SBRT radiation delivery is the main factor shaping the dose distribution around the target

(1,2,25). Rapid and uniform falloff of dose in all directions from the tumor is the consequence of noncoplanar method of stereotactic radiation delivery employed at both Karolinska Hospital and IU . The volume defined by the intersection of all beams is only slightly larger than PTV itself and it conforms closely to the shape of the target (24,28,36). The resulting isodose surface defined by full dose contributions from all beams matches closely, up to the margin defined by penumbra effects, the shape of the PTV. The speed of decrease of dose away from the tumor is defined under these circumstances primarily by the rate of decline in number of beams intersecting each other in subsequent shells that enfold the target. In turn, the rate of decline in number of beams intersecting in subsequent shells is correlated with the level of uniformity of used beams' directional distribution.

The above heuristic analysis indicates that shaping optimal dose distributions for SBRT treatments favor the use of large number of noncoplanar beams or arcs. However, practical considerations often limit the number of beam directions feasible to utilize in treatment. With limited number of directions, it is even more important to choose their directions so that they create the smallest possible volume of intersection. This usually involves finding directions that are maximally separated in the possible space of angles in three dimensions (24,28,36). The problem of separation of directions leads to counterintuitive results even in situations where there are no constraints imposed on the selection of angles (24). In real cases of SBRT irradiation, the additional limitations are added to avoid tissues of sensitive organs and to satisfy mechanical restrictions imposed by the equipment (25).

Implementing SBRT treatments with traditional linear accelerators and demanding that the total treatment time is less than 1 hour limits the number of beams per treatment to around seven to 12. When the prescribed dose is less than 20 Gy per fraction, seven or eight beam directions are satisfactory to achieve parameters of dose distributions appropriate for SBRT treatment. When dose prescribed is larger than 20 Gy per fraction, the number of beams directions needs to increase to nine or ten. The factor that is most influential in deciding the minimum number of beam directions per treatment as well as the relative beam weighting to isocenter is the dose at entrance (using dose at the beam's $d_{max}$) for each beam. In particular, it is prudent to keep each beam's $d_{max}$ dose to a modest amount (e.g., under 9 Gy per fraction times three fractions or the equivalent) and weight the beams to have relatively the same percent dose at each beam's $d_{max}$. These limitations prevent acute skin reaction while maintaining isotropic falloff dose gradients (31). Following the indication that seven to 12 is a practical number of beams for SBRT using the standard linear accelerator, calculations may be done to find their optimal placement (Table

▶ **TABLE 8.2   Couch and Gantry Relationships for Nonopposing, Noncoplanar Beams in SBRT.**

| Right-sided Lesion | Left-sided Lesion |
|---|---|
| (c, g) = (0,225) | (c, g) = (0,135) |
| (c, g) = (0,315) | (c, g) = (0,45) |
| (c, g) = (30,90) | (c, g) = (330,270) |
| (c, g) = (330,90) | (c, g) = (30,270) |
| (c, g) = (90,40) | (c, g) = (90,40) |
| (c, g) = (90,320) | (c, g) = (90,320) |
| (c, g) = (0,165) | (c, g) = (0,195) |

SBRT, stereotactic body radiation therapy; c, couch angle; g, gantry angle. Parameters above provide seven pairs of couch and gantry angles in degrees for noncoplanar SBRT treatment of lung and liver with Siemens KD2 accelerator (Munich, Germany). These beam positions relative to patient body optimize their angular space arrangement. Provided constraints limiting mutual positions of couch and gantry are satisfied (no collision ensured) the volume of intersection of all cylindrical beams irradiating a spherical tumor within the patient's body is minimized for these directions.

8.2) that simultaneously respects mechanical restrictions imposed by the equipment (collisions of couch and gantry, etc.) (25). These standard set of beam directions can, for each particular clinical case, be appropriately adjusted for obtaining the best possible dose distribution taking into account specific restrictions of individual patient geometry or anatomy.

## Target Dose Heterogeneity

Both SRS and SBRT generally are planned with nonuniformity throughout the target volume (1,2,15,25,38–40, 55). The nonuniform dose distribution inside the PTV volume intends to concentrate, similarly as it happens for Gamma Knife treatments, the highest dose to the central portion of the tumor where hypoxic cells potentially reside. For Gamma Knife treatments, the prescription at the outer edge of the tumor is customarily to 50% isodose surface whereas the prescription at the outer edge of the tumor for SBRT treatments is usually between 60% and 90%. The coincidence of beam aperture borders with the outline the PTVs for SBRT treatments means that portions of the PTV border will be located within penumbra region for certain beams. This in turn means that dose distribution will show a gradient near target edge (i.e., something less than 95%–100%), increasing in these regions toward the center of the PTV volume. For lung treatments, heterogeneous target dose deposition is partly related to tissue heterogeneity effects. These inherent physical as well as intended causes for dose heterogeneity will not necessarily result in the optimal desired distributions for tumor control. Such "painting" of dose can only be achieved by modulation of beam intensities. Delivery of such modulated intensities can be realized through various techniques; however, the most convenient method relies on the use of appropriately designed milled compensators. The advantage of milled compensators stems from the fact that they only slightly increase the number of monitor units utilized per each field (of the order of 10%). Moreover, they are not necessarily confounded by the time dependence of GTV/CTV target position leading to unintended "cold spots" within the target as with the multileaf collimator (MLC). In some situations, the use of MLC instead of compensators is acceptable as long as appropriate accounting of target motion is simultaneously realized. The number of monitor units for MLC intensity-modulated radiation therapy (IMRT) is generally larger than for compensator treated intensity modulated fields. For SBRT treatments, each fraction may require delivery of 4,000 to 6,000 monitor units without modulation of intensity. As such, any additional increases in number of monitor units per fraction must be seen as undesirable and potentially making the treatment unfeasible. Increases in number of monitor units are even larger when gating techniques are applied for compensation of respiratory motions to minimize volumes of tissue exposed. While combining compensator type delivery with gating may still be feasible for SBRT, combining MLC IMRT with gating for SBRT treatments is potentially unworkable.

## Tissue Heterogeneity Effects

One organ particularly suitable for treatments with SBRT techniques is the lung. One of the principal challenges for lung treatment is the evaluation of dose disturbance related to dramatic changes in tissue density also known as tissue heterogeneity effects. For lung treatments, beams have to first pass through chest wall, then penetrate low-density lung tissue, and finally deliver energy to cells of solid tumor. The chest wall is a combination of muscle and bone. Muscle has electron density close to the electron density of water, and bone has electron density somewhat higher than water. Overall, the disturbance of dose caused by the chest wall is negligible (5,65–67). On the other hand, dose disruption occurring at the tumor site caused by the low density of lung tissue (three to four times lower than density of muscle) can be significant (39,63,65,68–71). This dose variation can, to a degree, be compensated by the spectrum of beam used since lower average beam energies are relatively less affected by density changes. However, the variation in dose between homogenous and inhomogeneous media cannot be effectively compensated by modulation of beam intensity. Having reliable information relating to the limitations of accuracy for dose calculations employed is essential for proper prescription of dose. There are several dose correction algorithms used by commercially available planning systems. Existing algorithms

(equivalent tissue-air ratio [TAR] methods, collapsed cone, etc.) may lead to considerably different results as far as calculated dose is concerned. None of these algorithms is completely reliable for dose calculations in lung, especially when multiple, small fields are involved and when sharp changes of tissue densities in volumes of interest are present. On the other hand, the potential discrepancies between doses calculated and doses delivered are diminished by mutually compensating influences of electronic disequilibrium and altered photon fluence related to attenuation. First, when comparing actual measured dosimetry to a dosimetry plan assuming all tissues with water density, we notice that the decreased attenuation in the lung causes the increase in dose delivered to the target (i.e., higher photon fluence incident upon the target). However, the lack of electronic equilibrium in solid tissue due to decreased energy transfer in low-density tissue of the lung leads to decreased dose at the edge of the tumor. These two influences, one increasing and the other decreasing the dose at the surface of the target may in some situations cancel each other. As a result, a similar dose to the target outer edge in homogenous and inhomogeneous media may be expected so long as the dose is calculated and prescribed to the periphery of the target. Since delivery of the correct dose to the periphery of the tumor is more important in SBRT than any particular shape of dose inside the target, one may observe that the uncorrected for heterogeneity calculations of dose are suitable for most SBRT treatments. This observation is attractive from clinical point of view as it allows consistent dose prescription and dose delivery for all treated cases based on homogenous media dose calculations.

To verify this position relating to tissue heterogeneity correction, extensive data have been collected in the IU Department of Radiation Oncology. Multiple calculations of cases of lung SBRT treatment have been performed at our institution involving two treatment-planning systems (Render Plan 3D, Elekta, Stockholm, Sweden and CMS XIO Plan, CMS, St. Louis, MO) and Monte Carlo simulations. These calculations have been also verified against phantom measurements. The relevant anthropomorphic phantom of human chest has been provided for this purpose by Radiological Physics Center (RPC). The RPC lung phantom closely represents geometry of the upper trunk of the body, including relevant variations in densities for materials replicating muscles and lung tissue. Calculations and relevant measurements confirm the fact that using no corrections for lung density leads to adequate prescription dose target coverage of patients for typical beam arrangements in SBRT treatments as seen in Fig. 8.1. In other words, application of inhomogeneity corrections, although decreasing overall error between actual and calculated dose distributions throughout the entire plan does not generally improve the agreement of the dose prescribed to target's outer edge. At best, more computationally intensive algo-

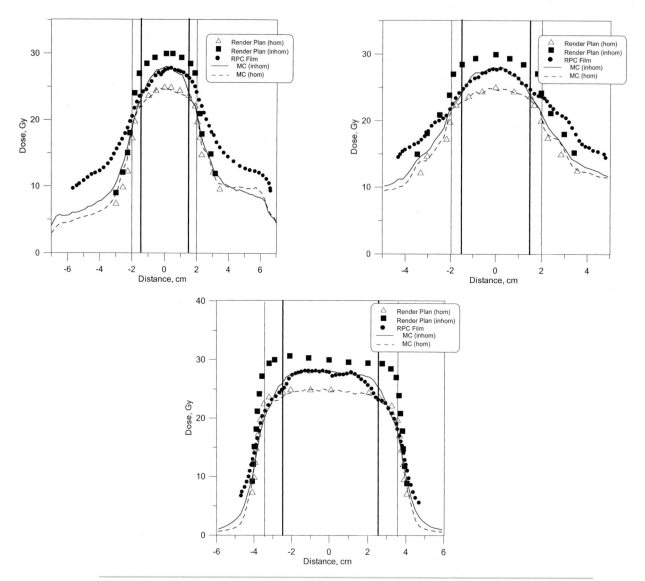

**FIGURE 8.1.** The comparison of dose distribution calculated and measured for typical stereotactic body radiation therapy (SBRT) treatment of the lung. Tumor [gross tumor volume (GTV)] is defined by a cylinder of diameter 3.0 cm and length 2.0 cm supplemented by two hemispheres of diameter 3 cm attached at each base of the cylinder. Thus total tumor length is 5.0 cm. Tumor has electron density 1 and is located at the center of the left lung that has electron density 0.26. Planning target volume (PTV) is a volume defined by union of two spatial volumes. First volume results from expanding surface of GTV by 0.5 cm in all directions in each axial plane. The second volume results from expanding surface of GTV by 1.0 cm in inferior–superior direction (direction perpendicular to axial plane). Treatment fields have outlines coincident with outlines of PTV projection on the plane of each field. Fields intensities are shaped to increase the dose (by 20 %) toward the center of the target and are higher by 25% to 35% at center than at the edge of each field. The arrangement of beams is noncoplanar and beam directions are distributed to minimize, within the range of angular space allowed by the gantry/table collision constraints, the volume of intersection of all beams. Dose of 20 Gy has been delivered to the outline of PTV (*thin vertical line*) according to plan calculated by Render Plan 3D (Elekta, Stockholm Sweden) for homogeneous phantom. Graphs **(A, B, and C)** show profiles along three main axes (x-axis, y-axis, and z-axis, appropriately) of the system of coordinates with origin at the center of the GTV. Axis x is coincident with line common to axial and coronal planes and describes right/left profile **(A)** axis y is coincident with line common to axial and sagittal planes and describes anterior/posterior profile **(C)** and axis z is coincident with line common to sagittal and coronal planes and describes inferior/superior profile **(D).** Each graph shows dose profile functions for (i) Render Plan homogeneous dose calculations (triangles), (ii) Render Plan inhomogeneous dose calculations (*squares*) based on monitor units calculated for homogeneous dose calculations , (iii) RPC TLD/film dose reading (*dotted line*), (iv) MC (PENELOPE) homogeneous dose calculations (dashed line), (v) MC (PENELOPE) inhomogeneous dose calculations (*continuous line*). MC homogeneous dose calculations have been normalized to 2,500 cGy at isocenter and MC inhomogeneous dose calculations have been normalized to dose measured at isocenter. Note that dose calculated, and delivered according to, by Render Plan homogeneous dose calculations (*triangles*) closely coincides with dose measured at the outline of PTV. Note also that if dose was delivered according to Render Plan inhomogeneous dose calculations (*squares*) it would require decrease of monitor units per field by 15% to 20% and would result in dose measured described by line that is shifted down from data displayed also by 15% to 20%. This dose would lead to considerable underdose at the edge of the PTV.

▶ **TABLE 8.3** Effect of Tissue Heterogeneity Correction on Monitor Unit Calculations.

| Beam No. (Energy) | No Correction | Inhomogeneity Correction (Convolution) | | | Inhomogeneity Correction (Superposition) | |
|---|---|---|---|---|---|---|
| | No. MU (20 Gy to PTV Outline) | No. MU (20 Gy to PTV Outline) | No. MU (25 Gy to Isocenter) | | No. MU (20 Gy to PTV Outline) | No. MU (25 Gy to Isocenter) |
| 1 (6 mV) | 407 | 349 | 397 | | 407 | 424 |
| 2 (15 mV) | 515 | 481 | 546 | | 515 | 591 |
| 3 (6 mV) | 405 | 335 | 381 | | 405 | 405 |
| 4 (6 mV) | 394 | 329 | 374 | | 394 | 398 |
| 5 (6 mV) | 481 | 360 | 409 | | 481 | 441 |
| 6 (15 mV) | 508 | 367 | 417 | | 508 | 463 |
| 7 (6 mV) | 368 | 318 | 361 | | 368 | 385 |
| Total No. MU | 3078 | 2539 | 2885 | | 3078 | 3080 |

MU, monitor unit; PTV, planning target volume.
The table compares treatments defined by seven beams (see beam angles in Table 8.1) and calculated with no inhomogeneity correction (column 2) and with two algorithms correcting for inhomogeneous tissue density (columns 2, 3, 4, and 5). Treatments defined by delivery of MU specified in columns 2, 3, and 5 are based on the prescription of 20 Gy to the outline of PTV (target). Notice that identical irradiation is defined in this case by no inhomogeneity correction calculation algorithm (column 2) and superposition inhomogeneity correction algorithm (column 5) and that considerably different irradiation is required (column 3) for identical prescription when inhomogeneity correction convolution algorithm is applied.

rithms (superposition, CMS XIO) lead to treatments equivalent to those that use no corrections for lung density while other less sophisticated algorithms correcting for tissue electron density may lead to treatments that are inconsistent with prescription (Table 8.3). Thus it seems reasonable to recommend that either sophisticated heterogeneity correction algorithms or no inhomogeneity corrections should be used for SBRT treatments of the lung.

## DOSIMETRY EXAMPLE CASE

What follows is a primer on approaching the dosimetry planning process for a typical patient with lung cancer. The patient has a left-sided, early-stage lung cancer. The computed tomography (CT) scans performed with accounting of respiratory motion are transferred to the three-dimensional (3D) treatment planning system. The outline of the GTV is identified using pulmonary windowing by the treating physician. This GTV is subsequently enlarged by 1.0 cm in the craniocaudal plane and 0.5 cm in axial plane as indicated in Fig. 8.2A and Fig. 8.2E. This enlarged volume is based specifically on the characteristics of the immobilization and respiratory inhibition system employed and constitutes the PTV. For this case, the GTV and CTV are the same target as no extra allowance for microscopic disease is used. An isocenter for beam and gantry rotation is placed at the center of mass of the PTV.

Standard normal tissue contouring for this pulmonary case would include the trachea, the proximal bronchial tree, the heart, the lungs (contoured as one structure), the esophagus, the spinal cord, and brachial plexus. Contouring the proximal bronchial tree is very important for SBRT as, in contrast to conventional ra-

diotherapy, injury to this structure may dramatically debilitate the patient.

Since the lesion is left sided, the table/gantry beam directions for source to axis distance (SAD) treatment are selected from Table 8.2. The relative directions of these seven beams are modified to avoid entrance dose through eloquent tissue like the spinal cord or proximal bronchial tree. The 3D arrangement of these seven beams is shown in Fig. 8.3. The entry points of these beams surround the patient on all sides and collectively cover a large solid angle.

All beams are shaped to coincide with the outline of the PTV along a beam's eye view projection. This is accomplished by focus blocks or MLC leaves with width of 5 mm or less. All beams are weighted to the isocenter, and total dose is normalized to the isocenter. As such, the periphery of the PTV is covered by an isodose line in the range of 60% to 90%. Beam weights are manipulated further to avoid excessive entrance dose as discussed above. At our center, such a lesion would receive 60 Gy to the margin of the PTV in three fractions given to the 80% isodose line. The target coverage in axial and coronal planes is shown in Fig. 8.2. Note how the lower isodose "spillage" lines are purposely diverted away from the large bronchi in the central chest. Dose falloff is rapid in all directions, particularly the craniocaudal plane on the superior and inferior aspects of the PTV.

Dose volume statistics for this plan indicate that 98% of the PTV volume is covered by the prescription isodose volume at the 60-Gy level. Ninety-nine percent of the PTV volume is covered by the 57-Gy volume (95% of the prescription dose). The 60-Gy volume is 1.1 times the PTV volume indicating excellent conformality. Doses greater than 105% of the prescription dose (63 Gy) occurring outside of the PTV only occupy a volume equal to 5% of the

*continued p. 66*

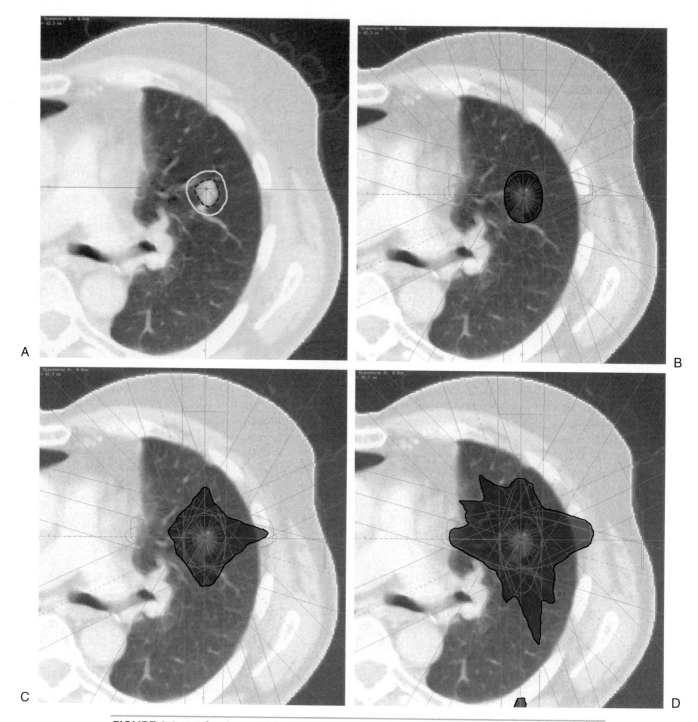

**FIGURE 8.2.** Axial and coronal target representation and resultant dose deposition from a seven-field stereotactic body radiation therapy treatment plan for an early-stage lung cancer. **A:** The axial enlargement of the planning target volume beyond the gross tumor volume as described in Section 2. The dose level depositions for the 60 Gy line **(B)**, 30-Gy line **(C)**, and 15-Gy line **(D)** for the same axial planes are shown.

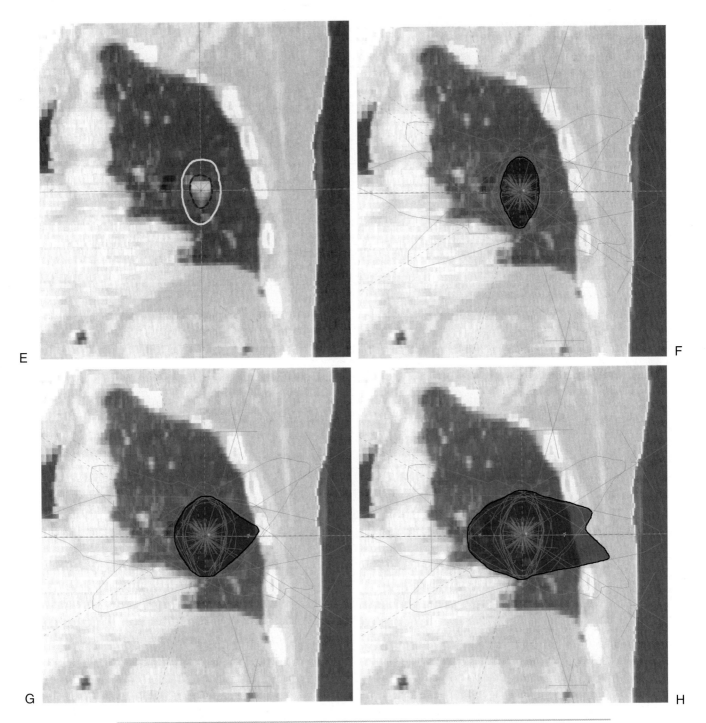

E

F

G

H

**FIGURE 8.2. (CONTINUED).** Axial and coronal target representation and resultant dose deposition from a seven-field stereotactic body radiation therapy treatment plan for an early-stage lung cancer. **E–H:** Same as frames **A–D,** except displayed in the coronal plane.

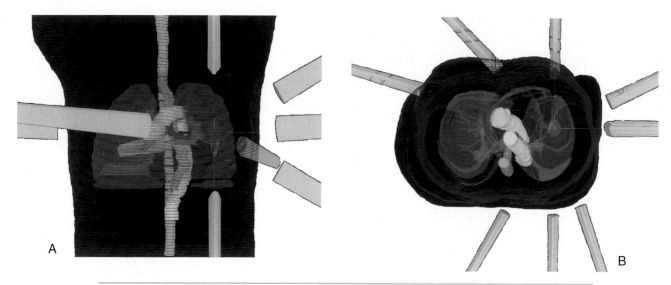

**FIGURE 8.3.** Three-dimensional representation of a typical beam arrangement for stereotactic body radiation therapy to a left-sided, early-stage lung cancer. **A:** The beams looking from a view directly in front of the patient. **B:** A view from the patient's feet. Contoured normal structures are shown as well as the tumor's planning target volume (*red*).

PTV volume. The maximum dose 2 cm anywhere from the edge of the PTV is less than 28.1 (Table 8.1), and the ratio of the 30-Gy volume to the PTV is less than 3.9. Normal tissue dose tolerance limits for this treatment dose fractionation are shown in Table 8.4.

▶ **TABLE 8.4** Normal Tissue Dose Tolerance for SBRT Delivered in Three Fractions.

| Organ | Volume | Dose (Gy) |
|---|---|---|
| Spinal cord | Any point | 18 Gy (6 Gy per fraction) |
| Esophagus | Any point | 27 Gy (9 Gy per fraction) |
| Ipsilateral brachial plexus | Any point | 24 Gy (8 Gy per fraction) |
| Heart | Any point | 30 Gy (10 Gy per fraction) |
| Trachea and Ipsilateral bronchus | Any point | 30 Gy (10 Gy per fraction) |
| Whole lung (right and left) | (See Table 8.1) | (See Table 8.1) |

SBRT, stereotactic body radiation therapy; RTOG, Radiation Therapy Oncology Group.
RTOG normal tissue dose constraints specifically for SBRT using a dose fractionation of three total fractions separated by 2 to 3 days. In the particular protocol (L-0236), the total dose used for treating early-stage non–small cell lung cancer was 60 Gy in three fractions.

## REFERENCES

1. Blomgren H, Lax I, Naslund I. Radiosurgery for tumors in the body. *Int J Radiat Oncol Biol Phys*1997;39:328–328.
2. Blomgren H, Lax I, Naslund I, Svanstrom R. Stereotactic high dose fraction radiation therapy of extracranial tumors using an accelerator: clinical experience of the first thirty-one patients. *Acta Oncologica* 1995;34:861–870.
3. Cardenes H, Timmerman R, Papiez L. Extracranial stereotactic radioablation: review of biological basis, technique and preliminary clinical experience. *Oncologica* 2002;25:193–199.
4. Gunven P, Blomgren H, Lax I. Radiosurgery for recurring liver metastases after hepatectomy. *Hepato-Gastroenterology* 2003;50:1201–1204.
5. Hadinger U, Thiele W, Wulf J. Extracranial stereotactic radiotherapy: evaluation of PTV coverage and dose conformity. *Zeitschrift fur Medizinische Physik* 2002;12:221–229.
6. Hara R, Itami J, Kondo T, et al. Stereotactic single high dose irradiation of lung tumors under respiratory gating. *Radiother Oncol* 2002;63:159–163.
7. Hara R, Itami J, Aruga T, et al. Development of stereotactic irradiation system of body tumors under respiratory gating. *Nippon Igaku Hoshasen Gakkai Zasshi* 2002;62:156–160.
8. Harada T, Shirato H, Ogura S, et al. Real-time tumor-tracking radiation therapy for lung carcinoma by the aid of insertion of a gold marker using bronchofiberscopy. *Cancer* 2002;95:1720–1727.
9. Herfarth KK, Debus J, Lohr F, et al. Extracranial stereotactic radiation therapy: Set-up accuracy of patients treated for liver metastases. *Int J Radiat Oncol Biol Phys* 2000;46:329–335.
10. Herfarth KK, Pirzkall A, Lohr F, et al. First experiences with a non-invasive patient set-up system for radiation therapy of the prostate. *Strahlenther Onkol* 2000;176:217–222.
11. Herfarth KK, Debus J, Lohr F, et al. Stereotactic radiation therapy of liver metastases. *Radiologe* 2001;41:64–68.
12. Herfarth KK, Debus J, Lohr F, et al. Stereotactic single-dose radiation therapy of liver tumors: Results of a phase I/II trial. *J Clin Oncol* 2001;19:164–170.
13. Herfarth KK, Hof H, Bahner ML, et al. Assessment of focal liver reaction by multiphasic CT after stereotactic single-dose radiotherapy of liver tumors. *Int J Radiat Oncol Biol Phys* 2003;57:444–451.

14. Hof H, Herfarth KK, Munter M, et al. Stereotactic single-dose radiotherapy of stage I non-small-cell lung cancer (NSCLC). *Int J Radiat Oncol Biol Phys* 2003;56:335–341.

15. Lax I, Blomgren H, Naslund I, et al. Stereotactic radiotherapy of malignancies in the abdomen. Methodological aspects. *Acta Oncologica* 1994;33:677–683.

16. Lohr F, Debus J, Frank C, et al. Noninvasive patient fixation for extracranial stereotactic radiotherapy. *Int J Radiat Oncol Biol Phys* 1999;45:521–527.

17. Nagata Y, Negoro Y, Mizowaki T, et al. Clinical outcome of 3D conformal radiotherapy for solitary lung cancer using a stereotactic body frame. *Radiology* 2000;217:140–141.

18. Nagata Y, Negoro Y, Aoki T, et al. Clinical outcomes of 3D conformal hypofractionated single high-dose radiotherapy for one or two lung tumors using a stereotactic body frame. *Int J Radiat Oncol Biol Phys* 2002;52:1041–1046.

19. Nakagawa K, Aoki Y, Tago M, et al. Megavoltage CT-assisted stereotactic radiosurgery for thoracic tumors: original research in the treatment of thoracic neoplasms. *Int J Radiat Oncol Biol Phys* 2000;48:449–457.

20. Negoro Y, Nagata Y, Aoki T, et al. The effectiveness of an immobilization device in conformal radiotherapy for lung tumor: reduction of respiratory tumor movement and evaluation of the daily setup accuracy. *Int J Radiat Oncol Biol Phys* 2001;50:889–898.

21. Nemoto K, Seiji K, Sasaki K, et al. A novel support system for patient immobilization and transportation for daily computed tomographic localization of target prior to radiation therapy. *Int J Radiat Oncol Biol Phys* 2003;55:1102–1108.

22. Onishi H, Kuriyama K, Komiyama T, et al. A new irradiation system for lung cancer combining linear accelerator, computed tomography, patient self-breath-holding, and patient-directed beam-control without respiratory monitoring devices. *Int J Radiat Oncol Biol Phys* 2003;56:14–20.

23. Papiez L. On the equivalence of rotational and concentric therapy. *Phys Med Biol* 2000;45:399–409.

24. Papiez L, Lu XY, Langer M. On the isotropic distribution of beam directions. *Math Models Meth Appl Sci* 2000;10:991–1000.

25. Papiez L, Timmerman R, DesRosiers C, et al. Extracranial stereotactic radioablation: physical principles. *Acta Oncologica* 2003; 42:882–894.

26. Ryu SI, Chang SD, Kim DH, et al. Image-guided hypo-fractionated stereotactic radiosurgery to spinal lesions. *Neurosurgery* 2001;49: 838–846.

27. Ryu S, Fang Yin F, Rock J, et al. Image-guided and intensity-modulated radiosurgery for patients with spinal metastasis. *Cancer* 2003; 97:2013–2018.

28. Sailer SL, Rosenman JG, Symon JR, et al. The tetrad and hexad: maximum beam separation as a starting point for noncoplanar 3D treatment planning: prostate cancer as a test case. *Int J Radiat Oncol Biol Phys* 1994;30:439–446.

29. Takai Y, Mituya M, Nemoto K, et al. Simple method of stereotactic radiotherapy without stereotactic body frame for extracranial tumors. *Nippon Igaku Hoshasen Gakkai Zasshi* 2001;61:403–407.

30. Thiele W, Hadinger U, Flentje M, et al. Stereotactic radiation for hepatic metastases: Reproducibility of risk organ doses during repeated CT simulations. *Strahlenther Onkol* 2002;178:11–11.

31. Timmerman R, Papiez L, McGarry R, et al. Extracranial stereotactic radioablation: results of a phase I study in medically inoperable stage I non-small cell lung cancer. *Chest* 2003;124:1946–1955.

32. Timmerman R, Papiez L, Suntharalingam M. Extracranial stereotactic radiation delivery: Expansion of technology beyond the brain. *Technol Cancer Res Treat* 2003;2:153–160.

33. Uematsu M, Shioda A, Tahara K, et al. Focal, high dose, and fractionated modified stereotactic radiation therapy for lung carcinoma patients: a preliminary experience. *Cancer* 1998;82:1062–1070.

34. Uematsu M, Shioda A, Suda A, et al. Intrafractional tumor position stability during computed tomography (CT)-guided frameless stereotactic radiation therapy for lung or liver cancers with a fusion of CT and linear accelerator (FOCAL) unit. *Int J Radiat Oncol Biol Phys* 2000;48:443–448.

35. Uematsu M, Shioda A, Suda A, et al. Computed tomography-guided frameless stereotactic radiotherapy for stage I non-small cell lung cancer: a 5-year experience. *Int J Radiat Oncol Biol Phys* 2001;51:666–670.

36. Webb S. The problem of isotropically orienting N converging vectors in space with application to radiotherapy planning. *Phys Med Biol* 1995;40:945–954.

37. Whyte RI, Crownover R, Murphy MJ, et al. Stereotactic radiosurgery for lung tumors: preliminary report of a phase I trial. *Ann Thorac Surg* 2003;75:1097–1101.

38. Wulf J, Hadinger U, Oppitz U, et al. Stereotactic radiotherapy of extracranial targets: CT-simulation and accuracy of treatment in the stereotactic body frame. *Radiother Oncol* 2000;57:225–236.

39. Wulf J, Hadinger U, Oppitz U, et al. Stereotactic radiotherapy of targets in the lung and liver. *Strahlenther Onkol* 2001;177:644–655.

40. Wulf J, Hadinger U, Oppitz U, et al. Impact of target reproducibility on tumor dose in stereotactic radiotherapy of targets in the lung and liver. *Radiother Oncol* 2003;66:141–150.

41. Etiz D, Marks LB, Zhou SM, et al. Influence of tumor volume on survival in patients irradiated for non-small-cell lung cancer. *Int J Radiat Oncol Biol Phys* 2002;53:835–846.

42. Hernando ML, Marks LB, Bentel GC, et al. Radiation-induced pulmonary toxicity: a dose-volume histogram analysis in 201 patients with lung cancer. *Int J Radiat Oncol Biol Phys* 2001;51:650–659.

43. Onimaru R, Shirato H, Shimizu S, et al. Tolerance of organs at risk in small-volume, hypofractionated, image-guided radiotherapy for primary and metastatic lung cancers. *Int J Radiat Oncol Biol Phys* 2003;56:126–135.

44. Madsen BL, Hsi RA, Pham HT, et al. Intrafractional stability of the prostate using a stereotactic radiotherapy technique. *Int J Radiat Oncol Biol Phys* 2003;57:1285–1291.

45. Meeks SL, Buatti JM, Bouchet LG, et al. Ultrasound-guided extracranial radiosurgery: technique and application. *Int J Radiat Oncol Biol Phys* 2003;55:1092–1101.

46. Murphy MJ, Adler JR Jr, Bodduluri M, et al. Image-guided radiosurgery for the spine and pancreas. *Comput Aided Surg* 2000;5:278–288.

47. Onishi H, Kuriyama K, Komiyama T, et al. CT evaluation of patient deep inspiration self-breath-holding: how precisely can patients reproduce the tumor position in the absence of respiratory monitoring devices? *Med Phys* 2003;30:1183–1187.

48. Shirato H, Shimizu S, Shimizu T, et al. Real-time tumour-tracking radiotherapy. *Lancet* 1999;353:1331–1332.

49. Schweikard A, Glosser G, Bodduluri M, et al. Robotic motion compensation for respiratory movement during radiosurgery. *Comput Aided Surg* 2000;5:263–277.

50. Shimizu S, Shirato H, Xo B, et al. Three-dimensional movement of a liver tumor detected by high-speed magnetic resonance imaging. *Radiother Oncol* 1999;50:367–370.

51. Shimizu S, Shirato H, Ogura S, et al. Detection of lung tumor movement in real-time tumor-tracking radiotherapy. *Int J Radiat Oncol Biol Phys* 2001;51:304–310.

52. Wagman R, Yorke E, Ford E, et al. Respiratory gating for liver tumors: use in dose escalation. *Int J Radiat Oncol Biol Phys* 2003;55:659–668.

53. Wong JW, Sharpe MB, Jaffray DA, et al. The use of active breathing control (ABC) to reduce margin for breathing motion. *Int J Radiat Oncol Biol Phys* 1999;44:911–919.

54. Schell M, Liu H, O'Dell W, et al. Analysis of targeting accuracy of a stereotactic camera system for the radiosurgery of extra-cranial lesions. *Med Phys* 2002;29:1369–1369.

55. Lax I. Target dose versus extratarget dose in stereotaxic radiosurgery. *Acta Oncol* 1993;32:453–457.

56. Wolbarst AB, Chin LM, Svensson GK. Optimization of radiation therapy: integral-response of a model biological system. *Int J Radiat Oncol Biol Phys* 1982;8:1761–1769.

57. Douglas BG, Fowler JF. The effect of multiple small doses of x rays on skin reactions in the mouse and a basic interpretation. *Radiat Res* 1976;66:401–426.

58. Yaes RJ, Kalend A. Local stem cell depletion model for radiation myelitis. *Int J Radiat Oncol Biol Phys* 1988;14:1247–1259.

59. vantRiet A, Mak ACA, Moerland MA, et al. A conformation number to quantify the degree of conformality in brachytherapy and external beam irradiation: application to the prostate. *Int J Radiat Oncol Biol Phys* 1997;37:731–736.

60. Knoos T, Kristensen I, Nilsson P. Volumetric and dosimetric evaluation of radiation treatment plans: radiation conformity index. *Int J Radiat Oncol Biol Phys* 1998;42:1169–1176.

61. Graham MV, Matthews JW, Harms WB Sr, et al. Three-dimensional radiation treatment planning study for patients with carcinoma of the lung. *Int J Radiat Oncol Biol Phys* 1994;29:1105–1117.
62. Graham MV, Purdy JA, Emami B, et al. Clinical dose-volume histogram analysis for pneumonitis after 3D treatment for non-small cell lung cancer (NSCLC)(see comment). *Int J Radiat Oncol Biol Phys* 1999;45:323–329.
63. Saitoh H, Fujisaki T, Sakai R, et al. Dose distribution of narrow beam irradiation for small lung tumor. *Int J Radiat Oncol Biol Phys* 2002;53:1380–1387.
64. Bortfeld T, Jokivarsi K, Goitein M, et al. Effects of intra-fraction motion on IMRT dose delivery: statistical analysis and simulation. *Phys Med Biol* 2002;47:2203–2220.
65. Butson MJ, Elferink R, Cheung T, et al. Verification of lung dose in an anthropomorphic phantom calculated by the collapsed cone convolution method. *Phys Med Biol* 2000;45:N143–N149.
66. Engelsman M, Damen EMF, Koken PW, et al. Impact of simple tissue inhomogeneity correction algorithms on conformal radiotherapy of lung tumours. *Radiother Oncol* 2001;60:299–309.
67. Moskvin V, DesRosiers C, Papiez L, et al. Monte Carlo simulation of the Leksell Gamma Knife, I: source modelling and calculations in homogeneous media. *Phys Med Biol* 2002;47:1995–2011.
68. Engelsman M, Damen EM, Koken PW, et al. Impact of simple tissue inhomogeneity correction algorithms on conformal radiotherapy of lung tumours. *Radiother Oncol* 2001;60:299–309.
69. du Plessis FC, Willemse CA, Lotter MG, et al. Comparison of the Batho, ETAR and Monte Carlo dose calculation methods in CT based patient models. *Med Phys* 2001;28:582–589.
70. Ahnesjo A. Collapsed cone convolution of radiant energy for photon dose calculation in heterogeneous media. *Med Phys* 1989;16:577–592.
71. Butts JR, Foster AE. Comparison of commercially available three-dimensional treatment planning algorithms for monitor unit calculations in the presence of heterogeneities. *J Appl Clin Med Phys* 2001;2:32–41.

## Chapter 9

# Quality Assurance in Stereotactic Body Radiation Therapy

*Ulrich Haedinger and *Jörn Wulf*

## INTRODUCTION

The primary goal of any quality assurance (QA) system used in clinical radiotherapy is to make certain that the prescribed dose distribution is delivered to the patient with highest possible accuracy. Published guidelines regarding QA for conventional radiotherapy are widely available (1–4). This chapter highlights the similarities and differences in QA for stereotactic body radiation therapy (SBRT) as opposed to conventional radiotherapy.

In the case of SBRT, the QA process assumes heightened importance. Because large fraction sizes and small planning target volume (PTV) margins are used, any small setup error risks not only geographic miss but also significant toxicity in adjacent normal tissue. Furthermore, the fact that SBRT is administered in a single, or at most a few, individual treatments does not allow for compensatory random error–driven averaging of the target dose coverage.

Unlike cranial radiosurgery, where the tumors are essentially immobile within a rigid anatomic structure, aspects of internal target mobility have to be taken into account carefully in SBRT. The level of geometric accuracy achievable in SBRT is limited by patient (re)positioning uncertainties with respect to the stereotactic reference system and the degree by which internal target motion can be controlled or accounted for. The clinical target volume (CTV) in SBRT is generally considered to be the gross tumor volume (GTV). The margin around the GTV used to create the PTV—hereafter referred to as the PTV margin—is usually approximately 5 mm radially and 5 to 10 mm in the superior–inferior direction (15–19). PTV margins in this range correspond to an expected repositioning accuracy of SBRT that lies between conventional radiotherapy and cranial radiosurgery (Table 9.1).

Klinik fuer Strahlen therapie und Radiologische Onkologie, St. Vincentius-Kliniken, Karlsruhe, Germany; and *Department of Radiotherapy, University of Würzburg, Würzburg, Germany

Several technical approaches to SBRT have been developed. The immobilization method may use a body frame (9,12,15,18,20) or may be frameless. Frameless approaches rely on computed tomography (CT) (21) or ultrasound guidance (22), infrared tracking procedures (23,24), or the insertion of radio-opaque markers (25–27) for target setup and verification. Abdominal compression, controlled inspiration, or gating techniques may be used to account for respiratory motion. Finally, there are different techniques to deliver the radiation to the patient, from using standard treatment units to robot-mounted systems (28). An overview of the various implementations of SBRT is presented elsewhere in this book. Because of the variety of methods available to administer SBRT, it is impossible to give detailed QA guidelines for every specific combination of stereotactic localization, respiratory motion adjustment, and delivery system. Instead, some general aspects relevant for achieving a high level of quality in SBRT are described.

## PATIENT POSITIONING AND REPOSITIONING

Accurate patient positioning in the stereotactic reference system is essential. The chosen patient support and fixation devices (head and neck supports, knee rolls, vacuum cushions, foam molds, etc.) will directly influence the resulting positioning accuracy. It is of the utmost importance that the patient is positioned as comfortably as possible. Especially when arms are raised into an overhead position (e.g., for targets in the lung or liver), it is necessary to support the shoulders and upper arms sufficiently. Because of long treatment times in SBRT in the order of 30 to 60 minutes (dose delivery including target verification), any uncomfortable patient positioning will lead to involuntary movements. Inevitably, the result is a loss of accuracy—although real-time target monitoring during treatment delivery may compensate to some extent for patient-related movements.

▶ **TABLE 9.1** Comparison of Key Aspects of Conventional Radiotherapy, Stereotactic Body Radiotherapy, and Cranial Radiosurgery.

| | *Conventional Radiotherapy* | *SBRT* | *Cranial Radiosurgery* |
|---|---|---|---|
| Target location | Cranial and extracranial | Extracranial | Cranial |
| Tumor volume | Moderate and large | Small and moderate | Small |
| External positioning reference | Skin markers for setup | Stereotactic setup | Stereotactic setup |
| Immobilization | Supporting devices (e.g., knee rolls, neck support, etc.) and/or firm patient immobilization | Firm patient immobilization and target motion minimization | Rigid fixation to the skull |
| Positional accuracy | 10–20 mm | 5–10 mm | ≤1 mm |
| Total treatment course | Many fractions | Single fraction or few fractions | Single fraction |

SBRT, stereotactic body radiation therapy.

The size of vacuum cushions, or alternatively the amount of mold material, has to be adapted the patient's dimensions to guarantee that the fixation device fits well to the patient's contour. Especially because most body frame systems are open in the craniocaudal axis, it is necessary to supply enough mold material around the waists to prevent patients from shifting in the craniocaudal direction. Newly purchased vacuum cushions should be evaluated prior to the first planned clinical use to check their integrity and the tightness of the valve. A vacuum loss during dose delivery may cause a considerable target miss and severe side effects in radiosensitive structures. Vacuum bags used for patient immobilization are vulnerable to punctures, and therapists assisting patients onto the treatment table must be careful to avoid damaging the bag with a fingernail, jewelry, or other sharp implement.

Fractionated treatment requires repeated positioning of the target with respect to the stereotactic coordinates of the isocenter. If a body frame is used, the patient has to be properly repositioned at each treatment within the frame. A sufficient number of setup markers have to be prepared at the patient's skin during initial simulation. These markers have to match with corresponding markers on the frame, when the patient is reinstalled. The skin markers must be prepared at locations where the skin is not very movable relative to the bony structure. Small tattooed dots at the chest and the tibias may be used to coincide with the lasers. Tattooing not only in the midline of the patient, but also on the right/left side of the chest, minimizes the chance of patient rotation very efficiently. If the immobilization device (e.g., vacuum pillow or synthetic mold) is not permanently fixed to the system, both components must be properly aligned with respect to each other.

Total target positioning uncertainty is always a superposition of two effects: (a) inaccuracy of patient positioning relative to the treatment machine's isocenter and (b) target motion (15). For a complete evaluation of the achievable treatment accuracy, it is important to consider both components.

## MINIMIZATION OF TARGET MOTION AND DETERMINATION OF PLANNING TARGET VOLUME MARGINS

Numerous studies have been conducted to evaluate target mobility and organ motion in conventional radiotherapy. Target movement primarily depends on the anatomic location of the tumor within the body of the patient. Bony targets, namely spine metastases, in principle should not move significantly, so that only setup uncertainties have to be covered by PTV margins (23,25). However, even bony targets might change their position due to pain or different muscle tension. Tumors near hollow organs like the stomach or urinary bladder can show large interfraction displacements due to variable organ fillings. For tumors in the lung and liver, movements in the order of 10 to 20 mm have been reported for free-breathing patients without any use of respiratory control devices (29,30). However, such large PTV margins, sufficient to cover this magnitude of uncontrolled target motion, are not feasible in SBRT, because the volume of irradiated normal tissue would become unacceptably large. Various methods, comprising mechanically increased abdominal pressure (15,17–19), oxygen-assisted shallow breathing (16), and more advanced techniques like jet-ventilation or gated therapy with or without breathing control systems (31–33), have been developed to reduce breathing-related target movement for lung and liver tumors to values in the order of 5 to 10 mm (Table 9.2).

The extent of target mobility depends on multiple patient- and method-related factors and is not necessarily predictable for an individual patient prior to a careful investigation. Targets in the liver and lower lung lobes are generally more prone to breathing-related motions than

▶ **TABLE 9.2** **Residual Target Motion Uncertainties for Stereotactic Body Radiotherapy after Application of Various Methods of Breathing Control.**

| Author | Target (No. of Lesions) | Method | Median or SD (mm) | Min–Max value (mm) |
|---|---|---|---|---|
| Lax et al. (15) | Lung, liver, abdomen, bone $n = 48$ | Abdominal pressure | AP: 3.1<br>Lateral: 3.1<br>Longitudinal: 5.5 | AP: 0.0–6.0<br>Lateral: 0.0–6.0<br>Longitudinal: 0.0–10.0 |
| Uematsu et al. (16) | Lung $n = 66$ | Oxygen assisted shallow breathing | <5.0<br><1.0 (76%)<br><1.0 (24%) | <0.5 (46%) |
| Herfarth et al. (17) | Liver $n = 26$ | Abdominal pressure | AP: 2.3<br>Lateral: 1.6<br>Longitudinal: 4.4 | AP: 0.0–6.3<br>Lateral: 0.2–7.0<br>Longitudinal: 0.0–10.0 |
| Wulf et al. (18) | Lung, liver, abdomen, pelvis bone $n = 32$ | Abdominal pressure | AP: 3.4<br>Lateral: 3.3<br>Longitudinal: 4.4 | AP: 0.0–11.0<br>Lateral: 0.2–10.0<br>Longitudinal: 0.0–12.0 |
| Negoro et al. (19) | Lung $n = 18$ | Abdominal pressure | | 2–11 |

SBRT, stereotactic body radiation therapy; AP, anteroposterior.

tumors fixed to the thoracic wall or mediastinum. Furthermore, breathing motions might differ significantly from patient to patient depending on respiratory function. It is therefore highly recommended to estimate target motion individually for each patient rather than rely exclusively upon published values.

The amount of diaphragm movement can be measured by fluoroscopy and provides an estimation of target mobility for tumors in liver or lung. For example, Blomgren et al. (5) apply abdominal pressure using a diaphragm control device if the diaphragm movement amplitude in fluoroscopy exceeds 5 mm. A three-dimensional (3D) assessment of tumor motion can be obtained by evaluating repeated CT scans, which are acquired asynchronously to the patients breathing rhythm without incrementing the CT couch (dynamic scans) (18,34). Additionally for small lung tumors, CT scans can be repeated at different states of the breathing cycle (deep inspiration, deep expiration, shallow breathing) to explore the whole range of target mobility. The introduction of modern-generation multislice CT scanners will provide improved possibilities for target motion analysis (36). Such devices allow the fast acquisition of complete volume data sets at different time coordinates. As a result, image series of target motion as a function of time will be available, which allow a more precise determination of individual PTV margins.

## TREATMENT PLANNING

The quality of a treatment plan for SBRT can be assessed by considering the following parameters:

PTV coverage
Conformality of the dose distribution

Steep dose gradients toward radiosensitive organs at risk (OARs)
Total time required for dose delivery
Accuracy of dose calculation

Limited dose coverage of the PTV may result in failure of local control thus questioning the whole treatment decision. On the other hand, if there are radiosensitive structures (e.g., large blood vessels, trachea, etc.) adjacent to the PTV, high conformality of the dose distribution with steep gradients toward the organs at OARs is valuable. Furthermore, dose should be quickly deliverable because the risk of patient movement due to limited tolerance in the stereotactic system—especially if abdominal pressure is applied for controlling breathing-related target motion—will increase with time, and the effectiveness of the radiation might diminish if there is opportunity for extensive intra-fraction repair.

Generally, not all requirements can be fulfilled simultaneously, and a compromise has to be reached. For example, when large hepatic tumors are treated, incomplete PTV dose coverage possibly has to be accepted, because otherwise the remnant functional reserve of normal liver tissue might be too small. The quality of dose distributions with respect to target coverage and dose conformality can be scored by evaluating dose volume histograms, as suggested by various authors. Knöös et al. (37) defined a radiation conformity index (RCI) as ratio of the PTV and $V_{treated}$ (defined as the volume enclosed by the isodose surface of the minimum relative PTV dose value). Optimal dose conformality (i.e., the surface of the minimum relative PTV isodose coincides with the PTV contour) results in RCI = 1. For stereotactic radiotherapy of brain tumors in seven patients using multiple individually collimated treatment fields they obtained RCI = 0.54 ±0.08.

Van't Riet et al. (38) introduced a conformation number (CN) as a product of two relative volumes:

$$CN = VPTV,ref / VPTV * VPTV,ref / Vref$$

The first factor, also called the PTV target coverage (TC), describes the fraction of the PTV that is encompassed by the reference isodose surface. TC = 1 if the PTV is completely surrounded by the reference isodose surface. On the other hand, TC = 0 would indicate the situation of a total geographical miss of the PTV. The second factor, also called the conformation index (CI), refers to normal tissue doses. Combining both factors results in the so-called conformation number (CN). CN = 1 only in the special case, if the PTV and the volume inside the reference isodose surface are identical. If CN is less than 1, there is either incomplete dose coverage of the PTV or suboptimal conformality (Fig. 9.1). According to the authors, a dose distribution should be considered as conformal if CN greater than 0.6.

An evaluation of treatment plans for 63 stereotactically treated targets in lung, liver, and abdomen/pelvis is summarized in Table 9.3 (39). Pulmonary or hepatic targets often have simple, convex shaped geometries, allowing highly conformal treatment with multiple coplanar static photon beams, which is reflected by large average conformation numbers. The situation might be more complex for targets in the abdomen or pelvis, because of sometimes-concave target shapes and nearby radiosensitive tissue, respectively. In such cases, SBRT can be used to achieve and ensure the steep dose gradients toward the

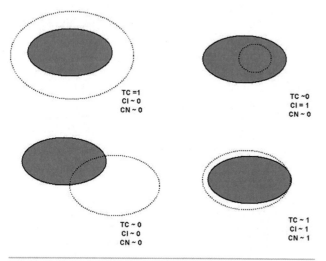

**FIGURE 9.1.** Visualization of the measures for characterizing the conformation number (CN) (38). Planning target volume (PTV) (*dark grey*); volume inside reference isodose surface $V_{ref}$ (*dotted*). Target coverage (TC) = PTV inside $V_{ref}$, or $V_{PTV,ref}$, divided by the volume of the PTV, or $V_{PTV}$. Conformation index (CI) = $V_{PTV,ref} / V_{ref}$. Conformation number (CN) = TCCI. **Top left:** Dose distribution too spacious. **Top right:** Dose distribution too tight. **Bottom left:** Geographic target miss. **Bottom right:** Dose distribution with adequate conformation.

radiosensitive structures rather than highly conformal dose distributions. The potential benefit of generally more time-consuming intensity-modulated radiotherapy techniques for improving conformality has to be weighed against a possible disadvantage due to enlarged patient motion during the longer radiation delivery times.

## Accuracy of Dose Calculation

A wide range of dose-prescribing and -normalization procedures has been used for SBRT. Some groups apply homogeneous dose distributions in concordance with International Commission on Radiation Units and Measurements publication number 50 (ICRU50) (40), while others prefer an inhomogeneous approach as suggested by Lax (41). Doses are prescribed either to the isocenter or to target circumscribing isodoses at levels from 65% to 100%. Perhaps surprisingly, the accuracy of the dose calculation itself is often neglected.

Calculations are mainly based on pencil beam (PB) algorithms, which are widely implemented in computerized treatment planning systems. This approach usually applies only one-dimensional density corrections in the direction along the beam's central axis, while ignoring lateral tissue inhomogeneities. Because pulmonary tumors are partially or completely surrounded by lower density lung tissue (0.1–0.3 g/mL), the secondary charged particle equilibrium is violated at the tumor–lung interface. This fact may lead to a significant underestimation of dose at the tumor edge, if lateral density variations are not properly accounted for.

The limitations of the PB model for tumors in the lung—currently one of the main applications of SBRT—have been recognized and reported (42). Point kernel-based superposition/convolution algorithms account for tissue inhomogeneities by a 3D density scaling of the energy deposition kernels, providing a more reliable prediction of doses in heterogeneous media. Insofar as they mathematically model the fundamental physical interaction processes, Monte Carlo approaches can enhance accuracy and might become the calculation option of choice in the future.

Various studies have evaluated the accuracy of different algorithms for slab geometries as well as in anthropomorphic phantoms by comparing the calculations with either thermoluminescent dosimeter (TLD) measurements or dosimetric films (43–51). The authors of those studies report significant reductions of dose at the tumor edge up to 25% to 50%, depending primarily on photon energy, target volume, and location with respect to the inhomogeneity. The use of low-energy photon beams (4–6 mV) can be advantageous, because penumbra broadening of the beam profiles increases with photon energy. For dose calculations in the lung, point kernel models are generally superior to the more simple PB algorithms. For tumors outside the lung, the accuracy achievable with PB algorithms may be sufficient.

▶ **TABLE 9-3** Volumetric and Dosimetric Data for Three Different Categories of Stereotactically Treated Tumors (39). Target Coverage and Conformation Number Are Defined in Text.

|  | Lung (n = 22) | Liver (n = 21) | Abdomen/Pelvis (n = 20) |
|---|---|---|---|
| Mean PTV, cc (range) | 144 (17–343) | 173 (42–772) | 207 (55–619) |
| Mean % PTV target coverage (range) | 96 (90–100) | 95 (83–100) | 92 (79–99) |
| Mean conformation number (range) | 0.73 (0.58–0.85) | 0.77 (0.45–0.91) | 0.70 (0.54–0.86) |

PTV, planning target volume.

Haedinger et al. (52) evaluated target dose coverage for 33 lung targets stereotactically treated in a body frame. Dose distributions were calculated with a PB algorithm (53) or a collapsed cone (CC) implementation of a point kernel model (54). Consistently, the PB algorithm calculated a higher dose to the target volumes than the CC algorithm. For example, the mean percentage of PTV coverage was 96% for PB and 89% for CC. The mean dose to the PTV was 137% of the nominal prescription dose with PB and only 125% with CC. These calculations were reflected also in the calculation of monitor units (MUs) required to administer the same given dose (i.e., a higher number of MUs was needed with CC calculations compared with PB). Differences between the results with different calculation algorithms were larger when the target volume was smaller (PTV <50 cc) and when higher energy photon beams (18 mV vs. 6 mV) were used.

## TARGET POSITION AND MOTION VERIFICATION

It is important to maintain a high level of confidence regarding the correct target location and its motion prior to each fraction of SBRT. A conventional verification method by comparison of port films with simulator images or digitally reconstructed radiographs (DRRs) is usually not sufficient for SBRT. Most tumors are not visible on high-energy–x-ray images, and the assumption that a correct position of bony structures correlates with a corresponding precise hit of the target is not generally valid. Especially during the developmental phase of an SBRT program, secondary verification of target position with CT imaging of the patient in the treatment position is advisable. As the treating team develops a solid idea of the magnitude of target position uncertainty expected given the immobilization system being used, it might be reasonable obtain a CT slice only through the isocenter or to forego the CT altogether after the first day of treatment.

In the case of any deviation of the target contour relative to the planning CT study, the longitudinal shift has to be determined by repeating scans cranially and caudally of the nominal isocenter plane. Abdominal compression, respiratory gating of planning CT acquisition and beam-on time, and breath-hold/breathing-control devices can all be used to minimize respiratory target motion. If these techniques are either unavailable or poorly tolerated by the patient, respiratory target motion can be checked by dynamic scans without couch movement as described previously. The action level for a correction of the longitudinal stereotactic coordinate depends on the target size and the applied geometrical margins. If 5- to 10-mm margins are used, deviations of more than 2 to 3 mm should be corrected by calculating a revised stereotactic coordinate. The patient should not be shifted relative to the stereotactic system.

Pre-SBRT verification CT simulation can be easily accomplished on the treatment couch if a mobile CT unit with gantry motion mode is available (Fig. 9.2). Other-

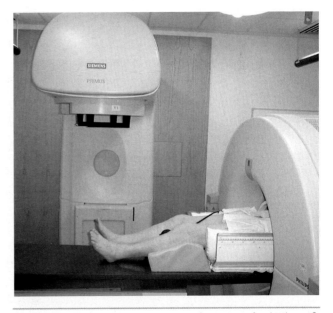

**FIGURE 9.2.** Pretreatment computed tomography (CT) verification of target position and residual breathing related mobility, using a mobile CT unit with gantry motion (Philips Tomoscan M, Philips, Best, The Netherlands). The patient is installed in an stereotactic body frame (Elekta, Norcross, GA) on a specifically designed carbon fiber couch of the treatment unit (Siemens Primus; Siemens Medial Solutions, Malvern, PA).

wise, after CT verification the patient has to be transported to the treatment unit with as little shift as possible relative to the stereotactic system. Nemoto and colleagues (55) developed a system for patient immobilization and transportation that allows a simple daily CT localization of targets prior to irradiation. To exclude transport-related patient movements or a setup of faulty stereotactic coordinates at the treatment unit, portal images can be recorded immediately prior to irradiation. A patient repositioning between verification CT and irradiation leads to a complete loss of information about the target position and should be avoided if possible.

Uematsu et al. (21) reported on frameless SBRT using an integrated system of a linear accelerator, CT scanner, kilovolt (kV) simulator, and a single carbon fiber treatment couch. The couch can be rotated for alignment with respect to the isocenter of either unit without moving or repositioning the patient. This feature allows for evaluation of intrafractional target position stability by repeated CT scans immediately before and after irradiation. Target motion was reduced using oxygen-assisted shallow breathing. The authors evaluated 50 targets in lung and liver (24 upper lung lobes, 14 lower lung lobes, 12 liver); most intrafractional tumor positioning errors were found to be less than or equal to 5 mm (24/24, 7/14, 3/12) or between 6 and 10 mm (0/24, 7/14, 9/12).

Nakagawa et al. (10) performed real-time lung target monitoring using a megavolt CT (MVCT) device attached to the treatment unit. After positioning the patient on the treatment couch, an MVCT scan is acquired and compared with the previously recorded CT planning study. Patient setup is corrected until a satisfactory match results. During treatment, the therapy beam is recorded by the detector array and superimposed to the MVCT image. The influence of the breathing motion on the MVCT image was evaluated by simulating a moving tumor with an oscillating acrylic pendulum.

Wulf et al. (34) studied the impact of target reproducibility on target dose in lung ($n = 22$) and liver ($n = 21$) tumors. A verification CT was performed over the complete target volume prior to each of three treatment fractions. The CTV was delineated in every verification CT image set. By using the stereotactic marker system of the body frame as a patient-independent reference for matching planning and verification CT studies, the CTV was correlated to the planned dose distribution. CTV dose coverage (defined as the fraction of the CTV within the reference isodose surface) was found to be less than 95% in three of 60 simulations for lung and seven of 58 for liver targets. While the results indicated that the accuracy of the procedure was sufficient in most patients, on some occasions the PTV margins were too tight. An analysis of the factors influencing the target coverage revealed different causes for lung and liver tumors. At higher risk of incomplete coverage were pulmonary targets with respiratory motion that could not be controlled by applying abdominal pressure and large hepatic tumors (CTV >100 cc), where the PTV margin had to be balanced against functional organ reserve (Fig. 9.3 and 9.4).

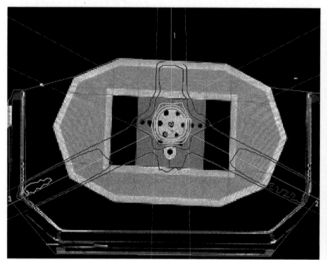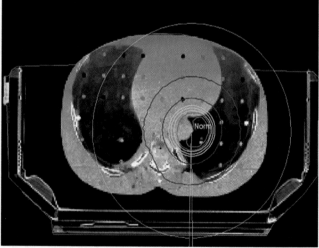

**FIGURE 9.3.** Computed tomography scans of a thoracic phantom **(left)** and a Rando-Alderson phantom **(right)** in a stereotactic body frame (Elekta, Norcross, GA). The thoracic phantom was equipped with an ionizing chamber at the center, while the Alderson phantom was loaded with thermoluminescent dosimeters. Measured absorbed doses were compared with TPS (Helax TMS; Nucletron BV, Veenendaal, The Netherlands) calculations for various beam configurations to evaluate the influence of the body frame's side walls and bottom plate (57).

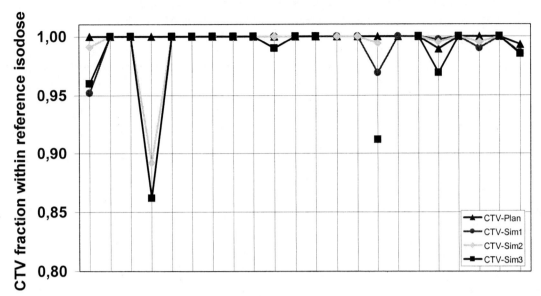

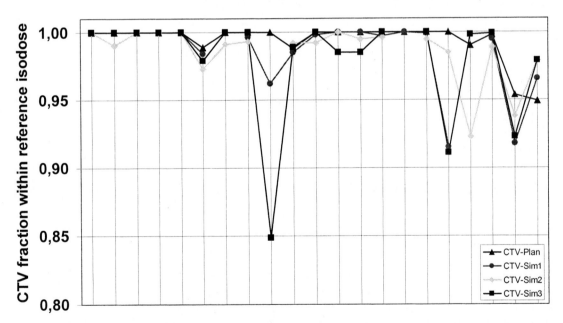

*FIGURE 9.4.* CTV dose coverage for liver targets.

O'Dell and colleagues (35) evaluated the influence of residual target position uncertainty on the dose distribution for small lung tumors and their surrounding normal tissue during fractionated irradiation using end expiration breath hold. They observed that radial and craniocaudal margins of 7 mm and 10 mm, respectively, were appropriate for treating tumors of 12-mm diameter.

## TREATMENT DELIVERY

At most centers where SBRT is administered, standard equipment (linear accelerators and treatment couches) is used in combination with a stereotactic reference system and dedicated methods or devices for patient immobilization and target motion control. The treatment units should be regularly checked and calibrated in accordance with prevailing regulatory standards. Because the maximum overall accuracy achievable in SBRT is limited by target position uncertainty to an order of around 5 mm, geometric requirements are usually not as rigid as in cranial stereotactic radiosurgery (SRS). Nevertheless, it has to be ensured that the specified stereotactic coordinates of the target point(s) are hit with sufficient accuracy during treatment delivery. While most commercially available treatment units provide the freedom to treat targets with noncoplanar beams and arcs across a wide range of treatment table angles and gantry positions, it should be remembered that the stereotactic system itself might limit the practical range of treatment beams because of potential collisions with the treatment head and stereotactic reference device. Prior to actual treatment, the combination of table angles and gantry positions should be checked to verify their feasibility relative to the stereotactic reference device(s) used.

## Mechanical Precision and Room Laser System

If the room laser system is used for coordinate setup at the treatment unit, the alignment of the laser lines to the isocenter has to be checked. The coincidence of opposing lasers can be verified on a daily basis using a translucent sheet of paper. Opposing lasers should not deviate more than 1 mm. In the case of a deviation, markers on the treatment room's walls (attached after the last laser adjustment) can help to decide very quickly which laser needs a readjustment. The mechanical precision of the machine isocenter should be checked regularly by performing "star shots" from different gantry angles on film. The diameter of the isocenter sphere as well as the deviation of the laser and radiation isocenter should be in the order of 1 mm (2 mm is considered to be sufficient for conventional radiotherapy). Similar measurements for collimator and table rotations might be appropriate.

Lax et al. (15) described a special check device used to measure the integrated uncertainty of the stereotactic coordinate setup. The device includes a small gold pellet that can be precisely positioned to predefined coordinates of a stereotactic body frame. The deviation of the nominal isocenter and the center of the pellet can be measured by exposing orthogonal films. The authors report setup uncertainties during repeated measurements within 1 mm. Kuriyama et al. (56) estimated the setup accuracy of a frameless stereotactic system by means of phantom studies. They reported an integrated positioning uncertainty of the entire system of 0.20 mm (lateral), 0.39 mm (longitudinal), and 0.18 mm (vertical).

## Monitor Chamber Linearity

The dose monitor system of linear accelerators is usually calibrated to 100 MUs per 1 Gy absorbed dose under calibration conditions. Due to the very large fraction doses in SBRT, several hundred MUs may be delivered per field. Deviations in dose output per MU should not exceed 1% to 2%.

## Treatment Planning System

The complete process of CT simulation, treatment planning, dose calculation, and dose delivery can be evaluated with phantoms, allowing measurements of the delivered dose. The influence of the stereotactic frame system itself on dose can be assessed. A comparison of calculated doses (Helax TMS, pencil beam algorithm; Nucletron BV, Veenendal, The Netherlands) and measurements with an ionizing chamber and TLD in two phantoms placed in an stereotactic body frame (Elekta, Norcross, GA) yielded differences between calculated and measured doses of up to 6% if the frame was not included into the CT density matrix (57). Additionally, integration of the stereotactic frame in the calculation model allows assessment of dose at the patients surface (e.g., hot spots at the skin).

### Digital Measurement Tools

Image-guided therapy approaches rely on the use of digital measurement tools that are incorporated into the software of CT scanners and treatment planning systems. Therefore, it is necessary to validate the accuracy of such tools, especially after software version updates. CT scans of dedicated phantoms with radio-opaque markers fixed at defined positions are adequate devices for checking digital measurement tools as well as the geometric accuracy of DRR calculation. Alternatively, a stereotactic body frame system itself, with its known distances between various coordinate points, is suitable for performing quality checks. At the same time, the integrity of the frame and its fiducial system can be verified.

Finally, it should be emphasized again that it is of urgent importance to elaborate the overall accuracy of the whole treatment process when an SBRT program is started. Patient (re)positioning uncertainties and the residual target motion after application of mobility reduction measures have to be carefully evaluated for a determination of appropriate PTV margins. The margins published in the literature can be used as guidelines but have to be reconciled with an evaluation of the accuracy achievable in a given institution.

# REFERENCES

1. Kutcher GJ, Coia L, Gillin M, et al. Comprehensive QA for radiation oncology: report of AAPM Radiation Therapy Committee Task Group 40. *Med Phys* 1994;21:581–618.
2. Thwaites D, Scalliet P, Leer JW, et al. Quality assurance in radiotherapy. *Radiother Oncol* 1995;35:61–73.
3. Leer JHW, McKenzie A, Scalliet P, et al. Practical guidelines for the implementation of a quality system in radiotherapy. ESTRO Booklet No.4.
4. Van Dyk J, Purdy JA. Clinical implementation of technology and the quality assurance process. In: Van Dyk J, ed. *The modern technology of radiation oncology*. Madison: Medical Physics Publishing, 1999:19–51.
5. Blomgren H, Lax I, Göranson H, et al. Radiosurgery for tumors in the body: Clinical experience using a new method. *J Radiosurg* 1998;1:63–74.
6. Hara R, Itami J, Kondo T, et al. Stereotactic single high dose irradiation of lung tumors under respiratory gating. *Radiother Oncol* 2002;63:159–163.
7. Herfarth KK, Debus J, Lohr F, et al. Stereotactic single dose radiation therapy of liver tumors: results of a phase I/II trial. *J Clin Oncol* 2001;19:164–170.
8. Hof H, Herfarht KK, Munter M, et al. Stereotactic single-dose radiotherapy of stage I non-small-cell lung cancer (NSCLC). *Int J Radiat Oncol Biol Phys* 2003;56:335–341.
9. Nagata Y, Negoro Y, Aoki T. Clinical outcomes of 3D conformal hypofractionated single high-dose radiotherapy for one or two lung tumors using a stereotactic body frame. *Int J Radiat Oncol Biol Phys* 2002;52:1041–1046.
10. Nakagawa Y, Aoki Y, Tago M, et al. Megavoltage CT-assisted stereotactic radiosurgery for thoracic tumors: original research in the treatment of thoracic neoplasms. *Int J Radiat Oncol Biol Phys* 2000;48:449–457.
11. Onimaru R, Shirato H, Shimizu S, et al. Tolerance of organs at risk in small-volume, hypofractionated, image-guided radiotherapy for primary and metastatic lung. *Int J Radiat Oncol Biol Phys* 2003;56: 126–135.
12. Timmerman RD, Papiez L, McGarry R, et al. Extracranial stereotactic radioablation: results of a phase I study in medically inoperable stage I non-small cell lung cancer. *Chest* 2003;124: 1946–1955.
13. Uematsu M, Shioda M, Suda A, et al. Computed tomography-guided frameless stereotactic radiotherapy for stage I non-small cell lung cancer: a 5-year experience. *Int J Radiat Oncol Biol Phys* 2001;51:666–670.
14. Wulf J, Haedinger U, Oppitz U, et al. Stereotactic radiotherapy of targets in the lung and liver. *Strahlenther Onkol* 2001;177:645–655.
15. Lax I, Blomgren H, Larson D, et al. Extracranial stereotactic radiosurgery of localized targets. *J Radiosurg* 1998;1:135–148.
16. Uematsu M, Shioda A, Tahara K, et al. Focal, high dose, and fractionated modified stereotactic radiation therapy for lung carcinoma patients. *Cancer* 1998;82:1062–1070.
17. Herfarth KK, Debus J, Lohr F, et al. Extracranial stereotactic radiation therapy: set-up accuracy of patients treated for liver metastases. *Int J Radiat Oncol Biol Phys* 2000;46:329–335.
18. Wulf J, Haedinger U, Oppitz U, et al. Stereotactic radiotherapy of extracranial targets: CT-simulation and accuracy of treatment in the stereotactic body frame. *Radiother Oncol* 2000;57:225–236.
19. Negoro Y, Nagata Y, Aoki T, et al. The effectiveness of an immobilization device in conformal radiotherapy for lung tumor: reduction of respiratory tumor movement and evaluation of the daily setup accuracy. *Int J Radiat Oncol Biol Phys* 2001;50:889–898.
20. Lohr F, Debus J, Frank C, et al. Noninvasive patient fixation for extracranial stereotactic radiotherapy. *Int J Radiat Oncol Biol Phys* 1999;45:521–527.
21. Uematsu M, Shioda A, Suda A, et al. Intrafractional tumor position stability during computed tomography (CT)-guided frameless stereotactic radiation therapy for lung or liver cancers with a fusion of CT and linear accelerator (FOCAL) unit. *Int J Radiat Oncol Biol Phys* 2000;48:443–448.
22. Meeks SL, Buatti JM, Bouchet LG, et al. Ultrasound-guided extracranial radiosurgery: technique and application. *Int J Radiat Oncol Biol Phys* 2003;55:1092–1101.
23. Ryu S, Fang Yin F, Rock J, et al. Image-guided and intensity-modulated radiosurgery for patients with spine metastasis. *Cancer* 2003;97:2013–2018.
24. Wang L, Solberg T, Medin PM, et al. Infrared patient positioning for stereotactic radiosurgery of extracranial tumors. *Comput Biol Med* 2001;31:101–111.
25. Ryu SI, Chang SD, Kim DH, et al. Image-guided hypofractionated stereotactic radiosurgery to spinal lesions. *Neurosurgery* 2001;49: 838–846.
26. Harada T, Shirato H, Ogura S, et al. Real-time tumor-tracking radiation therapy for lung carcinoma by the aid of insertion of a gold marker using bronchofiberscopy. *Cancer* 2002;95:1720–1727.
27. Madsen BL, Hsi RA, Pham HT, et al. Intrafractional stability of the prostate using a stereotactic radiotherapy technique. *Int J Radiat Oncol Biol Phys* 2003;57:1285–1291.
28. Whyte RI, Crownover R, Murphy MJ, et al. Stereotactic radiosurgery for lung tumors: preliminary report of a phase I trial. *Ann Thorac Surg* 2003;75:1097–1101.
29. Shimizu S, Shirato H, Ogura S, et al. Detection of lung tumor movement in real-time tumor-tracking radiotherapy. *Int J Radiat Oncol Biol Phys* 2001;51:304–310.
30. Shimizu S, Shirato H, Xo B, et al. Three dimensional movement of a liver tumor detected by high-speed magnetic resonance. *Radiother Oncol* 1999;50:367–370.
31. Wong JW, Sharpe MB, Jaffray DA, et al. The use of active breathing control (ABC) to reduce margin for breathing motion. *Int J Radiat Oncol Biol Phys* 1999;44:911–919.
32. Wagman R, Yorke E, Ford E, et al. Respiratory gating for liver tumors: Use in dose escalation. *Int J Radiat Oncol Biol Phys* 2003;55:659–668.
33. Onishi H, Kuriyama K, Komiyama T, et al. A new irradiation system for lung cancer combining linear accelerator, computed tomography, patient self-breath-holding and patient-directed beam-control without respiratory monitor devices. *Int J Radiat Oncol Biol Phys* 2003;56:14–20.
34. Wulf J, Haedinger U, Oppitz U, et al. Impact of target reproducibility on tumor dose in stereotactic radiotherapy of targets in the lung and liver. *Radiother Oncol* 2003;66:141–150.
35. O'Dell WG, Schell MC, Reynolds D, et al. Dose broadening due to target position variability during fractionated breath-held radiation therapy. *Med Phys* 2002;29:1430–1437.
36. Hof H, Herfarth K, Münter M, et al. The use of the multislice CT for the determination of respiratory lung tumor movement in stereotactic single-dose irradiation. *Strahlenther Onkol* 2003;179:542–547.
37. Knöös T, Kristensen I, Nilsson P. Volumetric and dosimetric evaluation of radiation treatment plans: radiation conformity index. *Int J Radiat Oncol Biol Phys* 1998;42:1169–1176.
38. Van't Riet A, Mak ACA, Moerland MA, et al. A conformation number to quantify the degree of conformality in brachytherapy and external beam irradiation: application to the prostate. *Int J Radiat Oncol Biol Phys* 1997;37:731–736.
39. Haedinger U, Thiele W, Wulf J. Extracranial stereotactic radiotherapy: evaluation of PTV coverage and dose conformity. *Z Med Phys* 2002;12:221–229.

40. International Commission on Radiation Units and Measurements. *Prescribing, recording and reporting photon beam therapy.* Bethesda, MD: International Commission on Radiation Units and Measurements; 1993. ICRU Report 50.
41. Lax I. Target dose versus extra-target dose in stereotactic radiosurgery. *Acta Oncol* 1993;32;453–457.
42. Knöös T, Ahnesjö A, Nilsson P, et al. Limitation of a pencil beam approach to photon dose calculation in lung tissue. *Phys Med Biol* 1995;40:1411–1420.
43. Butson MJ, Elferink R, Cheung T, et al. Verification of lung dose in an anthropomorphic phantom calculated by the collapse cone convolution method. *Phys Med Biol* 2000;45:143–149.
44. Francescon P, Cavedon C, Reccanello S, et al. Photon dose calculation of a three-dimensional treatment planning system compared to the Monte Carlo code BEAM. *Med Phys* 2000;27:1579–1587.
45. Butts JR, Foster AE. Comparison of commercially available three-dimensional treatment planning algorithms for monitor unit calculations in the presence of heterogeneities. *J Appl Clin Med Phys* 2001;2:32–41.
46. Engelsman M, Damen EMF, Koken PW, et al. Impact of simple tissue inhomogeneity correction algorithms on conformal radiotherapy of lung tumors. *Radiother Oncol* 2001;60:299–309.
47. Saitoh H, Fujisaki T, Sakai R, et al. Dose distribution of narrow beam irradiation for small lung tumor. *Int J Radiat Oncol Biol Phys* 2002;53:1380–1387.
48. Papiez L. Dosimetry of solid tumors in the lung and radioablative therapy: Proceedings of the Second Annual Extracranial Stereotactic Radioablation: Future Directions. Halifax June 6–8 2003:32.
49. Linthout N, Verellen D, van Acker S, et al. Evaluation of dose calculation algorithms for dynamic arc treatments of head and neck tumors. *Radiother Oncol* 2002;64:85–95.
50. Verellen D, Linthout N, van den Berge D, et al. Initial experience with intensity-modulated conformal radiation therapy for treatment of the head and neck region. *Int J Radiat Oncol Biol Phys* 1997;39:99–114.
51. Martens C, Reynaert N, De Wagter C, et al. Underdosage of the upper-airway mucosa for small fields as used in intensity-modulated radiation therapy: a comparison between radiochromic film measurements, Monte Carlo simulations and collapsed cone convolution calculations. *Med Phys* 2002;57:1528–1535.
52. Haedinger U, Krieger T, Flentje M, et al. Influence of the calculation model on dose distribution in stereotactic radiotherapy of pulmonary targets. Submitted for publication.
53. Ahnesjö A. A pencil beam model for photon dose calculation. *Med Phys* 1992;19:263–273.
54. Ahnesjö A. Collapsed cone convolution of radiant energy for photon dose calculation in heterogeneous media. *Med Phys* 1989;16:577–592.
55. Nemoto K, Seiji K, Sasaki K, et al. A novel support system for patient immobilization and transportation for daily computed localization of target prior to radiation therapy. *Int J Radiat Oncol Biol Phys* 2003;55:1102–1108.
56. Kuriyama K, Onishi H, Sano N, et al. A new irradiation unit constructed of self-moving gantry-CT and linac. *Int J Radiat Oncol Biol Phys* 2003;55:428–435.
57. Richter J, Hädinger U, Bratengeier K, et al. QA of stereotactic treatment techniques in the body region. *Radiother Oncol* 1998;48[Suppl 1]:S186.

# Initiating and Building a Clinical Stereotactic Body Radiation Therapy Program

## Chapter 10

### Clinical Operational Issues: Optimizing the Treatment Process

*Volker W. Stieber*
*and William H. Hinson*

Stereotactic body radiation therapy (SBRT) is far from being an automated process. As for conventional radiotherapy, numerous steps are involved from the time of first presentation of the patient for evaluation to the completion of treatment. Indeed, the more complex nature of SBRT typically necessitates additional stages in the process of treatment planning and delivery. It is helpful to create a well-organized clinical-throughput pathway, since there are expanded responsibilities and extra scheduled demands put upon the existing labor pool. For the process to function efficiently within the radiation oncology clinic, the treatment flow must be optimized to minimize eddies and maximize current.

From a logistics and operational aspect, the process of SBRT from initial patient consultation with the radiation oncologist to treatment can be broken down into modules running in serial fashion:

- Scheduling of consultation
- Consultation
- Determination of eligibility for treatment
- Simulation with imaging
- Treatment planning
- Verification/quality control
- Treatment

Two other components may run in parallel, and their insertion into the process is variable (although all must be completed before treatment):

- Additional testing [computed tomography (CT), magnetic resonance imaging (MRI), positron emission tomography (PET), or other laboratory studies)
- Consent

Each operational module requires a distinct set of personnel and equipment in order to function. Staff members who may typically be involved are:

- Physician
- Medical physicist
- Dosimetrist
- Therapist
- Nurse
- Scheduler
- Radiology services
- Engineering/other technical support personnel

To streamline the throughput of patients in a setting of maximum quality of delivered services, advance planning of each step and anticipation of potential issues is critical. Figure 10.1 outlines the suggested process integrating the various components, which are described in detail.

Department of Radiation Oncology, Wake Forest University
School of Medicine, Winston-Salem, NC 27157-1030

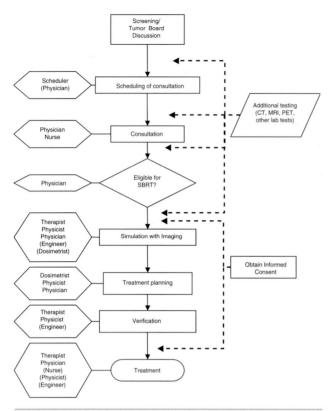

**FIGURE 10.1.** Flowchart of the process culminating in treatment. Modules with variable timing are shown at times where they may be best fit into the process. Optional personnel are shown in parentheses.

## STEPS IN THE CLINICAL OPERATIONS PROCESS

### Screening

Before scheduling a patient for consultation for SBRT, screening his or her records is advisable. Depending on the familiarity of the referring physician (or the patient, in the case of self-referral), expectations of what the new technology of SBRT can achieve may or may not be realistic. A multidisciplinary tumor board can be an ideal venue to discuss with referring physicians the risks and potential benefits of SBRT within the context of the patient's overall medical history, clinical findings, radiographic findings, and recent laboratory results. In addition, if it appears the patient is a potential candidate for treatment, review of available records may suggest that additional testing (typically radiographic imaging and/or laboratory evaluation such as pulmonary function testing or pertinent blood tests) may be useful to have at the time of consultation. Eligibility for participation in formal single- or multiinstitutional trials is generally dependent on a combination of clinical findings and laboratory test results. The consultation visit can be rendered

more productive if necessary studies are completed before the patient actually comes to the radiation oncology clinic.

### Scheduling the Consultation

Simply scheduling the patient is easy enough, but alert communication can often improve efficiency. Especially if the patient is traveling from a great distance and initial screening has suggested that he or she is a potential candidate for SBRT, it may be highly advantageous to schedule a simulation as well as any necessary additional studies on the same day or at least as close as possible to the time of the consultation. An experienced scheduler is extremely valuable here, where it is often necessary to coordinate the activities of numerous individuals within the radiation oncology department with scheduled testing to be accomplished in the diagnostic radiology or other hospital department.

### Consultation

The consideration of a patient for a novel, resource-intensive therapy will typically take 1 to 2 hours, depending on complexity of decision making required. Well-informed, intelligent patients will question the physician regarding their alternatives, which might include another form of radiotherapy, surgery, or systemic therapy. The physician should expect to review data the patients and their families might have obtained from the Internet or from patient-oriented printed publications.

Some patients will be ready to provide informed consent at the time of the initial consultation. In other instances, it might be advisable to defer the informed consent process until additional studies have been completed or even until after the treatment planning process is complete. Unforeseen clinical changes and technical limitations can arise, for example continued tumor growth since the most recent diagnostic imaging study that renders it impossible to administer SBRT without unacceptably high radiation doses to large volumes of adjacent normal tissues.

### Determination of Treatment Eligibility

Forthcoming results from the many ongoing single- and multiinstitutional phase 1 and phase 2 studies will inform decisions about patient selection. Offering eligible patients participation in an institutional review board–approved clinical trial is a legitimate application for SBRT. Outside of formal clinical studies, physicians would be wise to develop their own institutional guidelines in consideration of the equipment and expertise available locally. Determination of treatment eligibility might or might not be feasible at the time of initial consultation, depending on whether additional clinical or laboratory tests are needed. The final decision to offer SBRT might be delayed until key data are obtained.

## Simulation with Imaging

The simulation process is a critically important technical step in the process leading up to the actual treatment. The radiation therapist (or similarly qualified individual specially trained for radiotherapy simulation), a medical physicist, and the physician are generally present. Sometimes an engineer (depending on equipment used) is present during this process, and it can sometimes be helpful for the dosimetrist to observe the patient's setup. The simulation will include immobilization and imaging, sometimes several scans. Scans of different modalities (e.g. CT and MRI, CT/PET, etc.) can be used. The entire process of fashioning a customized immobilization device and obtaining scans, sometimes also involving patient education with regard to the use of respiratory gating or other special devices, will often last 2 hours or more.

## Treatment Planning

Treatment planning may include image fusion of different modality studies and contouring of all normal organs within the treatment volume. A dosimetrist usually performs a large share of the planning process, and significant physician interaction is needed to review proposed plans and suggest changes. In addition, the medical physicist should also review the treatment plan before final approval by the physician. Turnaround time may be as short as 1 day but should not take longer than 5 working days. Utilization of class solutions may considerably shorten the time for completion of the process (1–6).

## Verification

After completion of treatment planning, the patient is usually required to undergo a "dry-run" to verify that what was planned in virtual reality can be achieved in actual reality. Usually the same team used for simulation is present, although the radiation therapist delivering treatment is often a different one than was present during the simulation. In some instances, resimulation may be done on the same day as treatment. A wide assortment of Food and Drug Administration (FDA)–approved systems allows real-time verification and repositioning. If static beam apertures are used, it may be useful to film the fields without the patient and then plan for treatment the following day to allow for any necessary last-minute modifications.

## Treatment

Typically, SBRT should take less than 1 hour, unless multiple lesions are being treated in the same session and repeated treatment table shifts are required. Enough linear accelerator time must be allotted, and the team present is usually the same as that at the time of verification. Additionally, there might be a need for nursing support during all or part of the actual treatment. Some patients will benefit from premedication with antiemetics, analgesics, or antianxiety agents that will reduce the chance of upset stomach or promote patient comfort and relaxation during the treatment experience.

SBRT may be accomplished with any of numerous combinations of linear accelerators and peripheral support equipment. Chapter 7 includes descriptions of commercially available accessories and software to facilitate immobilization, repositioning, and relocalization. Figures 10.2 through 10.6 depict examples of linear accelerators designed with features well suited for SBRT applications.

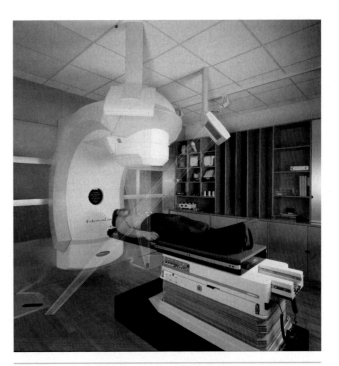

**FIGURE 10.2.** The Novalis Body System (BrainLAB, Inc., Westchester, IL) includes an accelerator and orthogonal x-ray cameras. The diagnostic energy x-ray beams, illustrated in yellow, are aimed from below and behind the patient to amorphous silicon flat panels mounted on the ceiling. The images obtained may be compared with digitally reconstructed radiographs constructed from the planning computed tomography scan to determine necessary patient position shifts. Also shown here are the ExacTrac surface markers that aid repositioning by an infrared tracking mechanism. (Courtesy of G. Cyranski, Brain-LAB, Inc.).

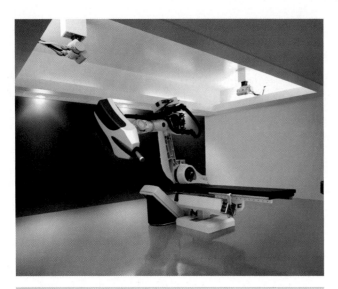

**FIGURE 10.3.** The CyberKnife (Accuray, Sunnyvale, CA) includes a lightweight linear accelerator mounted on a robotic arm. Diagnostic radiograph–based image guidance technology tracks patient and target position during treatment. Stereotactic body radiation therapy is performed without a stereotactic body frame. (Courtesy of P. Cardoza, Accuray).

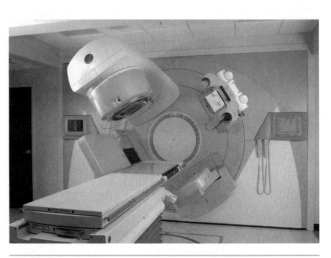

**FIGURE 10.5.** The Elekta Synergy combines x-ray imaging and treatment delivery into one integrated gantry-mounted system. Both planar images and cone-beam computed tomography three-dimensional volume reconstruction images may be obtained for position verification. (Courtesy of Elekta).

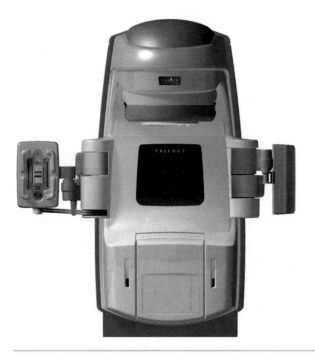

**FIGURE 10.4.** The Trilogy (Varian, Palo Alto, CA.) incorporates an image-guided treatment capability. An electronic portal imaging device is mounted on the same gantry as the treatment unit. The dose delivery rate is escalated relative to Varian's standard accelerators. (Courtesy of Varian).

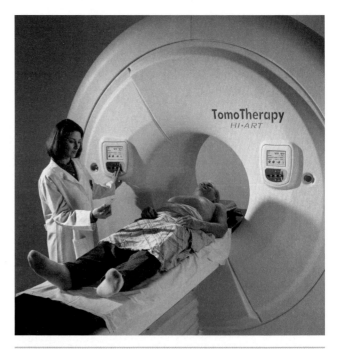

**FIGURE 10.6.** The TomoTherapy H•Art System (TomoTherapy, Madison, WI) combines computed tomography scanning capabilities with a linear accelerator mounted on a rotating gantry. Treatment is delivered as the gantry rotates, and the couch moves simultaneously so that the radiation effectively spirals around the patient. (Courtesy of TomoTherapy.)

## SUMMARY

In today's health care market, medical subspecialists compete for the patronage of patients and respect from referring physicians. The primary motivation for developing and implementing any new treatment delivery program within a department is the clinical benefit to patients. Delivery of SBRT is a complex, multistep process involving a multidisciplinary team. With careful planning and forethought, the process will run smoothly with maximum efficiency. Outcomes will be achievable in a fiscally responsible manner and will be beneficial to the patient. Ultimately, radiation oncologists must always remember that the goal of SBRT is to maximize patient comfort and quality of treatment while making the procedure affordable enough to be widely available to patients for whom it is helpful.

## REFERENCES

1. Arrans R, Gallardo MI, Rosello J, et al. Computer optimization of class solutions designed on a beam segmentation basis. *Radiother Oncol* 2003;69:315–321.
2. Bedford JL, Webb S. Elimination of importance factors for clinically accurate selection of beam orientations, beam weights and wedge angles in conformal radiation therapy. *Med Phys* 2003;30:1788–1804.
3. Khoo VS, Bedford JL, Webb S, et al. Class solutions for conformal external beam prostate radiotherapy. *Int J Radiat Oncol Biol Phys* 2003;55:1109–1120.
4. Chen Y, Michalski D, Houser C, et al. A deterministic iterative least-squares algorithm for beam weight optimization in conformal radiotherapy. *Phys Med Biol* 2002;47:1647–1658.
5. Hou Q, Wang J, Chen Y, et al. Beam orientation optimization for IMRT by a hybrid method of the genetic algorithm and the simulated dynamics. *Med Phys* 2003;30:2360–2367.
6. Hou Q, Wang J, Chen Y, et al. An optimization algorithm for intensity modulated radiotherapy—the simulated dynamics with dose-volume constraints. *Med Phys* 2003;30:61–68.

# Commissioning and Accreditation of a Stereotactic Body Radiation Therapy Program

*James M. Galvin and *Geoffrey S. Ibbott*

## INTRODUCTION

There are significant differences between cranial stereo-tactic radiosurgery (SRS) or radiation therapy (SRT) and stereotactic body radiation therapy (SBRT), and it is help-ful to view SBRT in relation to the technical advances that made cranial SRS possible so that the similarities and dif-ferences may be fully appreciated. Cranial SRS emerged as technology evolved to address three key aspects of the radiation treatment problem and thus allow a significant decrease in the planning target volume (PTV) margins needed around the gross tumor volume (GTV). First, to achieve precision in radiation beam positioning, mechan-ical tolerances for the treatment unit were tightened be-yond the levels previously considered the industry stan-dard. Second, techniques for immobilizing the cranium were devised to improve the accuracy of targeting of le-sions in the brain. Third, by tightly coupling imaging modalities with beam placement, it was possible to move through the imaging-to-delivery stages of the process with very little loss of accuracy as measured in relation to the resolution capabilities at the imaging step.

The overall accuracy with which the various mechani-cal components of a standard linear accelerator are posi-tioned has now improved to the point where many com-mercially available units will perform adequately for stereotactic dose delivery. This improved mechanical ac-curacy is driven by many factors. One example is the cur-rent trend of mounting imaging hardware and software directly on the treatment unit. This technology requires very tight control of the mechanical isocenter in order to produce artifact-free images.

Department of Radiation Oncology, Thomas Jefferson Univer-sity, Philadelphia, PA 19104; and *Department of Radiation Physics, The University of Texas MD Anderson Cancer Cen-ter, Houston, TX 77030

Although there are some SBRT immobilization tech-niques (e.g., stereotactic body frames) that closely mimic the approaches used for the cranial SRS, other stereotac-tic methods have deemphasized or sometimes supple-mented the immobilization part of the process with im-aging that is carried out in a nearly "real-time" fashion. Sophisticated imaging equipment may be incorporated as part of the treatment unit [e.g., cone-beam computed to-mography (CT)], or imaging devices may be placed within the treatment room (e.g., CT-on-rails). These two exam-ples illustrate a general trend whereby the imaging part of the treatment process is accomplished much nearer in time to actual treatment dose delivery.

One distinct advantage of moving the imaging nearer in time to the actual treatment is that it has been shown that some extracranial targets, for example the prostate, can move internally over time periods measured in min-utes. This could mean that using careful and exact immo-bilization to fix the patient in place might not be an effec-tive approach when there is a relatively long time between imaging and treatment. A good example of this situation is when there is a lengthy treatment planning time that could extend to a number of days that are inserted be-tween imaging and treatment. One obvious solution for this problem is to reimage to check the patient's position just prior to treatment. Some of the new built-in imaging capabilities offered by the various linear accelerators manufacturers make it possible to easily obtain such check images.

Much more important for SBRT than for cranial SRS is the problem of respiratory motion during treatment. For SBRT it has become common practice to control res-piratory motion as a method of minimizing the compo-nent of PTV margin required to account for motion of the tumor during the breathing cycle. Available methods in-clude variation of the breath-hold technique and gating methods that allow free breathing but effectively stop lung movement by switching the radiation beam on and off at fixed points in the patient's respiratory cycle; examples are provided in Chapter 7 and are further discussed below.

## WHAT DEFINES A STEREOTACTIC BODY RADIATION THERAPY SETUP?

There are many different ways of solving the problem of making the treatment of targets in the body more precise relative to older methods. It is currently common practice to attach the label "stereotactic" to any new idea that relates to patient immobilization or localization imaging. It is important for the user of any of these devices or approaches to determine whether they offer a real benefit relative to standard techniques and whether they do indeed allow, as determined by measurements, a reduction of PTV margins.

For the purposes of this chapter, SBRT is defined in terms of the results of a commissioning process and, when cooperative group protocols that use SBRT devices are entered, in terms of an accreditation process. We propose an operational definition of an SBRT treatment setup that involves connecting the initial imaging used for tumor targeting with the placement of the treatment beams (as determined by portal images or some accepted equivalent) with a mean deviation of 4.0 mm or less when treating lesions that are not influenced by physiologic motion (see the methodology for determining the mean deviation in reference 1). The mean deviation should remain within 7.0 mm for lesions that are influenced by either cardiac or some residual respiratory motion, or when bowel, rectum, or bladder changes are an issue.

## THE GENERAL COMMISSIONING PROBLEM

SBRT involves decreasing PTV margins relative to standard three-dimensional conformal radiation therapy (3DCRT) or intensity-modulated radiotherapy (IMRT) that do not use this added technology. SBRT systems rely on precisely integrated imaging to accomplish this goal, but different systems can use distinctly different ways of bringing the imaging into the process to solve the margin reduction problem. It has already been pointed out that there are two distinct ways of coupling the imaging to the treatment. First, rigid fixation of the patient's position allows the imaging to be performed, various other function carried out, and treatment accomplished with the assumption that the patient and reference system remained as a rigid body throughout the process or that the system can be reapplied to return the patient back to the original position used for imaging. Second, it is possible to use a daily imaging technique and to shorten the period be-

tween the imaging and treatment steps so that the likelihood of position change during the intervening time is reduced. Of course, some SBRT systems are hybrids of these two approaches in that they combine both the elements of improved immobilization and "on-line" imaging that is carried out just prior to treatment.

Given this variation in technique, the commissioning process should be aimed at verifying and quantifying the ability of a particular system to achieve the desired result of irradiating a target without having to use traditional margins to allow for possible beam misalignment. That is, that these traditional margins can be reduced by an amount that is determined by measurement. In the future, it might be possible to rely on values extracted from the peer-reviewed literature as a substitute for measurements performed at each institution starting an SBRT program, but this information is not readily available for most systems at this time. It is for this reason that a commissioning technique that includes a determination of the reproducibility of the SBRT system is recommended here.

For cranial SRS or SRT, commissioning tests are commonly restricted to mechanical alignment checks for both the immobilization/localization and treatment unit components of the overall system. At least for the case of head frames that are attached directly to the patient's skull, this method is useful because it is assumed that there is little possibility of movement of the cranium relative to the frame once this device is fixed in place. Mechanical checks should also be carried out for SBRT systems, but additional checks must be added to the procedure when the rigidity of the immobilization does not duplicate what is possible when a patient's cranium is fixed directly to the patient support system. While there is a system for spinal SBRT that involves rigid fixation of the vertebral bodies to the patient support system when treating lesions in or around the spinal canal, the additional tests described here should be used for all other SBRT systems.

The commissioning process that is recommended in this chapter for SBRT systems involves a patient study to determine that the system goes beyond achieving simple basic mechanical precision. A patient study is required because there is no phantom study, simulation, or modeling technique that can answer the question of the reproducibility of an SBRT system when the patient is included in the process. Suggestions on how this might be done are given here.

### Verification of Patient Repositioning and Tumor Relocalization

In many cases, it is possible to reimage the patient at the time of treatment, or soon after the treatment ends, as a method of gathering quantitative information on the performance of a particular SBRT system. Reimaging here means the obtaining of a secondary image data set that checks the imaging used initially for patient setup. The recommendation here is that some reimaging technique be used to check the reproducibility of the SBRT system. This reimaging can be inserted at various points in the overall process, and care must be taken to guarantee that an approach that checks the overall process is adopted. For example, imaging for the patient at the final stage of setup just before treatment accomplishes this objective. An alternative is to use imaging to check the reproducibility of the patient's setup in whatever immobilization device is used, but this method must also include some mechanical check to prove that the coupling between the immobilization device and the treatment unit does not add additional unacceptable setup uncertainty.

As pointed out, taking additional images of the patient is the easiest way to provide the needed information. However, depending on local institutional regulations, institutional review board (IRB) approval might be required when additional radiation is to be delivered to a patient for research purposes. For Radiation Therapy Oncology Group (RTOG) protocols that use SBRT, this approval should be specifically requested as part of the IRB application if added radiation will be given for this purpose. An example of an approach that will have the patient receive additional radiation is the use of serial CT studies performed on different days to determine patient setup error within an immobilization device. RTOG Protocol L-0236 ("A Phase 2 Trial of Extracranial Stereotactic Radioablation in the Treatment of Patients with Medically Inoperative Stage 1 Non–Small Cell Lung Cancer") states all positioning systems must be validated and accredited by the study committee prior to enrolling or treating patients on the trial. While it might well be argued that the repeated imaging studies are an integral component of quality assurance—and, further, that the radiation is expected to be clinically inconsequential for a patient with cancer already slated for therapeutic irradiation involving much higher doses than the position-verification images—investigators will need to determine the prevailing opinion locally if they intend to carry out serial CT on some initial small group of patients as a commissioning step that can then be used for credentialing when an RTOG or other protocol group study is being considered.

Another technique that does not give additional radiation to the patient can also be used, and it might not need IRB approval. The technique simply introduces an FDA-approved immobilization system as a new device without attempting to decrease margins at the same time. It is then possible to use the standard port films obtained on a weekly basis to commission the device for use as part of an SBRT program where margins will be reduced. Again, this procedure could be done for a small group of patients, perhaps five or six. If an electronic portal imaging device (EPID) system is available, images can be obtained daily without increasing the patient's dose, and the entire process of gathering commissioning information can be accelerated as a result of the daily imaging. This approach might not be suited for all systems. For example, if very small fields are used for treatment and/or the particular treatment device is restricted in field size, it may not be possible to see sufficient bony anatomy to draw any useful conclusions about the equipment's performance in terms of field position relative to visible anatomy.

It is important to study a group of patients for each disease site that will be treated with SBRT. One approach might be to restrict the initial commissioning study to patients in the appropriate disease site category that have lesions that are not overly challenging. That is, it is not advisable to undertake this part of the commissioning process with patients who have lesions that directly abut or even surround a critical structure. Instead, to ensure safety in the initial use of a new SBRT system with small margins before its setup reproducibility has been demonstrated, patients with some reasonable distance between the target and critical structures should be studied.

## Commissioning a Stereotactic Body Frame

There are a number of companies now manufacturing stereotactic body frames (SBFs), and examples are discussed in Chapter 7. Only one of these devices will be discussed here, but it is assumed that the method suggested for commissioning for this equipment can be applied to the other devices. The Elekta stereotactic body frame (Norcross, GA) consists of a wood and plastic frame that surrounds the patient on three sides with a beanbag-type insert that molds to the patient's body as a vacuum is drawn. One feature of this device is that it has two laser lights mounted directly on the frame that can be adjusted along calibrated scales to place reference marks on the patient at positions that are selected to give good reproducibility. That is, they can be located away from regions where the patient's skin is loose and easily moved. For example, two places where the reference marks might be placed are near the sternum and on the anterior portion of either leg at about the level of the mid calf.

The SBF also contains a complex arrangement of radio-opaque fiducials that allow a target center as determined by CT imaging to be precisely translated to positions on either side of the frame. Thus, one method of using the SBF is to use its extra features (special laser marker lights and vacuum cushion) to position the patient reproducibly within the frame, and then treat the frame using reference marks placed on its surface or special adjustable scales that highlight the positioning points. For SBF systems that include embedded fiducial markers, it is also possible to use this capability to take daily CT images to determine the offset of the target center on a particular day so that this deviation can be corrected. Some systems provide the software needed to calculate these offsets so that the correction can be made quickly.

Verifying the performance of the SBF as an immobilization device requires an analysis of images taken in the treatment position. In some cases, it is possible to examine orthogonal portal images to determine the setup uncertainty of the body frame system. Using this approach depends on having reliable landmarks in the images to help determine the variation of the target position relative to the treatment fields. The reliability of the landmarks depends on their visualization and on their maintaining a fixed geometric relationship relative to the target. If fusion software is available to aid in the process of quantifying shifts in the landmarks, the process might be simplified considerably. In situations where no reasonable landmarks are available or where the target can change positions with time, using serial CT images might be a better way of determining setup uncertainty for the SBF. If respiration is a consideration, some type of gated CT imaging might be necessary.

### Marker Seeds Viewed with Orthogonal Radiographs

Placing gold marker seeds in the prostate and viewing its position (actually using the seeds as a surrogate for the prostate) on a daily basis with an EPID is now becoming a relatively routine procedure. EPIDs that use amorphous silicon flat panels give excellent images that can easily detect the seeds when transmission images through the patient's pelvis are obtained. The technique uses two orthogonal views and commonly uses special software that allows the user to mark the seeds in each image and returns a set of coordinates for treatment unit adjustment when the setup does not agree with the planning information.

Commissioning seed marker systems is relatively straightforward, because the seeds are directly visible without using either bony anatomy or other anatomic landmarks as a surrogate for target position. As long as the seeds do not migrate within the tissue, their position can be used to determine target position even if the tissue containing them moves. Of course, the assumption is that the seeds can be readily visualized with the detector used to find them. Some aspects of the system can give incorrect results, but the performance of the overall system can usually be checked with phantom measurements without resorting to a patient study.

The phantom used for evaluating the system can be a block made up of slabs of plastic. Three seeds can be placed between different slabs (it is best to scribe the surface of the slabs and place the seeds so that they do not separate the slabs) to create a three-dimensional pattern, and three additional seeds can be placed on the surface to

simulate lateral and anterior setup points. With the seeds in place, CT scans of the phantom are obtained and some field arrangement is selected to represent a treatment plan. The phantom is then placed on the treatment couch and positioned using the same surface marks used at the time of CT simulation. EPIDs or port films are obtained for one of the lateral fields and an anterior projection. These images can be compared to digitally reconstructed radiographs (DRRs) made from the CT data obtained at the time of CT simulation. Any differences represent the inherent setup error for the system.

Seed marker systems usually include software for correcting the patient's position relative to the treatment unit's mechanical isocenter when deviation from the desired setup position is detected. Simple experiments can be performed to check the operation of the software used to make these corrections. Moving the phantom by known amounts and making sure that the software can effectively direct compensatory adjustment back to the starting point will provide performance verification. When a Lucite tray with embedded markers is used as a reference for the field center for the portal image, the placement of these markers must also be verified. Another technique is to use software that is often available with the EPID system to reference to a multileaf field outline. If rigorous quality assurance (QA) is routinely performed for the multileaf collimator, only the performance of the software that performs the field outline matching need be checked.

### Kilovoltage X-ray–Based Repositioning

The BrainLAB ExacTrac technology is an infrared (IR) external marker tracking system that consists of IR-sensitive markers placed on the patient's skin that are viewed with two IR cameras and a conventional video camera. The IR system is useful for initial patient setup and can be combined with a complementary BrainLab kilovoltage x-ray system for more precise positioning. The x-ray localization system uses two diagnostic energy x-ray generators with opposed amorphous silicon panels for imaging. The center axes of the two x-ray beams intersect at a 90-degree angle. Daily images as recorded by the two amorphous silicon panels can be used to determine if the patient is in the same position each day relative to the planning CT data set. This determination is made by using the CT information to generate DRRs corresponding to the geometry of the two flat panel images. Software is provided to compare the DRRs to the amorphous silicon images, and coordinates can be generated when it is necessary to shift the patient support system to adjust for any misalignment.

The x-ray method of adjusting the patient's position is similar to the use of a standard radiation therapy EPID to view orthogonal images of the patient. However, major differences are that EPIDs usually work with the higher energy treatment beam and that there is a time delay between images as the gantry rotates by 90 degrees. Independent of these differences, the procedure for commissioning a kilovoltage x-ray system is in general the same as the procedure that is used to commission a system that tracks the movement of gold marker seeds placed in the prostate (see last section). Phantom studies similar to the ones described above have been performed and indicate excellent reproducibility for this type of device (2).

Even when treating targets near the vertebral bodies, the precision obtainable with phantoms that have embedded markers is not expected to apply to actual patient situations because the vertebral bodies do not provide clear point objects for matching. Sophisticated fusion techniques can be used to attempt to solve this problem, but this approach is limited by the fact that a full 3D representation of the anatomy is not available for registration of images. It is for this reason that a patient study is recommended.

Special attention should be paid to the problem of having a limited field of view of surrounding anatomy when conducting x-ray–based studies to determine field placement reproducibility. The vertebral bodies are a good reference for fusion of imaging information, but often when treating lesions in the liver no bony anatomy falls within the field of view of the imaging devices. One solution to this problem is the use of a "virtual isocenter" for a patient setup selected in a location within the body such that there will definitely be bony structures visible within the orthogonal x-ray images. Once the x-ray images and DRRs of the virtual isocenter are compared to determine the x, y, and z distances to move for proper matching, it is then necessary to translate the additional x, y, and z distances known to separate the virtual isocenter from the true isocenter within the patient. This technique can be very helpful in clinical practice (B. Kavanagh, personal communication, July, 2004).

## Techniques for Addressing Respiratory Motion

Commissioning and accreditation of an SBRT system when respiratory motion is an issue adds another level of complication that is dependent on the exact method of breathing control to be combined with any of the immobilization/localization systems presented above. For example, if a patient can hold his or her breath for the required time period and in exactly the same way (i.e., stop breathing at exactly the same point in the breathing cycle) for each treatment fraction, the commissioning process does not need to consider breathing control any further. However, if the patient is asked or forced to adopt shallow breathing during treatment, the added uncertainty in the target position must be quantified in order to properly represent the overall setup reproducibility so that the PTV

margin can be correctly assigned. In the first example, where the patient's respiration is effectively halted, the commissioning process might be simplified, but the techniques required for gaining the imaging information to be used for treatment planning will usually be more complicated. Taking the example of using CT images for planning, these images will have to be acquired under the same conditions of suspended respiration. Since not all of the image information can normally be acquired during a single breath hold, it might be necessary to use different breath holds and to "sew" the imaging data together at the end of the process. This is not a trivial process, and many CT or planning systems may not be able to accomplish this task.

Complete and exact suspension of respiration is not achievable. This is due to the difficulty of having a patient do the same thing each day. This problem can be partially overcome by teaching or coaching the patients, but some amount of variability must always be expected. Some of the methods described below expect the patient's respiration to remain constant and regular during the period that extends from the start to the end of dose delivery. However, it might take considerable vigilance or the introduction of certain measuring devices to make sure that this is actually accomplished.

Several different approaches for controlling respiratory motion were discussed in Chapter 7. Techniques now in common clinical practice for SBRT include an external compression-based approach to force shallow breathing, use of a device to regulate the depth of inspiration during breath-holding, and gating the linear accelerator output to the breathing cycle.

Each approach has different features that influence the way in which an institution's particular system would be evaluated prior to clinical implementation. Although the external compression-based method is the simplest, the compression device itself can create imaging artifacts that can mask the target that is being treated. Commissioning an SBRT system that uses depth-regulated inspiration requires considerable operator experience on the part of the therapists operating the accelerator to turn it on and off properly in concert with breathing regulation. Gating techniques that use some surrogate to follow the patient's breathing (e.g., a spirometer, a temperature-sensitive resistor placed under the patient's nose, or markers placed on the patient's chest that can be followed with a pair of cameras as the chest rises and falls) likewise involve turning the treatment unit on only during preselected portions of the respiratory cycle. Commissioning of a SBRT system that uses gating to suspend respiration requires a good understanding of the stability of the patient's respiratory cycle. Any drifting of this pattern relative to the patient's breathing during the treatment planning process can be important and should be taken into account during the evaluation of the overall SBRT system reproducibility.

## ACCREDITATION PROGRAMS

Before allowing participation in some clinical trials, cooperative groups may require a demonstration of the relevant treatment delivery and treatment planning capabilities. The purpose of this demonstration is to assure that the institutions planning to participate in the trial have the capabilities and understanding necessary to comply with the trial. The Radiological Physics Center (RPC) was established as a resource in radiation dosimetry and physics for cooperative clinical trial groups and all radiotherapy facilities that deliver radiation treatments to patients entered onto cooperative group protocols. The primary responsibility is to assure the National Cancer Institute (NCI) and the cooperative groups that the participating institutions have adequate quality assurance procedures and no major systematic dosimetry discrepancies, so that they can be expected to deliver radiation treatments that are clinically comparable to those delivered by other institutions in the cooperative groups. To fulfill this responsibility, the RPC monitors the basic machine output and brachytherapy source strengths, the dosimetry data used by the institutions, the calculation algorithms used for treatment planning, and the institutions' quality control procedures.

The RPC's methods of monitoring include on-site dosimetry review and a variety of remote audit tools. During the on-site evaluation, the institution's physicists and radiation oncologists are interviewed, physical measurements are made on the therapy machines, dosimetry and quality assurance data are reviewed, and patient dose calculations are evaluated. The remote audit tools include the following: (a) mailed dosimeters evaluated on a periodic basis to verify output calibration and simple questionnaires to document changes in personnel, equipment, and dosimetry practices; (b) comparison of dosimetry data with RPC "standard" data to verify the compatibility of dosimetry data; (c) evaluation of reference and actual patient calculations to verify the validity of treatment planning algorithms; and (d) review of the institution's written quality assurance procedures and records. Anthropomorphic phantoms are also used to verify tumor dose delivery for special treatment techniques.

The prerequisites vary from one trial to another. In some cases, completing a questionnaire about the facilities and technologies available is sufficient. For other trials, the completion of representative benchmark treatment plans is adequate, whereas in other cases benchmark plans specific to the particular trial are required. However, in circumstances where the technology used for treatment is complex and critical to the successful completion of the trial, more demanding requirements for credentialing are set. In the case of SBRT, the RTOG has determined that credentialing will require the completion of several questionnaires, demonstration of adequate patient immobilization and positioning, the irradiation of an anthropomorphic phantom, and the electronic submission of a representative treatment plan.

Accreditation of institutions to participate in cooperative group trials is managed by a quality assurance office (QAO). For trials managed by the RTOG, the RPC participates in credentialing of institutions. When electronic data submission is required, the RPC's involvement is coordinated through the Advanced Technology QA Consortium (ATC), an NCI-funded consortium of QAOs established to support the use of advanced technologies, including electronic data exchange, by cooperative groups. The ATC provides the infrastructure for electronic submission and review of treatment planning data, including CT and MRI images. The RPC then uses the ATC's evaluation tools to review and compare an institution's treatment plan with other data, including measurements. For SBRT, as is described below, the RPC uses these capabilities to compare the treatment plan submitted by an institution with the measured dose distribution determined by dosimeters embedded in an anthropomorphic phantom.

The RPC will evaluate the questionnaires submitted by each institution, in preparation for credentialing for the SBRT protocol. Review of the institution's procedures and technologies for patient immobilization and positioning will be reviewed by the study committee, defined by the protocol as being composed of the study cochairs.

### Facility Inventory Questionnaire

As part of accreditation for specific clinical trials, institutions may be asked to complete a questionnaire describing the equipment and procedures in place that are relevant to SBRT. The questionnaire also asks the institution to identify the personnel who will be participating in the procedure. In particular, the participating staff must be have the knowledge and skill necessary to identify the target volumes and organs at risk, understand the tumoricidal doses and tolerance doses of normal tissues, and the technical understanding of the immobilization and treatment techniques to be used. These staff include the radiation oncologist, the medical physicist, the dosimetrist, and the data manager.

The equipment to be used will be identified and its characteristics described. For SBRT this will include the immobilization devices, and the procedures used for

The Advanced Technology QA Consortium (ATC) is funded through PHS grant CA81647 awarded by the NCI, DHHS, to James Purdy, Ph.D., at Washington University. The members of the consortium include the RPC, the Image-guided Therapy QA Center (ITC), the Resource Center for Emerging Technologies (RCET), the Quality Assurance Review Center (QARC) and the RTOG's Headquarters Dosimetry Group.]

compensating for respiratory and other motion. These are to be described so that they may be considered for the acceptability by the study chair but also to enable retrospective review of the performance of the immobilizing devices. The questionnaire will include a description of the treatment equipment and any necessary accessories, as these may introduce variations in treatment from one facility to another. In the specific case of SBRT, a description of the collimator system is required, as differences among standard multileaf collimators, micromultileaf collimators, and detachable cones may be significant when considering the small fields used for SBRT.

Finally, the questionnaire will ask details about the imaging and treatment planning systems to be used by the facility. With regard to the imaging system, the study chairs will want to be assured that the equipment is state-of-the-art and capable of providing the image quality needed for the study. In particular, as small volumes are to be treated with small fields, very thin CT image slices are necessary. Not all CT scanners have this capability. The method used to transfer images to the treatment planning system is of interest, in case there are difficulties in receiving and interpreting the images at a central review facility.

## Knowledge Assessment Questionnaire

A second questionnaire has been used for credentialing for advanced technologies such as SBRT. This questionnaire functions as an informal examination of the key staff members at the institution, and asks them to answer questions about the protocol. The purpose is to ensure that the staff have read, and are familiar with, key provisions of the protocol. This questionnaire has proven useful in the past, by prompting staff to examine the protocol more carefully before implementing it in their departments.

## Evaluation of Positioning and Immobilization

As indicated in the sections above, SBRT requires extraordinary attention to patient immobilization and positioning. The RTOG protocol requires that institutions document

their ability to account for motion of internal organs. The SBRT protocol will not require evaluation of these techniques for credentialing, although a dynamic phantom is under development and will be used in credentialing programs for subsequent protocols (see below).

## Irradiation of Standard Phantom

The approach of the RPC when conducting credentialing is to investigate the result rather than individual steps in the process of treatment delivery. To assist with credentialing for clinical trials, the RPC has developed a family of anthropomorphic phantoms that are used to evaluate treatment delivery. These phantoms include a stereotactic brain phantom that has been used to evaluate the quality of stereotactic radiosurgery at nearly 200 institutions (3), a head and neck phantom for IMRT, a thorax phantom, and a pelvis phantom. The head and neck phantom has been irradiated more than 60 times, in most cases for credentialing purposes. The pelvis phantom and thorax phantom are newer and less experience has been obtained to date. However, the thorax phantom is expected to be used to evaluate the ability of institutions to deliver SBRT to lung lesions.

The thorax phantom is shown in Fig. 11.1. It consists of a plastic water-fillable shell of approximately lifelike dimensions. The shell contains a right lung, made of lung tissue–equivalent material (CIRS, Norfolk, VA). The left lung, also made of tissue-equivalent material, is separated into a fixed portion and a removable portion. The removable portion contains a target volume, 3 cm diameter by 5 cm long, constructed of high-impact polystyrene. The removable portion can be dismantled and loaded with capsules containing thermoluminescent dosimeters (TLDs) composed of lithium fluoride. This portion also has slits that accommodate sheets of radiochromic film. Also shown in Fig. 11.1 is a CT image of the phantom through the target volume. The image also demonstrates the location of heart structure and a spine. Both the heart and the spine contain TLDs.

To demonstrate the value of this phantom in determining dose distributions, a treatment plan was designed that consisted of several 6 MV accelerator beams of small di-

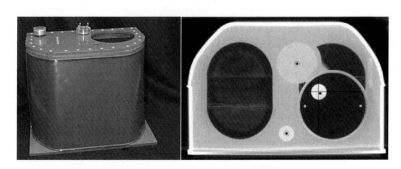

**FIGURE 11.1.** Left, the Radiological Physics Center (RPC) thorax phantom, shown fully assembled. A CT image of the RPC thorax phantom, showing the target volume located in the medial aspect of the left lung **(right).**

mensions. The plan corrected for the tissue densities and was designed to deliver 20 Gy to the periphery of a PTV drawn around the target. Figure 11.2 shows a comparison between the calculated dose distribution and the distribution measured with the TLDs and the radiochromic film. The TLDs indicated doses that were slightly higher than those predicted by the treatment plan. The radiochromic films displayed a dose distribution that showed a great deal of similarity with the calculated dose distribution, but also showed regions exhibiting differences of greater than 5% or 5 mm distance to agreement. On the basis of these data, and a number of measurements of simpler dose distributions, the phantom was considered suitable for use as a credentialing tool.

When an institution indicates interest in becoming credentialed to participate in a protocol requiring SBRT, the institution is instructed to first complete the knowledge assessment questionnaire and the facility inventory questionnaire. Once the institution has demonstrated sufficient familiarity with the protocol and has indicated that their equipment and procedures meet the minimum standard established by the protocol, the phantom is sent to the institution. The institution is instructed to treat the phantom as they would a patient. The institution is to perform imaging procedures, develop a treatment plan, conduct their standard QA procedures, and then deliver the treatment, just as they would to a patient. Finally, the phantom is to be returned to the RPC for evaluation. Details of the treatment delivery are to be returned with the phantom, including a description of the QA procedures performed, the results of those procedures, and the manner in which those results were used. For example, if the QA procedures indicated that the treatment plan overestimated the dose to the target, were the monitor unit settings reduced?

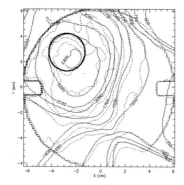

**FIGURE 11.2.** A comparison of calculated isodoses (*straight line*) with measured data (*dotted line*) from radiochromic film inserted into the Radiological Physics Center thorax phantom.

Institutions are expected to deliver a dose to the phantom that agrees with their treatment plan within 7% or 4-mm distance-to-agreement in steep dose gradient regions. These relatively relaxed criteria were adopted to reflect the difficulty in correcting for low-density heterogeneities, particularly with the small fields to be used for SBRT.

Modifications are under way to introduce motion to simulate respiration of this phantom. A reciprocating table has been constructed that moves the phantom back and forth in the longitudinal dimension. The range of motion and the parameters of the respiratory cycle can be altered to simulate actual patient breathing. Gated CT images of this phantom have been obtained and used for treatment planning. A method of predicting structure position at points during the respiratory cycle has been developed (4). The reciprocating table is being modified to induce motion of the phantom in two dimensions (superior-inferior and anterior-posterior). Additional developmental work is being performed on a phantom with internal moving parts to more realistically simulate respiratory motion. Preliminary tests have been conducted to evaluate the dose distribution delivered to the phantom when the beam is gated in synchrony with the phantom motion. It is anticipated that this system will be used to evaluate gating and target tracking procedures used at participating institutions.

## Electronic Submission of Treatment Plan Data

As the complexity of radiotherapy clinical trials increases, it has become impractical to review the data from hard copies. The complex dose distributions that are typical of IMRT and SBRT demand the ability to view multiple distributions, in many axial planes as well as coronal, sagittal, and arbitrary planes. More important, clinical trials involving such advanced treatment technologies require the use of advanced tools to evaluate. Tools such as dose-volume histograms (DVHs) are known to be calculated inconsistently from one treatment planning system to another. To ensure consistency, DVHs should be recalculated using a single method. Finally, it is increasingly difficult to maintain high quality of clinical trials involving large numbers of patients. To perform the type of comprehensive review demanded by such a trial is not possible with traditional methods.

To address these difficulties, electronic means of data transfer and quality assurance are under development (5,6). The ATC was established to provide the infrastructure to enable Internet-based submission and evaluation of treatment planning data for clinical trials. Today, many treatment planning systems support electronic submission of treatment plan data to the Image-guided

Therapy QA Center (ITC), a member of the ATC. Treatment plans developed for dose delivery to the RPC phantom are submitted electronically to the ITC for evaluation by the RPC.

Tools developed by the ATC enable review of the treatment plans over the Internet. Thus, the study chair or another reviewer can evaluate the treatment plans for patients submitted to the trial from any location with Internet access. The tools also provide the ability to redraw contours, so that the study chair can redefine target volumes and organs at risk. DVHs can be recalculated based on the re-drawn contours so that the calculations are consistent across the population of patients enrolled in the study.

## References

1. Rosenthal SA, Galvin, JM, Goldwein JW, et al. Improved methods for determination of variability in patient positioning for radiation therapy using simulation and serial portal film measurements. *Int J Radiat Oncol Biol Phys* 992;23:621–625.
2. Yan H, Yin FF, Kim JH. A phantom study on the positioning accuracy of the Novalis Body System. *Med Phys* 2003;30:3052–3060.
3. Stovall M, Balter P, Hanson WF, et al. Quality audit of radiosurgery dosimetry using mailed phantoms. *Med Phys* 1995;22:1009.
4. Zhang G, Guerrero T, Huang T-C, et al. *3D optical flow method implementation for mapping of 3D anatomical structure contours across 4D CT data.* Seoul, Korea: ICCR, 2004.
5. Palta JR, Frouhar VA, Dempsey JF. Web-based submission, archive, and review of radiotherapy data for clinical quality assurance: a new paradigm. *Int J Radiat Oncol Biol Phys* 2003;57:1427–1436.
6. Low DA, Dempsey JF, Markman J, et al. Toward automated quality assurance for intensity-modulated radiation therapy. *Int J Radiat Oncol Biol Phys* 2002;53:443–453.

## Chapter 12

# Personnel Training for Stereotactic Body Radiation Therapy

*Lucien Nedzi, Robert A. Sanford, Elly Zakris, \*Scott Alleman, Alichia White, and Anna Hall*

## INTRODUCTION

The coordination and preparation of the stereotactic body radiation therapy (SBRT) team is essential for safe and effective treatment. While the previous chapter addressed the issue of efficient clinical operations from a systems perspective, here we expand on the roles of individual members of the clinic team, with particular attention to important aspects of staff development and training.

## PHYSICIANS

As much for SBRT as for any other medical service provided to a patient, the ultimate responsibility for ensuring the quality of care rendered falls squarely upon the physician's shoulders. In addition to understanding clinical applications and recognizing the range of radiation doses that can be administered safely to tumors and normal tissues around the body, the radiation oncologist launching an SBRT program should first inventory current staffing to assure that there is adequate administrative and technical support for the program.

Appropriate, conservative patient selection at the initial stages of a program helps promote understanding and confidence among staff as all progress on the learning curve. In addition, it creates credibility among referring physicians because the chances of a good result are maximized. Physicians must understand that the planning process is lengthy (sometimes more than 1 week) and that the patient must be motivated to cooperate with a lengthy treatment that may involve discomfort related to prolonged immobilization. Patients with a poor performance status or patients with significant symptoms will be diffi-

Department of Radiology, Tulane University, New Orleans, LA 70112; and \*Radiation Therapy Program, Willis-Knighton Cancer Center, Shreveport, LA 71103

cult or impossible to treat, especially in the start-up phase of a program.

## MEDICAL PHYSICISTS

In 2003, the American Association of Physicists in Medicine (AAPM) formed a Task Group (TG 101) specifically charged with the following goals:

- To review the literature and identify the range of historical experiences, reported clinical findings, and expected outcomes
- To review the relevant commercial products and associated clinical findings for an assessment of system capabilities, technology limitations, and patient-related expectations and outcomes
- To determine required criteria for setting up and establishing an SBRT facility, including protocols, equipment, resources, and quality assurance (QA) procedures
- To develop consistent documentation for prescribing, reporting, and recording extracranial stereotactic radiation therapy (SBRT) treatment delivery

SBRT clearly requires medical physicist efforts well beyond what is typically needed for other forms of radiotherapy, and at a minimum, there should be at least one properly trained physicist at each center where SBRT is administered. AAPM TG 101 guidelines are expected to be forthcoming within the next few years, as published clinical experiences accumulate. In the meantime, it is advisable to comply with American Society for Therapeutic Radiology and Oncology (ASTRO) guidelines for cranial radiosurgery, which specify that a board-eligible or board-certified medical physicist be directly involved.

The institution-specific training for SBRT depends on the available equipment to be used but should cover the three general categories of QA: the patient immobilization and positioning systems; the therapy delivery machine and related hardware; and the treatment planning and delivery software. Physicist education should include vendor training for all commercial hardware and software, and the physicist should have a firm familiarity with any in-house system(s). The physicist should be well versed in the issues of cranial radiosurgery QA, as detailed in the AAPM report number 54 (1), as well as the complex aspects of QA for therapy and treatment planning equipment discussed in AAPM report number 46 (2). Other resources for the medical physicist are AAPM report numbers 74 (3) and 82 (4) detailing QA aspects for diagnostic imaging and intensity-modulated radiotherapy (IMRT), respectively. The QA requirements of SBRT demand that each step in the imaging, planning, and delivery process is thoroughly understood and checked by at least one knowledgeable physicist.

## DOSIMETRISTS

An SBRT program requires careful acquisition of patient computed tomography (CT) data and transfer of this information into a treatment planning system. Registration of this CT data with the stereotactic positioning system may not be supported in the same software, and cross-registration of coincident images must be ensured. In addition, fusion of data acquired from multiple CTs, magnetic resonance images, or positron emission tomography (PET) may be required for target definition. Developing proficiency with these components will greatly facilitate implementation in the first case. Practice with a few more conventional treatments is a good step in ensuring a smooth transition to the first SBRT case. If new software is acquired to facilitate SBRT planning, there should always be manufacturer training for the dosimetrist as well as physician and physicist involved.

## THERAPISTS

Therapists should be trained in correct construction of the immobilization device and positioning of the stereotactic body frame or other external fiducial marker system, under the supervision of a physician and physicist. The therapist must be taught that stereotactic techniques require reference to points external to the patient rather than skin tattoos. Tattoo marks may still serve as references to this external coordinate system. This conceptual transition can require a period of adjustment and reinforcement. Prior experience with cranial stereotaxy using a removable frame can be helpful in departments with this capability.

The therapist must understand the importance of pretreatment position verification supervised by physician

and physicist prior to each fraction of SBRT. At Tulane, we initiated a daily position shift chart that therapists complete at each treatment to reinforce and track daily verification.

Therapists must also be trained in the monitoring of the respiratory control device or monitor during therapy. Whenever new immobilization or respiratory gating equipment is obtained to facilitate SBRT, on-site presence of the manufacturer's technical support representative is strongly recommended for the first few treatments, both to educate the therapists and to troubleshoot problems and assure optimal performance. At Tulane, we have two therapists operating the machine so that one may ensure that real-time position monitoring parameters remain within acceptable tolerance. The therapist must also be prepared for a lengthy treatment, during which the patient must be coached to comply with treatment position or respiratory control device.

## NURSES

Educating nurses about the additional needs of a patient undergoing SBRT promotes a satisfied patient and a smooth transition to treatment. Preparing the patient with realistic estimates of the time-consuming treatment planning, verification, and delivery process is important to allay fears and promote confidence. Nurses provide invaluable assistance when they are educated about the process and have the opportunity to contribute by ensuring the comfort of the patient during the simulation and treatment process.

Side effects, particularly nausea and fevers related to hepatic SBRT, should be reviewed with the nurse. Information about prophylactic antiemetics and antipyretics prior to hepatic treatments should be incorporated into patient education. The demands of a lengthy treatment, sometimes in an uncomfortable position, should also be discussed with the nurse. Occasional patients benefit from pretreatment anxiolytics or opiates, particularly if the patient has discomfort in the stereotactic device at initial simulation. Educating patients about possible skin reactions a few weeks following treatment and the importance of avoiding sun exposure to irradiated areas is important.

## ADMINISTRATORS

The forever-changing nature of charge code definitions and fee-for-service reimbursement scales is challenging for radiation oncologists and their departmental administrators. ASTRO has been proactively involved in the process to consolidate many of the special activities of SBRT into a new current procedural terminology (CPT) code definition. Until the new code definitions have been endorsed by the Centers for Medicare and Medicaid Services, the professional activities and technical services associated with SBRT are billed under the various existing codes that represent individual aspects of the entire complicated process. Depending on the specific technique used, the treatment itself might or might not be categorized as a form of IMRT, with IMRT planning and treatment codes applicable. A special physics consultation is a separately billable professional item that can cover the physicist's involvement in the process. The initial complex simulation and associated immobilization devices may be billed when properly documented, as can a verification simulation. For courses of treatment of three fractions or more, a weekly treatment management charge is appropriate; shorter courses are covered under the 77431 code.

Hospital administrators must be educated about the special nature of SBRT and understand the additional demands this high-precision therapy places on radiation on-cology department resources. At the same time, providing this new service to patients also frequently involves the utilization of numerous other revenue-generating activities within the institution outside the radiation oncology department, namely additional imaging studies and laboratory testing. It is important for administrators to understand SBRT in this context so that they will be more supportive of the physician's efforts to bring this novel therapy to a community.

## REFERENCES

1. Stereotactic Radiosurgery (1995) Radiation Therapy Committee Task Group #42, AAPM, College Park, MD.
2. AAPM. Comprehensive QA for radiation oncology. *Med Phys* 1994;21:37.
3. Quality Control in Diagnostic Radiology (2002) Diagnostic X-Ray Imaging Committee Task Group #12, AAPM, College Park, MD.
4. AAPM. Guidance document on delivery, treatment planning, and clinical implementation of IMRT: report of the IMRT Subcommittee of the AAPM Radiation Therapy Committee. *Med Phys* 2003;30:27.

# Stereotactic Body Radiation Therapy for Lung Tumors

*Danny Y. Song and Henric Blomgren\**

## INTRODUCTION

The application of stereotactic body radiotherapy (SBRT) for tumors within the lung presents both unique challenges as well as opportunities for improving clinical outcomes. Targeting difficulties in delivering radiotherapy to lung tumors derive from both interfractional setup errors presented by the relative independence of lung position from bony anatomy as well as intrafractional movement due mainly to respiration. Conventional radiotherapy methods have compensated for these factors with the use of generous margins around clinical target volumes (CTVs), leading to the treatment of significant amounts of surrounding normal lung tissues to the target dose. The ability to accurately target the tumor while reducing the volume of lung irradiated opens the possibility of improved tumor control via dose escalation or shortened overall treatment durations (acceleration via hypofractionation), while maintaining or decreasing current levels of treatment morbidity. Reports of SBRT in lung to date have included patients treated for primary non–small cell lung cancer (NSCLC) as well as metastases to lung from tumors originating at other sites. This chapter will briefly cover the theoretical benefits of SBRT in these settings and summarize the published experience while also including some description of the variety of targeting methods utilized.

## OVERVIEW OF TECHNIQUES FOR LUNG STEREOTACTIC BODY RADIATION THERAPY

Unlike cranial radiosurgery, lung position cannot be fixed in reference to an external bony structure. Many authors have treated patients using a stereotactic body frame, an apparatus designed to more precisely reposition the patient daily for each treatment compared to conventional setup techniques by the use of an external stereotactic fiducial system and patient immobilization. Preliminary studies have demonstrated the accuracy of stereotactic body frames to be in the 3- to 6-mm range for reproduction of target position (1,2). Respiratory motion during radiation delivery can be accounted for using either abdominal pressure to limit diaphragmatic excursion, breath-hold devices (3), or respiratory gating to selectively activate the beam during a portion of the breathing cycle (4). Others have taken the simpler approach of measuring respiratory variation with separate computed tomography (CT) scans at inspiration and expiration and incorporated the differences in tumor position into their planning target volume (PTV).

An alternative method for achieving precise daily tumor localization as well as compensation for respiratory movement is to implant a radio-opaque marker visible on a linear accelerator. Shimizu et al. (5) placed gold spheres via bronchoscopy into airways of 20 patients with lung tumors. A real-time tumor tracking system consisting of dual fluoroscopic detectors was used to activate the beam when the marker was within a certain positional range. Fourteen of 16 peripherally located tumors were successfully localized with this technique, whereas all spheres placed for centrally located tumors were displaced during the treatment course, as they lacked physical properties to resist displacement from coughing and respiration. Thirteen primary or metastatic lung tumors in 12 patients were successfully treated with this technique using 5-mm PTV margins, and local control maintained in all but one patient.

## RATIONALE FOR USE OF STEREOTACTIC BODY RADIATION THERAPY

Lung cancer is the most common cause of death from malignancy within the United States (6). Eighty percent of lung cancer is of non–small cell histology (7), and radia-

Department of Radiation Oncology and Molecular Radiation Sciences, the Sidney Kimmel Comprehensive Cancer Center at Johns Hopkins, Baltimore, MD 21231 and *Karolinska University Hospital and Karolinska Institute, Stockholm, Sweden.

tion is the primary treatment for most patients with non–small cell lung cancer who have localized disease without hematogenous metastasis (8). For purposes of treatment selection, NSCLC is generally divided into early stage and advanced stage depending on local extent of the primary and involvement of draining lymph nodes. The standard radiation dose for NSCLC in both early and advanced stages is 60 to 66 Gy. These dose levels are based on studies reported in the 1980s (9). However, at this dose level it has been shown that 30% to 50% of patients with advanced-stage disease will develop radiographically evident isolated local failure within the irradiated primary tumor (10), and local failure has been correlated with subsequent distant metastases and death (11). The same is true for patients treated for early-stage disease. In a review of the literature for medically inoperable early-stage NSCLC, Sibley et al. (12) found a 30% rate of isolated local failure. Krol et al. (13) reported a 66% local failure rate in patients treated for early-stage NSCLC with 60 to 65 Gy in 2.5- to 3-Gy fractions, with a higher rate of distant metastasis in patients failing to achieve local control. Cheung et al. (14) found a component of local failure in 53% of patients treated with 48 Gy in 12 fractions, and 69% in patients treated with 52.5 Gy in 20 fractions. Using a more stringent histologic evaluation of tumor responses after treatment to 65 Gy (2.5 Gy per fraction), Arriagada et al. (15) reported tumor control in only 20% of patients.

There are several reports showing that there is a radiation dose-response relationship in NSCLC and that local tumor control is associated with improved survival (16–21). On the basis of tumor control probability calculations applied to data from a dose escalation study, Martel et al. (22) predicted a dose of 84 Gy would achieve tumor control for longer (>30 months) local progression-free survival. Currently used doses are substantially less than those predicted to achieve 50% long-term progression-free survival (22). Although increasing the dose of radiation using conventional techniques may provide improved tumor control, increasing doses to normal lung are also associated with higher complication rates (23,24). Radiation pneumonitis is a potentially fatal complication of lung irradiation, and its occurrence is proportional to the volume of lung irradiated. Current radiotherapy techniques result in symptomatic pneumonitis in 14% to 30% of patients (26,27). Other frequent complications include radiation fibrosis and reduced pulmonary function. Given that most patients with NSCLC have marginal lung function due to smoking-related pulmonary disease, these effects are clinically relevant, limiting possibilities for dose escalation (28).

These factors have led to clinical trials evaluating dose escalation using three-dimensional (3D) conformal radiotherapy (CRT), often in combination with chemotherapy for patients with advanced-stage disease (29). However,

some early results indicate unexpected late toxicity. Maguire et al. (30) found a 17% incidence of late grade ≥3 pulmonary toxicity following 3D radiotherapy given in a twice-daily schedule to 73.6 to 80 Gy. Preliminary results of a Radiation Therapy Oncology Group (RTOG) dose escalation study (RTOG 9311) indicate late pulmonary toxicity in 15% of patients treated to doses of 70.9 to 77.4 Gy in 2.1-Gy daily fractions (31). Further follow-up is needed to assess whether dose escalation with these methods is tolerable. With regard to early-stage disease, although 3DCRT doses of 60 to 66 Gy to fields limited to the primary tumor alone are generally not associated with radiation pneumonitis, a study by Langendijk et al suggests that 3DCRT may negatively affect quality of life. Patient-reported quality-of-life was assessed at intervals starting prior to radiotherapy in 46 patients, and showed worsening trends in dyspnea, appetite, and fatigue up to 24 months after therapy (32). Despite the fact that progression of medical comorbidities is common in this population, the worsening trend was seen to begin at 2 weeks into therapy. Some patients received treatment to nodal areas, but dysphagia was the only symptom that was statistically different between patients treated to locoregional fields versus those receiving treatment to the lung primary alone.

Reports of SBRT in NSCLC generally describe doses that are biologically higher and more accelerated than those used in 3DCRT. Any dose escalation scheme using conventional fractionation requires an increase in overall treatment time, which has been negatively correlated with tumor control rates and patient outcomes (33). Randomized clinical evidence supports the use of a shortened treatment duration (accelerated fractionation) in NSCLC, albeit at a cost of increase pneumonitis with 3DCRT (34). Due to the large differences in fraction sizes between SBRT and conventional treatment, direct comparison of total nominal doses is not feasible. The linear quadratic method is a generally accepted method for drawing comparisons between different fractional schemes. Table 13.1 compares the biologic effective dose (BED) of several SBRT series with conventional fractionation, assuming an $\alpha/\beta$ ratio of ten. One can readily see that the BEDs for SBRT are higher than the standard 60 to 66 Gy for conventional therapy. The use of similar dose fractionation regimens with conventional therapy may lead to increased toxicity. Cheung et al. reported a study where a hypofractionated regimen (48 Gy in 12 fractions) was used for patients with early-stage NSCLC. Although no serious pulmonary complications were reported, 30% of patients had acute dermatitis and 24% developed late subcutaneous fibrosis where the beams entered skin. Such toxicities are less frequently encountered in patients treated with SBRT, likely due to the multiple beam or conformal arc field arrangements used (36).

▶ TABLE 13.1 Comparison of Biologic Equivalent
Doses (Linear Quadratic Method,
$\alpha/\beta = 10$) of Representative Dose
Regimens Used in Stereotactic Body
Radiation Therapy Versus
Conventional Radiotherapy for Early-
stage Non–Small Cell Lung Cancer.

| Author | Dose | Biologic Equivalent Dose |
|---|---|---|
| Standard radiotherapy | 2 Gy × 30–33 fx | 72–79 Gy |
| Hara (58) | 30 Gy × 1 fx | 120 Gy |
| Nagata (50) | 12 Gy × 4 fx | 105 Gy |
| Timmerman (51) | 20 Gy × 3 fx | 180 Gy |

The ability to deliver higher doses to tumor without increasing doses to surrounding lung tissue would improve the therapeutic ratio, leading to better control rates and survival. For example, median tumor size for NSCLC is in the range of 4 to 6 cm (37,39). For a tumor measuring 6 cm in diameter, a reduction from 2.0 to 0.5 cm of margin results in a 66% decrease in volume of lung treated to prescription dose level. The relative reduction in lung volume irradiated is even greater for smaller tumors. Using risk models for predicting pneumonitis, Hanley et al. estimated a possible 16-Gy increase in total dose without increased risk if modest reductions in margin were used (38). As dose escalation would occur on the steep portion of the dose-response curve, tumor control probability models predict approximately 30% to 50% improvement in tumor control (39). The benefits of SBRT for patients with lung cancer also extend to reducing the potential for missing the target volume. With conventional methods, most patients are treated with 2.0- to 2.5-cm circumferential block margins around tumor; even so, daily positioning errors have been demonstrated to result in suboptimal tumor dosing for a portion of treatments. Engelsman et al. (40) performed phantom studies using similar margins and found a reduction in effective dose to tumor due to setup errors, correlating with a 41% tumor control probability as opposed to 50% for the prescribed dose. In summary, the potential improvements in radiation tumor targeting and dose conformality of SBRT offers the potential for increased local control rates and survival for patients with NSCLC without increasing complications.

## EARLY-STAGE NON–SMALL CELL LUNG CANCER

The best survival outcomes in early-stage NSCLC are seen following surgical tumor resection. Surgery alone may produce a 5-year survival of 60% to 80% in patients with stage I, 30% to 40% in stage II, and less in stage III (41–43). However, a proportion of patients with technically operable lung cancer are medically inoperable due to comorbidities such as emphysema and cardiac disease. In the past, these patients and those with operable cancers who refused surgery have been offered conventional radiation therapy alone. Disease-free and overall survival rates for patients who receive 3DCRT are generally inferior to those of surgery, even beyond what could be accounted for by differences in staging. Since patients referred for 3DCRT usually have significant intercurrent illnesses, selection bias may play some role in the observed differences in outcome, but many patients treated with radiotherapy die with local recurrence (13).

Early-stage NSCLC lends itself to the use of SBRT because of the need to treat only the primary site. Retrospective analyses strongly suggest that elective irradiation of regional lymph nodes does not markedly change the rate of regional tumor relapses following 50 to 70 Gy of conventional or hyperfractionated irradiation. Bradley et al. (44) found only two nodal failures of 33 patients who received treatment to only the primary tumor without elective nodal coverage. Similarly, Krol et al. (13) reported only 4% incidence of regional failure in patients treated to the primary tumor site alone. A comprehensive review by Sibley (45) of the results of CRT for patients with T1-2, N0 tumors found elective nodal irradiation to be unwarranted and higher doses to be associated with improved tumor control and disease-free survival.

A variety of techniques has been used for treatment of patients with early-stage NSCLC. All series have in common an attempt to account for or limit respiratory movement, as well as to use high conformal dose distributions by employing multiple beams, often in noncoplanar arrangements.

The initial report of clinical results from the Karolinska institute contained five patients who were treated for metastatic disease, but subsequent patients with primary lung cancer have been treated. A high dose per fraction technique directed against the CTV with a margin of 5 to 10 mm (PTV) was used. Heterogeneous target dose distributions were used with a 50% higher dose in the center of the targets. The doses per fraction and number of fractions were dependent on factors like tumor size, histologic type, and the tumor location within the lung (46).

From March 1996 through April 2001, 65 patients with NSCLC with an adequate clinical follow-up received SBRT. Most patients were deemed medically inoperable mostly due to severe emphysema. They received 8 to 20 Gy per fraction to the margin of the PTV. Two to five such fractions were delivered at 1- to 2-day intervals. The clinical effects of the treatments were recorded 25 to 85 months after stereotactic radiotherapy (SRT).

The overall 5-year survival of 35 stage I patients was around 35% (Fig. 13.1). One patient had a local recur-

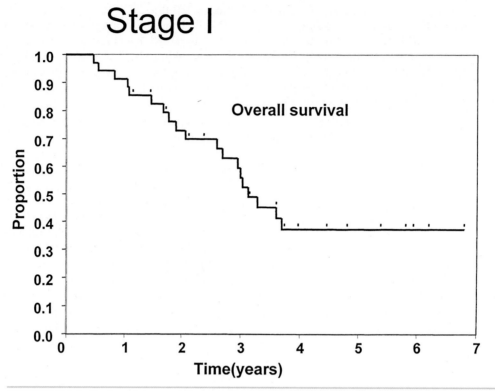

**FIGURE 13.1.** Kaplan-Meier overall survival for patients with stage I non–small cell lung cancer treated at the Karolinska Hospital with stereotactic body radiation therapy. The 5-year survival is around 35%.

rence (within the CTV), four patients developed regional recurrences, and in seven patients, the first relapse represented by distant metastases. Seven of the patients died without evidence of cancer.

Only two stage II patients were treated. The overall 2-year survival of 25 stage III patients was around 40% (Fig. 13.2). Eleven of them developed locoregional recurrences and the first appearance of recurrent disease represented distant metastases in six patients. Five died without evidence of cancer. There were no serious acute or late side effects except for one patient who died of a pulmonary hemorrhage.

Uematsu et al. (47) treated 50 patients with T1-2, N0 disease who were either medically inoperable (21 patients) or refused surgery. The treatment unit consisted of a combined linac, CT scanner, and x-ray simulator with coaxial gantry axes and a shared couch such that the patient is scanned, positioned, and treated without getting off the table. Respiratory movement was limited by having patients perform shallow respirations with oxygen and/or use of an abdominal pressure belt. The dose prescribed was 50 to 60 Gy in five to ten fractions; 18 patients also received conventional therapy with 2-cm margins, and SBRT doses were sometimes reduced to 30 to 45 Gy in these patients. Beam arrangements consisted of six to 15 noncoplanar arcs. With a median follow-up of 36

months, the 3-year actuarial cause-specific survival was 88% and overall survival was 66%.

Hof et al.(48) used a stereotactic body frame to treat ten patients with stage I NSCLC with single-dose radiotherapy. Jet ventilation was used in five patients, while in the remaining patients respiratory motion was measured fluoroscopically and an abdominal pressure device used if motion exceeded 1 cm. Doses ranged from 19 to 26 Gy, prescribed to the 80% isodose line. Five to six coplanar shaped beams were distributed along a 180-degree gantry rotation. At a median follow-up of 14.9 months, eight of ten patients were locally controlled, with actuarial overall survival of 80% and 64% at 12 and 24 months, respectively.

The largest series of SBRT for early-stage NSCLC was reported by Onishi et al, who summarized the results of 241 patients treated at 13 institutions in Japan using a variety of techniques, all with noncoplanar arcs or multiple static beams and mechanisms to reduce respiratory movement. Total doses of 18 to 75 Gy in one to 22 fractions were delivered with 20% homogeneity in the PTV. During a median follow-up of 18 months, pulmonary complications greater than National Cancer Institute (NCI) grade 2 were noted to occur in only 2.1% of patients. Local recurrence occurred in only 10.4% of patients, and a higher local failure rate was found in pa-

# Stage III

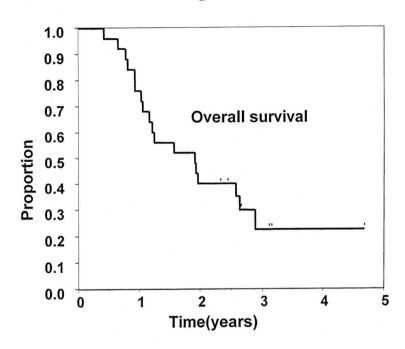

*FIGURE 13.2.* Kaplan-Meier overall survival for patients with stage III non–small cell lung cancer treated at the Karolinska Hospital with stereotactic body radiation therapy. The 2-year survival is around 40%.

tients who had received biologic equivalent doses of less than 100 Gy. The 3-year cause-specific and overall survival rates were 72% and 56%, respectively, with cause-specific survival significantly better in the patients receiving BEDs greater than 100 Gy (49).

In their experience using a stereotactic body frame with a regimen of 40 Gy in four fractions (BED = 80 Gy), Nagata et al. (50) had of one of three patients experience a local recurrence. Following dose escalation to 48 Gy in four fractions (BED = 105.6 Gy), no local failures occurred in 16 patients with T1 N0 tumors. No treatment-related complications were found in either group.

Given that a dose-response relationship appears to exist for NSCLC treated with SBRT, dose escalation studies are warranted. Timmerman et al. (51) have performed the only dose-finding study for SBRT thus far. Thirty-seven patients with medically inoperable stage I NSCLC were treated on a phase 1 study using a three-fraction regimen, starting at 8 Gy per fraction. The technique was the same as that of the Karolinska Institute using a stereotactic body frame with abdominal pressure. Beam arrangements consisted of seven noncoplanar static fields. Despite dose escalation to 20 Gy per fraction (total dose 60 Gy, BED = 180 Gy), maximal tolerated dose as defined in the study was not reached. Major toxicity consisted of one incidence of grade 3 pneumonitis and one incidence of grade 3 hypoxia. Interestingly, both were patients treated to less than 18 Gy per fraction, and other patients treated at those dose levels did not have dose-limiting toxicity.

Radiographic response was seen in 87% of patients. At a median follow-up of 15 months, there were six local failures, all occurring in patients treated with less than 18 Gy per fraction (which equals a BED of 154 Gy). However, other series have demonstrated excellent control rates with lower doses, albeit in smaller numbers of patients and with short follow-up. Some of these disparities may also be due to differences in dosimetric calculation and inhomogeneity correction algorithms between various treatment planning systems. Further experience may allow determination of optimal dosing.

In summary, numerous series have documented efficacy and safety of SBRT in the treatment of early-stage NSCLC (summary of results in Table 13.2). Although median follow-up durations are short, local control and overall survival rates are high and compare favorably with those for conventional treatment.

## LUNG METASTASES

Multiple series describing SBRT for lung tumors include patients treated for metastatic disease as well as primary lung cancer. Dose-fractionation schemes and techniques used are identical to those for treating primary lung tumors. Although radiotherapy has not traditionally been used in curative fashion for these patients due to general poor prognosis, data exist to support aggressive surgical therapy for selected patients (52,53). Resection for metas-

▶ TABLE 13-2  Results of Stereotactic Body
Radiation Therapy for Early-stage
Non–Small Cell Lung Cancer.

| Author | No. of Patients | Median Follow-up | Local Control | Survival |
|---|---|---|---|---|
| Timmerman (57) | 37 | 15 m | 83% | 54% |
| Uematsu (47) | 43 | 20 m | 100% | 3-yr 66% |
| Nagata[a] (50) | 16 | 16 m | 100% | 2-yr 79% |
| Wulf[b] (62) | 12 | 8 m | 85% | 2-yr 40% |
| Hara (58) | 5 | 20 m | 100% | |
| Hof (48) | 10 | 15 m | 80% | 2-yr 64% |
| Onishi[c] (49) | 241 | 18 m | 90% | 3-yr 56% |
| Lee (59) | 9 | 18 m | 90% | 100% |

[a]Only T1 N0 patients shown.
[b]Included some patients with T3 N0 and recurrent disease.
[c]Multiinstitutional study; may contain overlapping patients from other authors.

tases from sarcomas and colorectal carcinomas is generally accepted, but patients with other histologies may also benefit (54,55).

The International Registry of Lung Metastases reported the largest series of surgical metastasectomy on 5,206 cases from 18 institutions in Europe and North America. Primary histology was epithelial in 2,260 cases, sarcoma in 2,173, germ cell in 363, and melanoma in 328. With a median follow-up of 35 months, actuarial survival after complete metastasectomy (achieved in 88% of patients) was 36% at 5 years and 26% at 10 years. Multivariate analysis showed better prognoses for patients with single metastases, disease-free intervals of 36 months or more, and germ cell tumors, although long-term survivors were seen in all histologic types (56). Some series of surgical metastasectomy have also found tumor size and nonmelanoma histology to be of prognostic significance, although others report no differences (53,57).

Hara et al. (58) treated 23 lung tumors in 19 patients, including 17 metastatic tumors. Their technique consisted of placing the patient in a custom vacuum mold with a verification CT scan on the day of treatment. Patient position was verified and adjusted if needed, followed by transfer of the patient in the mold to the treatment machine. Treatment was delivered in a single fraction of 20 to 30 Gy using ten or more noncoplanar fixed beams with respiratory gating. Local regrowth was seen in four of the 17 metastatic tumors, with three failures occurring in patients treated with less than 30 Gy.

Using a stereotactic body frame system with diaphragmatic pressure, Lee et al. (59) treated 34 lung tumors in 28 patients, including 19 metastatic tumors. Beam arrangements consisted of four to eight coplanar or noncoplanar static fields. Doses were relatively modest, 30 to 40 Gy in three or four fractions, but in contrast to many other institutions treatment was delivered on consecutive

days. With a median follow-up of 18 months, local control rates were 90% overall and 88% within the patients treated for metastatic disease. No patients developed symptomatic complications.

SBRT holds promise for translating into clinically meaningful benefits for patients with metastatic lung tumors. A recent RTOG study has demonstrated a survival benefit for patients receiving radiosurgery for brain metastases (60), and further experience with SBRT may allow the identification of subsets of patients with lung metastases who will similarly benefit from aggressive local therapy. Control rates with SBRT range from 66% to 100% with minimal reported toxicity (Table 13.3). Given the high rates of local control and low toxicity demonstrated for SBRT, similarly selected patients who are not otherwise eligible for surgery may receive comparable benefit from treatment with SBRT and should be considered for treatment.

There may also be a role for SBRT in the palliation of patients with symptomatic lung or chest wall tumors. Most patients treated by Nakagawa et al. (61) had metastatic tumors involving the lung or pleural surface. Using a linear accelerator (linac) equipped with a megavoltage CT scanning detector for isocenter positioning and shallow respiratory effort supplemented by abdominal pressure and oxygen in select patients with large respiratory variation, they treated 22 tumors in 15 patients, with all but one tumor being of metastatic origin. The median dose was 20 Gy in a single fraction, with ten patients also receiving conventional fractionated radiotherapy following SBRT. Local failure occurred in one patient. The median survival time was 9.8 months following treatment, with only one patient reporting symptomatic decline due to the treatment. The unique aspect of this report is that of 11 patients who were symptomatic due to tumor prior to treatment, improvement in symptoms was reported as "excellent" in seven, "good" in two, and "fair" in two patients. Symptomatic improvement was noted within 1 to 2 weeks of treatment.

▶ TABLE 13-3  Results of Stereotactic Body
Radiation Therapy for Metastatic
Lung Tumors.

| Author | No. of Targets | Median Follow-up | Local Control |
|---|---|---|---|
| Blomgren (63) | 14 | 8 m | 92% |
| Uematsu (47) | 23 | 20 m | 100% |
| Nakagawa (61) | 21 | 10 m | 95% |
| Nagata (50) | 9 | 18 m | 66% |
| Wulf (62) | 11 | 8 m | 85% |
| Hara (58) | 18 | 12 m | 78% |
| Lee (59) | 19 | 18 m | 88% |

## NORMAL TISSUE REACTION TO STEREOTACTIC BODY RADIATION THERAPY

Despite the use of higher doses than typically given with conventional radiotherapy, SBRT has not been associated with an increased rate of lung complications, and many have reported no pulmonary symptomatology in their series (59). Radiographic changes suggestive of fibrosis are commonly seen after SBRT, but without clinical symptoms. Hof et al. (48) noted perifocal lung reaction in 70% of patients occurring at a median of 4.8 months following SBRT. Lee et al. (59) reported all patients developing grade 1 pneumonitis within 3 months of treatment. This fibrosis may continue to evolve for years after treatment, with the potential for being mistaken as tumor recurrence (62).

Table 13.4 summarizes the incidence of grade 3 or greater pulmonary toxicities described in the literature for SBRT in lung tumors (both NSCLC and metastatic), with toxicities generally less than 5%. Studies where pulmonary function testing has been performed have not shown permanent declines in measured function. Fukumoto et al. (36) performed routine pulmonary function testing before and after treatment and found no decline in median forced expiratory volume (FEV$_1$) or carbon monoxide diffusing capacity (DLCO) values following 48 to 60 Gy in eight fractions. Of 37 patients treated on their protocol, Timmerman et al. (51) reported ten patients with greater than 10% decline in one measured parameter (DLCO, FEV$_1$, etc.) approximately 6 weeks after treatment, but seven of the ten subsequently returned to baseline levels. No statistically significant changes in any of the parameters were seen, but six patients did develop worsening shortness of breath and nonproductive cough, although not severe enough to meet dose-limiting criteria. Hof et al. (48) noted a mild increase in dyspnea in several patients, but no pulmonary function studies were performed to quantitate the change. Of 19 patients treated with single dose radiation by Hara et al. (58), one patient developed grade 2 pneumonitis and another grade 3 pneumonitis, although the latter patient had a history of active tuberculosis and idiopathic interstitial pneumonia. Some insight into the histologic evaluation of changes following SBRT are available from Nakagawa et al. (61), who performed autopsy on a patient who died of progressive metastases from hepatocellular carcinoma. The treated area revealed necrosis and hemorrhage as well as macrophage infiltration. Although tumor cells persisted in islands of hemorrhage and necrosis, they differed markedly from those in untreated areas, displaying nuclear degeneration, multinucleation, and vacuolar degeneration.

The high doses delivered in SBRT may lead to complications in nonlung tissues, however. Uematsu et al. (47) described no symptomatic pulmonary complications even

**TABLE 13-4** Complications of Lung Stereotactic Body Radiation Therapy.

| Author | No. of Patients | Dose | Grade 3 Toxicity |
|---|---|---|---|
| Uematsu (47) | 66 | 30–76 Gy, 5–15 fx | 0% |
| Nakagawa (61) | 22 | 15–24 Gy, 1 fx | 0% |
| Nagata (50) | 40 | 40–48 Gy, 4 fx | 0% |
| Wulf (62) | 61 | 26–37.5 Gy, 1–3 fx | 3% |
| Hara (58) | 23 | 20–30 Gy, 1 fx | 4% |
| Hof (48) | 10 | 19–26 Gy, 1 fx | 0% |
| Onishi[a] (49) | 241 | 18–75 Gy, 1–22 fx | 2% |
| Lee (59) | 28 | 30–40 Gy, 3–4 fx | 0% |
| Blomgren (63) | 13 | 15–45 Gy, 1–3 fx | |
| Timmerman (51) | 37 | 24–60 Gy, 3 fx | 5.4% |

Fx, fraction.
[a]Multiinstitutional study; may contain overlapping patients from other authors.

in patients who had severe chronic obstructive pulmonary disease, but did report two patients who developed bony fractures, one in a rib and the other in a vertebral body. Both fractures occurred within the 80% isodose prescription line. Another six patients who received conventional radiotherapy followed by SBRT had temporary pleural pain that did not require medication. Mediastinal organs such as esophagus and airways, which have serial arrangement of functional subunits, may be sensitive to high doses. Wulf et al. (62) reported a patient who developed grade 3 esophageal ulceration 3 months after treatment, and another patient who had a fatal bleed 9 months following SBRT for a lesion located adjacent to the pulmonary artery, which had been previously irradiated to 63 Gy. Timmerman et al. (51) reported one patient who developed an asymptomatic pericardial effusion following treatment, and all patients treated in that series were noted to develop fatigue. Hara et al. (58) reported two patients who developed transient skin erythema after treatment for peripheral tumors.

## CONCLUSIONS

In summary, the advantages of spatial accuracy, high conformality, and accelerated dose regimens of SBRT for the treatment of primary and metastatic lung tumors appear to be realized in early clinical results seen thus far. A variety of specific treatment methods appears to achieve reasonably similar outcomes. Conflicting data exist with regard to the need to escalate doses beyond those at the lower end of the ranges currently used, and large-scale studies may be needed to elucidate small differences in tumor control and complication rates with higher doses. Longer term follow-up will be useful to fully assess risks of late toxicity in lung and other thoracic organs.

## REFERENCES

1. Herfarth KK, Debus J, Lohr F, et al. Extracranial stereotactic radiation therapy: set-up accuracy of patients treated for liver metastases. *Int J Radiat Oncol Biol Phys* 2000;46:329–335.
2. Wulf J, Hadinger U, Oppitz U, et al. CT-simulation and accuracy of treatment in the stereotactic body frame. *Radiother Oncol* 2000;57:225–236.
3. Cheung PC, Sixel KE, Tirona R, Ung YC. Reproducibility of lung tumor position and reduction of lung mass within the planning target volume using active breathing control (ABC). *Int J Radiat Oncol Biol Phys* 2003;57:1437–1442.
4. Keall PJ, Kini VR, Vedam SS, et al. Potential radiotherapy improvements with respiratory gating. *Australas Phys Eng Sci Med* 2002;25:1–6.
5. Shimizu S, Shirato H, Ogura S, et al. Detection of lung tumor movement in real-time tumor-tracking radiotherapy. *Int J Radiat Oncol Biol Phys* 2001;51:304–310.
6. Parker SL, Tong T, Bolden S, et al. Cancer statistics. *Cancer J Clin* 1996;65:5–27.
7. Ries LAG, Hankey BF, Miller BA, et al. *National Cancer Institute: Cancer statistics review.* Bethesda, MD: National Institutes of Health, 1991:1973–1988.
8. Bulzebruck H, Bopp R, Drings P, et al. New aspects in the staging of lung cancer: prospective validation of the International Union Against Cancer TNM classification. *Cancer* 1992;70:1102–1110.
9. Perez CA, Stanley K, Grundy G, et al. Impact of radiation technique and tumor extent on tumor control and survival of patients with unresectable non-oat cell carcinoma of the lung: report by the RTOG. *Cancer* 1982;50:1091–1099.
10. Sibley GS, Jamieson TA, Marks LB, et al. Radiotherapy alone for medically inoperable stage I non-small-cell lung cancer: the Duke experience. *Int J Radiat Oncol Biol Phys* 1998;40:149–154.
11. Malissard L, Nguyen TD, Jung CM. Localized adenocarcinoma of the lung: a retrospective study of 186 non-metastatic patients from the French Federation of Cancer Institutes—the Radiotherapy Cooperative Group. *Int J Radiat Oncol Biol Phys* 1991;21:369.
12. Sibley GS. Radiotherapy for patients with medically inoperable stage I nonsmall cell lung carcinoma. *Cancer* 1998;82:433–438.
13. Krol ADG, Aussems P, Noordijk EM, et al. Local irradiation alone for peripheral stage I lung cancer: could we omit the elective regional nodal irradiation? *Int J Radiat Oncol Biol Phys* 1996;34:297–302.
14. Cheung PCF, Mackillop WJ, Dixon P, et al. Involved-field radiotherapy alone for early-stage non-small-cell lung cancer. *Int J Rad Oncol Biol Phys* 2000; 45:703–710.
15. Arriagada R, Le Chevalier T, Quoix E, et al for the ASTRO Plenary. Effects of chemotherapy on locally advanced non-small cell lung cancer: a randomized study of 353 patients. *Int J Radiat Oncol Biol Phys* 1991;20:1183–1190.
16. Coy P, Kennelly GM. The role of curative radiotherapy in the treatment of lung cancer. *Cancer* 1980;45:698–702.
17. Kaskowitz L, Graham MV, Emami B, et al. Radiation therapy alone for stage I nonsmall cell lung cancer. *Int J Radiat Biol Phys* 1993;27:517–523.
18. Perez CA, Stanley K, Hanson W, et al. Impact of radiation technique and tumor extent in tumor control and survival of patients with unresectable non-oat cell carcinoma of the lung. *Cancer* 1982;50:1091–1099.
19. Talton BM, Constable WC, Kersh CR. Curative radiotherapy in non-small cell carcinoma of the lung. *Int J Radiat Biol Phys* 1990;19:15–21.
20. Würschmidt F, Bünemann H, Benemann C, et al. Inoperable nonsmall cell lung cancer: a retrospective analysis of 427 patients treated with high dose radiotherapy. *Int J Radiat Biol Phys* 1994;28:583–588.
21. Zhang HX, Yin WB, Zhang LJ, et al. Curative radiotherapy of early operable nonsmall cell lung cancer. *Radiother Oncol* 1989;14:89–94.
22. Martel MK, Ten Haken RK, Hazuka MB, et al. Estimation of tumor control probability model parameters from 3D dose distributions of non-small cell lung cancer patients. *Lung Cancer* 1999;24:31–37.
23. Armstrong JG, Zelefsky MJ, Leibel SA, et al. Strategy for dose escalation using 3-dimensional conformal radiation therapy for lung cancer. *Ann Oncol* 1995;6:693–697.
24. Cox JD, Azarnia N, Byhardt RW, et al. A randomized phase I/II trial of hyperfractionated radiation therapy with total doses of 60.0 Gy to 79.2 Gy: possible survival benefit with greater than or equal to 69.6 Gy in favorable patients with Radiation Therapy Oncology Group stage III non-small-cell lung carcinoma—Report of Radiation Therapy Oncology Group 83-11. *J Clin Oncol* 1990;8:1543–1555.
25. Emami B, Lyman J, Brown A, et al. Tolerance of normal tissue to therapeutic irradiation. *Int J Radiat Oncol Biol Phys* 1991;15:109–122.
26. Sunyach MP, Falchero L, Pommier P, et al. Prospective evaluation of early lung toxicity following three-dimensional conformal radiation therapy in non-small-cell lung cancer: preliminary results. *Int J Radiat Oncol Biol Phys* 2000;48:459–463.
27. Monson JM, Stark P, Reilly JJ, et al. Clinical radiation pneumonitis and radiographic changes after thoracic radiation therapy for lung carcinoma. *Cancer* 1998;82:842–850.
28. Seppenwoolde Y, Lebesque JV. Partial irradiation of the lung. *Sem Radiat Oncol* 2001;11:247–258.
29. Hayman JA, Martel MK, Ten Haken RK, et al. Dose escalation in non-small-cell lung cancer using three-dimensional conformal radiation therapy: update of a Phase I trial. *J Clin Oncol* 2001;19:127–136.
30. Maguire PD, Marks LB, Sibley GS, et al. 73.6 Gy and beyond: hyperfractionated, accelerated radiotherapy for non-small-cell lung cancer. *J Clin Oncol* 2001;19:705–711, 2001.
31. Bradley JD, Graham MV, Winter KW, et al. Acute and late toxicity results of RTOG 9311: a dose escalation study using 3D conformal radiation therapy in patients with inoperable non-small cell lung cancer [Abstract]. *Int J Radiat Oncol Biol Phys* 2003;57[Suppl 1]:137–138.
32. Langendijk JA, Aaronson NK, de Jong JMA, et al. Quality of life after curative radiotherapy in stage I non-small cell lung cancer. *Int J Radiat Oncol Biol Phys* 2002;53:847–853.
33. Fowler JF, Chappell R. Non small cell lung tumors repopulate rapidly during radiation therapy. *Int J Radiat Oncol Biol Phys* 2000;46:516–517.
34. Saunders M, Dische S, Barrett A, et al. Continuous, hyperfractionated, accelerated radiotherapy (CHART) versus conventional radiotherapy in non-small cell lung cancer: mature data from the randomized multicentre trial. *Radiother Oncol* 1999;52:137–148.
35. Cheung PCF, Yeung LTF, Basrur V, et al. Accelerated hypofractionation for early-stage non-small-cell lung cancer. *Int J Radiat Oncol Biol Phys* 2002;54:1014–1023.
36. Fukumoto S, Shirato H, Shimzu S, et al. Small-volume, image-guided radiotherapy using hypofractionated, coplanar and non-coplanar multiple fields for patients with inoperable stage I non-small cell lung carcinomas. *Cancer* 2002;95:1546–1553.
37. Rosenman JG, Halle JS, Socinski MA, et al. High-dose conformal radiotherapy for treatment of stage IIIA/IIIB non-small-cell lung cancer: technical issues and results of a phase I/II trial. *Int J Radiat Oncol Biol Phys* 2002;54:348–356.
38. Hanley J, Debois MM, Mah D, et al. The potential value of target immobilization and reduced lung density in dose escalation. *Int J Radiat Oncol Biol Phys* 1999;45:603–611.
39. Willner J, Baier K, Caragiani E, et al. Dose, volume, and tumor control predictions in primary radiotherapy of non-small-cell lung cancer. *Int J Radiat Oncol Biol Phys* 2002;52:382–389.
40. Engelsman M, Damen EMF, Jaeger KD, et al. The effect of breathing and set-up errors on the cumulative dose to a lung tumor. *Radiother Oncol* 2001;60:95–105.
41. Nesbitt JC, Putnam JB, Walsh GL et al. Survival in early stage non-small cell lung cancer. *Ann Thorac Surg* 1995;60:466–472.
42. Fry WA, Menck HR, Winchester DP. The National Cancer Data Base report on lung cancer. *Cancer* 1996;77:1947–1955.
43. Wingo PA, Tong T, Bolden S. Cancer statistics. *CA Cancer J Clin* 1995;45:8–30.
44. Bradley JD, Wahab S, Lockett MA, et al. Elective nodal failures are uncommon in medically inoperable patients with stage I non-small-cell lung carcinoma treated with limited radiotherapy fields. *Int J Radiat Oncol Biol Phys* 2003;56:342–347.
45. Sibley GS. Radiotherapy for medically inoperable stage I non-small cell lung carcinoma: smaller volumes and higher doses—a review. *Cancer* 1998;82:433–438.

46. Lax I, Blomgren H, Näslund I, et al. Stereotactic radiotherapy of malignancies in the abdomen: methodological aspects. *Acta Oncol* 1994;33: 677–683.
47. Uematsu M, Shioda A, Suda A, et al. Computed tomography-guided frameless stereotactic radiotherapy for stage I non-small-cell lung cancer: a 5-year experience. *Int J Radiat Oncol Biol Phys* 2001;51: 666–670.
48. Hof H, Herfarth KK, Munter M, et al. Stereotactic single-dose radiotherapy of stage I non-small-cell lung cancer. *Int J Radiat Oncol Biol Phys* 2003;56:335–341.
49. Onishi H, Nagata Y, Shirato H, et al. Stereotactic hypofractionated high-dose irradiation for patients with stage I non-small cell lung carcinoma: clinical outcomes in 241 cases of a japanese multi-institutional study [Abstract]. *Int J Radiat Oncol Biol Phys* 2003; 57[Suppl 1]:142.
50. Nagata Y, Negoro Y, Aoki T, et al. Clinical outcomes of 3D conformal hypofractionated single high-dose radiotherapy for one or two lung tumors using a stereotactic body frame. *Int J Radiat Oncol Biol Phys* 2002;52:1041–1046.
51. Timmerman R, Papiez L, McGarry R, et al. Extracranial stereotactic radioablation: results of a phase I study in medically inoperable stage I non-small cell lung cancer. *Chest* 2003;124:1946–1955.
52. Mountain CF, McMurtrey MJ, Hermes KE. Surgery for pulmonary metastasis: a 20-year experience. *Annals Thor Surg* 1984;38: 323–330.
53. Venn GE, Sarin S, Goldstraw P. Survival following pulmonary metastasectomy. *Eur J Cardio-thorac Surg* 1989;3:105–110.
54. Ishida T, Kaneko S, Yokoyama H, et al. Metastatic lung tumors and extended indications for surgery. *Int Surg* 1992;77:173–177.
55. Wright JO, Brandt B, Ehrenhaft JL. Results of pulmonary resection for metastatic lesions. *J Thorac Cardiovasc Surg* 1982;83:94–99.
56. Pastorino U, Buyse M, Friedel G, et al. Long-term results of lung metastasectomy: prognostic analyses based on 5206 cases. *J Thorac Cardiovasc Surg* 1997;113:37–49.
57. Ishida T, Kaneko S, Yokoyama H. Metastatic lung tumors and extended indications for surgery. *Int Surg* 1992;77:173–177.
58. Hara R, Itami J, Kondo T, et al. Stereotactic single high dose irradiation of lung tumors under respiratory gating. *Radiother Oncol* 2002;63:159–163.
59. Lee SW, Choi EK, Park HJ, et al. Stereotactic body frame based fractionated radiosurgery on consecutive days for primary or metastatic tumors in the lung. *Lung Cancer* 2003;40:309–315.
60. Sperduto PW, Scott C, Andrews D, et al. Stereotactic radiosurgery with whole brain radiation therapy improves survival in patients with brain metastases: report of Radiation Therapy Oncology Group Phase III study 95-08 [Abstract]. *Int J Radiat Oncol Biol Phys* 2002;54[Suppl 1]:3.
61. Nakagawa K, Aoki Y, Tago M, et al. Megavoltage CT-assisted stereotactic radiosurgery for thoracic tumors: original research in the treatment of thoracic neoplasms. *Int J Radiat Oncol Biol Phys* 2000;48:449–457.
62. Wulf J, Hadinger U, Oppitz U, et al. Stereotactic radiotherapy of targets in the lung and liver. *Strahlenther Onkol* 2001;177:645–655.
63. Blomgren H, Lax I, Naslund I, Svanstrom R. Stereotactic high dose fraction radiation therapy of extracranial tumors using an accelerator. *Acta Oncologia* 1995;34:861–870.

# Case Studies

## Case Studies in Lung SBRT: Application of the FOCAL Unit

Minoru Uematsu and *James R. Wong

## CASE 1

### Clinical Presentation

A 54-year-old man who had previously undergone a right middle lobe wedge resection for a T1 N0 M0 adenocarcinoma of the lung was noted to have a local recurrence approximately 1 year later (Fig. 13.3). He began a course of conventionally fractionated external beam radiation therapy at another institution and received a dose of 10 Gy in five fractions before electing to obtain a second opinion at the National Defense Medical College. Here he was offered treatment with lung stereotactic body radiation therapy (SBRT), and the patient elected to complete his definitive therapy with this form of therapy.

### Stereotactic Body Radiation Therapy Treatment Planning and Dose Delivery

Treatment planning and dose delivery were accomplished using the FOCAL unit (Fusion of CT and Linear Accelerator) developed by Uematsu and colleagues (1–3). During simulation and treatment, the patient was given supplemental oxygen and instructed to keep shallow and rapid respiration (about 30–40 respirations per minute). The x-ray simulator was used to evaluate the respiratory motion of the tumor or the lung.

After it was established that the lung motion was acceptable, specifically less than 5 mm superior–inferior movement, computed tomography (CT) scanning was performed. To include the respiratory motion and its partial volume effects within the CT images, images were obtained at a slow rate (4 seconds per scan). The isocenter of the tumor or target was ascertained by using the CT images. The planning target volume has a 5-mm margin around the clinical target volume. SBRT was administered via a multiple noncoplanar arc plan. The dose given was 50 Gy in ten fractions prescribed to the 80% isodose line.

### Discussion

The treatment of this patient was performed safely without any acute toxicity. A comparison of pre- and post-SBRT CT images

Department of Radiation Oncology, National Defense Medical College, Tokorozawa Saitama, 359-8513, Japan; and *Department of Radiation Oncology, Morristown Memorial Hospital, Morristown, NJ 07960

revealed a sustained complete response and only mild fibrosis in the treated region. Eight and one-half years after SBRT, he was alive and well without any adverse effects or tumor recurrence by chest CT, brain magnetic resonance imaging, and whole-body positron emission tomography scan.

More recently, the lung SBRT prescribed dose has been 50 to 55 Gy prescribed to the 80% isodose, given in five fractions over a week. Body-fixation devices are found not to be necessary using this technique, because the treatment time is short and positioning is reproducible. Repeated CT scans after the completion of each treatment have confirmed minimal movements of the patient and the isocenter (3).

Very favorable clinical outcomes have been achieved. The median follow-up period of the initial 50 patients with pathologically proven stage I non–small cell lung cancer was already over 6 years, and the 5-year overall survival and 5-year cause-specific survival rates were 60% and 84%, respectively (4). The treatment was performed safely without any acute symptoms, and the chronic adverse effects observed were pleural pain (15%) and minor bone fractures (4%).

## CASE 2

### Clinical Presentation

A 68-year-old man had undergone surgical resection of a lung cancer approximately 2 years prior to presenting to our facility. A routine follow-up computed tomography (CT) scan of the chest showed a 2.0-cm lesion in the right upper lobe. A positron emission tomography (PET) scan showed uptake at this right upper lobe lesion consistent with malignancy, and CT-guided biopsy proved the presence of non–small cell lung cancer. The patient declined surgical resection and was therefore offered definitive treatment with stereotactic body radiation therapy (SBRT) to the lung at the Morristown Memorial Hospital (Morristown, NJ).

### Stereotactic Body Radiation Therapy Treatment Planning and Dose Delivery

The method of treatment planning and dose delivery was very similar to what was described for the previous case. A commercially available combination CT scanner–linear accelerator unit (Primatom; Siemens Medial Instruments, Malvern, PA) similar to the FOCAL system was used.

On the day of treatment, the patient was set up on the treatment couch, with the skin marks set up by the cross-hair laser system. Radio-opaque markers were placed over these skin marks to delineate the central axis planes. The treatment couch was rotated 180 degrees for CT scanning. Supplemental oxygen was given to ensure shallow breathing, and the patient was scanned three consecutive times by the CT unit, which moves along a pair of horizontal rails. The exact positions of the lung lesion and the metallic markers were identified and compared

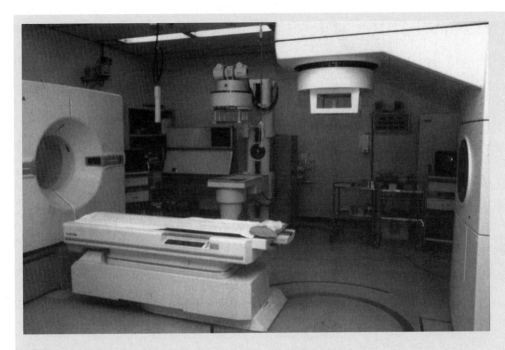

FIGURE 13.3. The FOCAL (fusion of CT and linear accelerator) unit at the National Defense Medical College, Japan. A computed tomography scanner, linear accelerator, and x-ray simulator are located in the same treatment room.

with the planned positions. Each of these positions was mapped out on the beam's eye views (BEVs) of the anterior and lateral fields.

Superimposed on these BEVs were the contours of lung lesion obtained from the initial treatment planning CT study. Variations of the lung lesion from the central axis planes determined the daily position variation of the target lesion in the anteroposterior, left–right, and cephalic–caudal directions. The treatment isocenter was shifted to correct for the daily variations. The treatment table was then rotated 180 degrees back to the treatment position, with the cross-hair laser beam now placed on the corrected, newly derived isocenter. The patient was treated at 5 Gy per fraction for a total of 50 Gy in ten fractions, with treatment accomplished by a series of arc rotations and different table/couch positions.

## Discussion

This patient tolerated the treatment extremely well and reported no side effects or discomforts from this treatment. The follow-up CT scan obtained more than 2 years after SBRT revealed a sustained complete response with only asymptomatic pulmonary fibrosis in the region (Fig. 13.5). A PET scan obtained shortly thereafter revealed no residual active tumor.

## Acknowledgment

We thank our teams at Division of Radiation Oncology at the National Defense Medical College, Japan, and at Department of Radiation Oncology, Morristown Memorial Hospital for their technical, clinical, and professional support. We especially thank Jackie Vizoso and Elizabeth Rodriquez for their technical support.

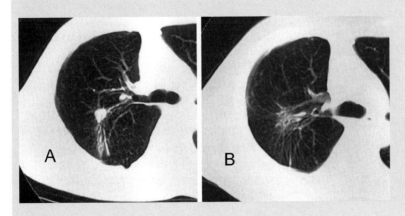

FIGURE 13.4. **A:** Recurrent cancer in the right lung after prior wedge resection. **B:** Computed tomography scan appearance 36 months after stereotactic body radiation therapy showing only residual fibrosis at the site of the treated lesion.

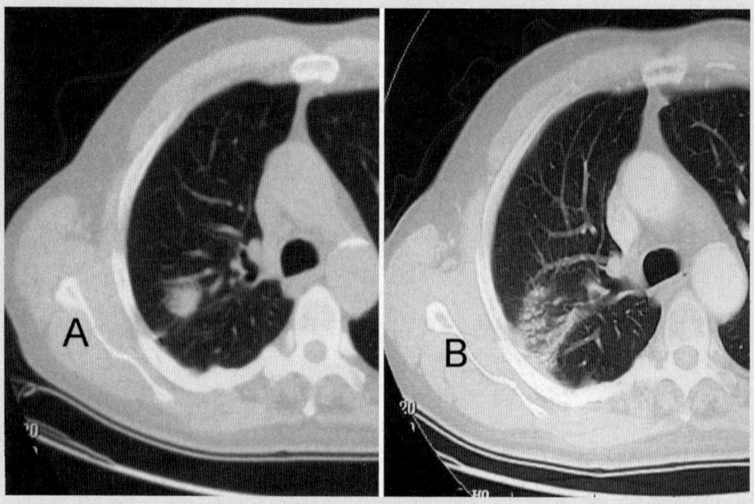

FIGURE 13.5. **A:** Pretreatment image demonstrating the 2-cm lesion in the right lung. **B:** Follow-up computed tomography scan 25 months after stereotactic body radiation therapy showing sustained complete response and fibrosis in the high-dose region.

## References

1. Uematsu M, Fukui T, Shioda A, et al. A dual computed tomography and linear accelerator unit for stereotactic radiation therapy: a new approach without cranially fixated stereotactic frame. *Int J Radiat Oncol Biol Phys* 1996;35:587–592.
2. Uematsu M, Shioda A, Tahara K, et al. Focal, high dose, and fractionated modified stereotactic radiation therapy for lung carcinoma patients: a preliminary experience. *Cancer* 1998;82:1062–1070.
3. Uematsu M, Shioda A, Suda A, et al. Interfractional tumor position stability during computed tomography (CT)-guided frameless stereotactic radiation therapy for lung or liver cancers with a fusion of CT and linear accelerator (FOCAL) unit. *Int J Radiat Oncol Biol Phys* 2000;48:443–448.
4. Uematsu M, Shioda A, Suda A, et al. Computed tomography-guided frameless stereotactic radiotherapy for stage I non-small-cell lung cancer: a 5-year experience. *Int J Radiat Oncol Biol Phys* 2001;41:666–670.

## Case Study in Lung SBRT: The Indiana University Phase II Protocol for Medically Inoperable Lung Cancer

Ronald C. McGarry

### CLINICAL PRESENTATION

The patient was a 55-year-old man with cough and increasing shortness of breath of several weeks' duration. He was admitted to hospital for an exacerbation of his chronic obstructive pulmonary disease with associated right-sided heart failure. The medical history was significant for hypertension, previous congestive heart failure, and alcohol dependence. He had a 35 pack-year smoking history and continued to smoke.

Pulmonary function tests revealed a forced expiratory volume (FEV$_1$) of 0.9 L (27% predicted) with a force vital capacity (FVC) of 1.74 L (42% predicted). Diffusion capacity was 18% pre-

Department of Radiation Oncology, Indiana University School of Medicine, Indianapolis, IN 46260

dicted. Chest radiograph revealed a lesion in the right upper lung. Computed tomography (CT) scan of the chest revealed a 2-cm irregular, noncalcified nodule in the right upper lobe with no evidence of adenopathy or other masses (Fig. 13.6A). Mild cardiomegaly with small pericardial effusion was noted. The 18-fluorodeoxy glucose ($^{18}$FDG)–positron emitted tomography (PET) showed uptake in the nodule with no other abnormalities, consistent with a solitary lung cancer (Fig. 13.7). CT-guided biopsy revealed non–small cell lung carcinoma, most likely adenocarcinoma. Due to his poor pulmonary reserve and history of congestive heart failure, the patient was considered a poor candidate for surgical excision. The patient was offered potentially curative nonsurgical treatment with stereotactic body radiation therapy (SBRT), and he gave informed consent to participate in the Indiana University phase 2 trial of SBRT. No chemotherapy was included in the treatment plan.

### STEREOTACTIC BODY RADIATION THERAPY TREATMENT PLANNING AND DELIVERY

The patient was immobilized in the stereotactic body frame (Elekta, Norcross, GA) with a custom vacuum mold (Vac-Loc; Med-Tec, Orange City, IA). Once setup fiducial markers were recorded, radio-opaque markers were placed on two physician-defined sternal points and abdominal compression was applied. Movement of the nodule was monitored by fluoroscopy in the simulator room and compression was applied as tolerated to decrease the movement of the nodule to less than 1.0 cm. Planning CT scan was performed.

The gross tumor volume (GTV) was contoured by the physician and did not include obvious atelectasis. The planning target volume (PTV) was manually determined by adding 0.5-cm laterally and 1.0 cm in the axial plane to the GTV. Seven beams were used with custom compensators and blocks to provide a prescribed tumor dose of 2,000 cGy to the 80% dose line per frac-

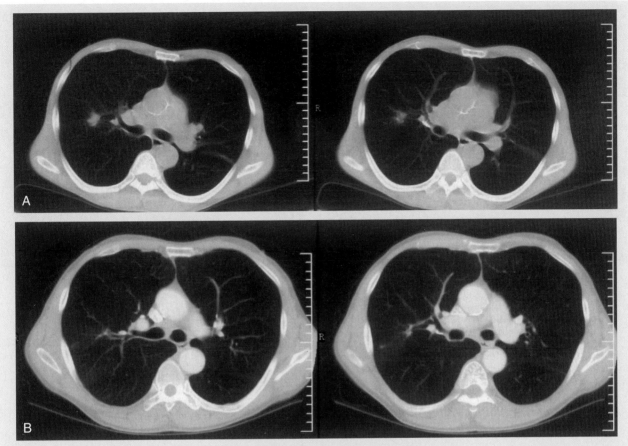

**FIGURE 13.6.  A:** Pretreatment computed tomography (CT) scan showing speculated mass in right mid-lung field. **B:** CT scan 7 months after stereotactic body radiotherapy. Slight atelectasis is noted.

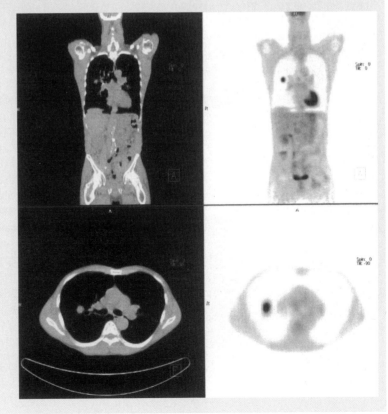

**FIGURE 13.7.**  Fluorodexoy glucose positron emission computed tomography scan demonstrating lesion in right mid lung.

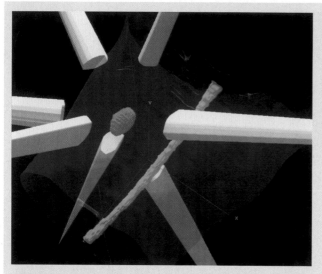

**FIGURE 13.8.** Three-dimensional representation of patient setup. Planning target volume in right mid lung (*red*) and spinal cord (*blue*). Note orientation of seven noncoplanar beams (*yellow*).

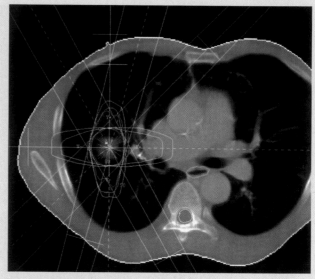

**FIGURE 13.9.** Axial computed tomography slice showing coverage of planning target volume by 80% isodose line.

tion for three fractions (Figs. 13.8–13.10). Total tumor dose prescribed was 6,000 cGy to the 80% line. Daily setup included verification anteroposterior and lateral films to confirm position of bony landmarks relative to the digitally reconstructed radiograph. Two or more days were allowed between fractions.

## DISCUSSION

The patient tolerated treatment well with no reported acute side effects. The patient was followed up every 3 months with complete pulmonary function testing and alternating CT scans of the chest or chest radiograph. The patient quit smoking by the third month post treatment. Seven months following therapy, pul-

monary function tests showed an $FEV_1$ of 1.47l (45% predicted), an FVC of 2.74l (66% predicted), and a diffusion capacity of 29% predicted. The improvement was attributed to his nonsmoking. No pneumonitis has been noted either clinically or radiologically. Follow-up CT scan obtained 14 months after SBRT showed local consolidation in the treated areas, no mediastinal adenopathy or other nodules, and a decrease in the overall size of the residual radiographic irregularity to approximately 1.5 cm in diameter. He remains with no evidence of disease.

This case illustrates that patients considered poor candidates for conventional therapy due to either chronic obstructive airways disease or other medical comorbidities can be good candidates for SBRT. Previous work from our group shows that expectant management with supportive care alone is generally a poor option for patients. In a review of approximately 100 patients with stage I non–small cell lung cancer followed by observation only at the Richard L. Roudebush Veteran's Administration Hospital, the 3-year survival was only 8% with approximately 63% of patients having lung cancer as their reported cause of death (1). Half of these patients eventually received palliative radiation therapy for progression of their disease. It thus appears that lung cancer is not a benign disease that is amenable to a policy of observation.

SBRT offers an option for curative therapy in early-stage disease despite significant patient comorbidities. The results presented here are consistent with the preliminary results reported for the Indiana University phase 1 study of SBRT showing it to be an option for these patients with low risk of side effects. The local control rates appear to be very high with good long-term survival (2). This approach is being tested in an ongoing phase 2 study. Aoki et al. (3) likewise report their results of three-dimensional conformal stereotactic radiation therapy for solitary lung

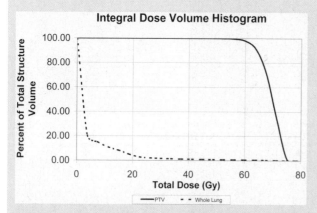

**FIGURE 13.10.** Integral dose volume histogram for the planning treatment volume and the whole lung (**right** and **left**). Ninety-eight percent of the PTV is covered by the prescription dose of 60 Gy. The mean lung dose is 5 Gy and the percent volume of lung receiving 20 Gy or more ($V_{20}$) is 4%.

tumors receiving 48 Gy in four fractions. In their series of 27 patients, patchy consolidation was noted with late changes appearing more solid and possibly representing fibrosis. This makes the issue of response rates difficult to interpret; however, they reported either complete or partial responses in 93% of patients. While all patients in this study demonstrated radiographic changes in the treated areas, none developed grade II or higher pneumonitis requiring steroid treatment.

In summary, patients who are considered high risk for surgical resection for early-stage lung cancer may be treated by carefully planned SBRT. Current trials continue to assess radiotherapy doses, safety, and cure rates. Long-term follow-up to monitor recurrence rates after SBRT will be important to record and evaluate.

## References

1. McGarry RC, Song G, Desrosiers P, et al. Observation-only management of early stage medically inoperable lung cancer: poor outcome. *Chest* 1999;121:1155–1158.
2. Timmerman R, Papiez L, McGarry RC, et al. Extracranial stereotactic radioablation: results of a phase I study in medically inoperable stage I non-small cell lung cancer. *Chest* 2003;124:1946–1955.
3. Aoki T, Nagata Y, Negoro Y, et al. Evaluation of lung injury after three dimensional conformal stereotactic radiation therapy for solitary lung tumors: CT appearance. *Radiology* 2004;230:101–108.

## Case Study in Lung SRBT: Long-term Follow-up in a Patient with a History of Tuberculosis

Yasushi Nagata, Kenji Takayama, *Takashi Mizowaki, Tetsuya Aoki, Takashi Sakamoto, Masato Sakamoto, Yukinori Matsuo, Yoshitsugu Norihisa, Shinsuke Yano, and Masahiro Hiraoka.

## CLINICAL PRESENTATION

A 70-year-old man had a chest computed tomography (CT) scan as a follow-up study several years after suffering an empyema

Department of Therapeutic Radiology and Oncology, Kyoto University, Sakyo, Kyoto, Japan; and *Department of Radiology, Tenri Hospital, Nora, Japan

of the right lung several years previously. The patient's medical history also included tuberculosis when he was a teenager. The CT scan revealed changes consistent with his prior diagnoses and a new 3-cm pulmonary nodule in his left lung (Fig. 13.11). Bronchoscopically directed biopsy proved the lesion to be a squamous cell carcinoma.

The review of systems revealed substantial compromise in pulmonary function. The patient's dyspnea with exertion prevented him from walking more than 200 m. Pulmonary function tests revealed a forced vital capacity (FVC) and forced expiratory volume (FEV) (1.0 second) both less than 60% of the predicted values for his height and weight. For medically inoperable T1 N0 M0 non–small cell lung cancer, the patient was offered stereotactic body radiation therapy (SBRT).

## STEREOTACTIC BODY RADIATION THERAPY TREATMENT PLANNING AND DOSE DELIVERY

The patient was positioned during the CT simulation and treatment within a stereotactic body frame. Typically, we use an abdominal compression device to minimize the degree of respiratory motion during simulation and treatment (1). However, in this particular case, because the amount of respiratory motion of the tumor was noted to be only a few millimeters, no additional means of respiratory gating or breathing modulation were used. The gross tumor volume (GTV) defined by the planning CT images was considered to be the clinical target volume(CTV). The planning target volume (PTV) was created from the CTV by adding a margin of 5 mm radially and 10 mm superiorly and inferiorly.

A multiple noncoplanar beam arrangement was used. The prescribed dose was 12 Gy per fraction at the isocenter for each of four fractions. The $V_{20}$ (percent of uninvolved lung volume that received more than 20 Gy) was 11.6%, which was the highest of all cases we have treated to date. The maximum point dose per fraction to the left bronchus was 4.6 Gy per fraction, and the volume over 4 Gy per fraction was 0.3 cc. The maximum point dose per fraction to the left pulmonary artery was 11.2 Gy, and the volume over 10 Gy per fraction was 0.9 cc. The SBRT was given on 2 days per week over 2 weeks. The setup position was verified each day with orthogonal anteroposterior and lateral portal images of the isocenter.

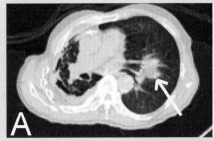
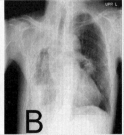

**FIGURE 13.11. A:** Computed tomography scan reveals a new pulmonary nodule (*arrow*) in the left lung. **B:** The chest radiograph reveals the tumor in the left hilar region as well as pleural thickening and significant volume loss in the right side from the prior empyema.

## DISCUSSION

Although the degree of underlying pulmonary disease in this case raised concerns, the patient did not experience any new respiratory symptoms related to the SBRT. No other treatment-related toxicity has been observed. Follow-up CT scans showed very mild radiation-induced pulmonary changes and sustained tumor control (Fig. 13.12). The pulmonary function did not significantly change after radiotherapy, and the patient was alive with no evidence of active lung cancer 5 years after SBRT.

The very favorable clinical outcome overall is consistent with what we have previously reported. Among forty patients treated for primary (31) or metastatic (nine) neoplasms of the lung between July 1998 and November 2000, the overall radiographic response rate was 94%, including an 18% complete response rate. All patients received four fractions 10 to 12 Gy within a total treatment time of 1 to 2 weeks. No grade 3 pulmonary toxicity was observed (2). We are usually able to constrain the $V_{20}$ to less than 10%, and we record doses to the bronchus and major vessels—although the tolerance of these organs to SBRT is not well established. A multiinstitutional clinical trial of SBRT using a regimen of 48 Gy in four fractions is ongoing in Japan.

### References

1. Negoro Y, Nagata Y, Aoki T, et al. The effectiveness of an immobilization device in conformal radiotherapy for lung tumor: reduction of respiratory tumor movement and evaluation of daily set-up accuracy. *Int J Radiat Oncol Biol Phys* 2001;50:889–898.
2. Nagata Y, Negoro Y, Aoki T, et al. Clinical outcomes of 3-D conformal hypofractionated single high dose radiotherapy for one or two lung tumors using a stereotactic body frame. *Int J Radiat Oncol Biol Phys* 2002;52;1041–1046.

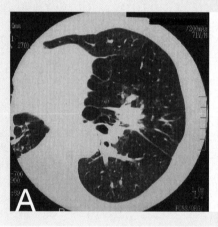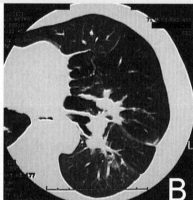

**FIGURE 13.12.** Follow-up computed tomography images 2 months after treatment **(A)** and 30 months after treatment **(B)**.

# Stereotactic Body Radiation Therapy for Liver Tumors

*Tracey E. Schefter, *Higinia R. Cardenes, and Brian D. Kavanagh*

## INTRODUCTION

Stereotactic body radiation therapy (SBRT) offers the potential to provide safe, effective treatment for primary and metastatic tumors of the liver. The clinical rationale for considering SBRT to the liver, reported experiences to date, and technical considerations will be discussed in this chapter.

## STEREOTACTIC BODY RADIATION THERAPY FOR LIVER METASTASES

### Scope of the Problem

Secondary spread of cancer to the liver is an important clinical problem. Colorectal cancers are the most common source of hepatic metastases and colorectal cancer accounts for the third most common cause of death in the United States, with most patients having liver metastases (1). Furthermore, it is estimated that 20% to 50% of patients with stages II and III colorectal cancer will develop liver metastases within 5 years of treatment of their primary diagnosis (2). Observational studies of patients with hepatic metastatic colorectal cancer have shown that the natural history of untreated patients, whether they had technically resectable disease or not, was uniformly poor, with 5-year survivals less than 3% (3,4). In selected operable colorectal cases where complete surgical extirpation of hepatic disease is achieved, average 5 year survival rates of 30% have been reported (5–8), suggesting that aggressive local therapies truly confer a benefit, even though randomized trials with an untreated control group have not been performed.

Department of Radiation Oncology, University of Colorado Comprehensive Cancer Center, Aurora, CO, 80010; * Department of Radiation Oncology, Indiana University School of Medicine, Indianapolis, IN 46202

Hepatic metastases due to hematogenous dissemination from breast cancer, melanoma, sarcoma, renal cell carcinoma, head and neck carcinoma, and neuroendocrine cancer further increase the overall incidence of hepatic metastases. It has been observed that more than half of all patients with breast cancer develop hepatic metastases. When minimal-volume disease isolated to the liver is present, aggressive local therapies have been associated with improvements in long-term outcome (9).

### Surgical Resection

Retrospective single-institution reports have formed the basis for considering surgery for patients with resectable metastases confined to the liver. Patients are typically considered eligible for surgery if they meet certain criteria: (a) they are medically fit for general anesthesia and recuperation after laparotomy; (b) they have disease limited to the liver; (c) they have adequate reserve of normal liver parenchyma for full recovery; and (d) they have technically resectable disease such that the resection safely encompasses all clinically apparent liver disease. There has never been a randomized, prospective trial to compare the efficacy of surgery with nonsurgical therapy for patients with isolated liver metastases, and the retrospective reports documenting outcomes after surgery are subject to inherent selection bias because patients selected for surgery are likely to be a highly favorable subset of the group with hepatic metastases.

Fong et al. (10) from Memorial Sloan-Kettering Cancer Center reported the largest surgical experience to date (n = 1,001). Multivariate analysis established risk factors for recurrence. These include positive margin, extrahepatic disease, node-positive primary, disease-free interval from primary to metastases less than 12 months, more than one hepatic tumor, largest hepatic tumor greater than 5 cm, and carcinoembryonic antigen (CEA) level above 200 ng/mL. Importantly, the latter six variables are available preoperatively and could be used to limit surgery or aggressive local therapy such as SBRT to those most likely to benefit. They observed that no patient with a score of five was a long-term survivor. Overall, they observed 5- and 10-year survivals of 37% and 22%, respectively.

Hepatic metastasectomy is associated with significant operative morbidity and mortality. Dimmick reported the results of a United States observational population-based study of 2,097 patients who underwent hepatic resections at more than 200 centers (11). Despite refinements in patient selection and improvements in operative techniques and perioperative management reported in recent years, considerable morbidity and mortality remain. Operative mortality was 5.8 % overall; the rate was slightly lower (3.9%) in higher volume hospitals than lower volume hospitals (7.6%). Only a minority of patients meets all the criteria for surgical eligibility, anyway, leaving most patients with hepatic metastases better suited for nonsurgical therapy.

It is possible to maintain normal liver function while surgically removing 75% to 80% of the total hepatic parenchyma or the equivalent of six of eight hepatic segments, as long as the remaining liver is normal and non-cirrhotic (12). This supports the concept that the liver is organized into functional subunits that are arranged in a parallel fashion and that normal function will be maintained as long as there is sufficient volume (subunits) remaining in the case of surgical resection and untreated or minimally treated in the case of local ablative therapies such as radiotherapy.

## Nonsurgical Therapy

Potential nonsurgical therapeutic options for this patient population include radiofrequency thermal ablation (RFA), cryotherapy, systemic chemotherapy, intrahepatic chemotherapy, yttrium-90 ($^{90}$Y) microsphere brachytherapy, chemoembolization, fractionated external beam radiation therapy, and SBRT.

RFA and cryotherapy are moderately invasive procedures performed percutaneously, laparoscopically, or via open laparotomy. Widely variable results are reported, with median survival after RFA or cryotherapy ranging from 12 to 32 months, depending on patient selection for tumor size and other prognostic factors (13). Systemic chemotherapy alone for hepatic metastases rarely results in complete responses, and median survivals in the range of 10 to 15 months have been reported.

The combination of hepatic artery chemotherapy plus $^{90}$Y microspheres was compared with hepatic artery chemotherapy alone in a randomized trial of patients with liver metastases from colon cancer. A higher radiographic response rate was observed with the combination therapy (44% vs. 17%, $p = 0.001$). The higher response rate was reflected in a higher 2-year survival (39% vs. 29%) (14). In a prospective phase 2 trial of chemoem-

bolization for the treatment of metastatic colorectal carcinoma to the liver, investigators at Northwestern University observed a median survival of 8.6 months, a result that is representative of other reported series (15).

## Fractionated Whole- and Partial-liver Radiation Therapy

The limitations of whole-liver radiation therapy were discussed earlier in the book, in the chapter addressing liver dose constraints in SBRT. The Radiation Therapy Oncology Group (RTOG) trials conducted in the 1980s confirmed that the maximum safe dose to the entire liver is approximately 30 Gy, even with hyperfractionation (16). Doses in this range are unlikely to result in durable tumor control, but there is good chance of palliative effect, even with a short, hypofractionated course of treatment (17).

University of Michigan investigators reported the results of a phase 1 trial of partial liver radiation and concurrent hepatic artery fluorodeoxyuridine for unresectable intrahepatic malignancies (18). A total of 43 patients were treated between 1996 and 1998, 27 of whom had primary hepatic tumors [mostly hepatocellular carcinoma (HCC)] and 16 were colorectal liver secondaries. The median radiation dose was 58.5 Gy (range, 28.5–90 Gy), given in twice-daily 1.5-Gy fractions along with concurrent continuous-infusion hepatic arterial fluorodeoxyuridine (0.2 mg/kg/d) during the first 4 weeks of radiation. Fourteen of the colorectal patients were evaluable, and 12 (86%) had responses. On multivariate analysis for the entire group, escalated radiation independently correlated with improved survival.

As noted earlier in the book, the risk of radiation-induced liver disease (RILD) was analyzed for a large cohort of patients treated at the University of Michigan with partial liver radiation and intrahepatic chemotherapy (19). Patients were selected for this analysis if they had long enough follow-up (at least 4 months) without hepatic progression, so that they were assessable for RILD. During the study period, approximately 75% were eligible and selected for this analysis ($n = 203$). Forty-one patients received whole-liver radiation, 20 received whole-liver radiation followed by a partial liver boost, and 142 were treated with partial-liver radiation alone. The median total dose was 52.5 Gy (range, 24–90 Gy) for the entire group and was delivered in twice-daily fractions of 1.5 to 1.65 Gy per fraction. Dose–volume histograms (DVHs) were obtained for normal liver [total liver volume minus cumulative gross tumor volumes (GTVs)] for all patients. Nineteen of 203 patients developed grade 3 or higher RILD. A strong volume effect was observed and there was significant correlation of mean dose to normal liver and incidence of RILD. No patient developed RILD at mean doses below 30 Gy; mathematical modeling predicted that

RILD increased by 4% for every increase of 1 Gy mean dose.

The risk of radiation hepatitis was higher in the patients with primary hepatic tumors compared with those with metastases (mean liver dose associated with a 5% risk of RILD for patients with primary hepatobiliary cancer and metastases were 32 Gy and 37 Gy, in 1.5 Gy twice daily, respectively), which is likely due to the higher incidence of baseline liver dysfunction in this group (viral hepatitis and cirrhosis). While this study provides useful information on hepatic tolerance to radiotherapy, stringent guidelines based on these results might be overly conservative when applied to SBRT without concurrent hepatic arterial chemotherapy.

## Stereotactic Body Radiation Therapy: Fractionated and Radiosurgical

A resurgence of interest in radiation therapy for liver tumors occurred as European investigators explored the application of stereotactic radiation treatment techniques,

initially developed for the brain, to the body (liver and lung) (20). It was hypothesized that higher doses to focal lesions would result in improvements in local control, while limiting toxicity by not treating the entire liver. Clinical experience to date is summarized in Tables 14.1 and 14.2. Most of these initial reports grouped lung and liver tumors together in the same reports.

Blomgren et al. (21) reported their initial pilot data of 31 patients with lung, liver and retroperitoneal tumors. Fourteen patients had 17 liver metastases (11 colorectal primaries), and eight patients had primary hepatic tumors. For the metastases group, the total minimum dose to the planning target volume (PTV) varied from 7.7 to 45 Gy in one to four fractions (7.7–20 Gy per fraction). Nausea and fever occurred a few hours after radiotherapy in most patients, but only one case of more severe toxicity (hemorrhagic gastritis in a patient with a pretreatment history of gastritis) possibly caused by radiotherapy occurred. There was no other major acute or late toxicity attributable to radiation therapy. Tumor regression rates were based on computed tomography (CT) evaluation and

▶ **TABLE 14-1** Single-institution Reports of Stereotactic Radiotherapy for Liver Metastases: Technical Details.

| Author (Institution) | Blomgren (Karolinska Hospital, Sweden) (21) | Blomgren (Karolinska Hospital, Sweden) (22) | Herfarth (University of Heidelberg, Germany) (26) | Wulf (University of Wuerzburg, Germany) (28) |
|---|---|---|---|---|
| Time | 1991–1995 | 1991–1996 | 1997–1999 | 1997–2001 |
| Systemic therapy | Not reported | Not reported | All breast patients had failed systemic therapy | 11 of 23 patients, within 3 mo of radiotherapy |
| No. of patients | 14 | 17 | 29 | 23 |
| No. of liver metastases | 17 | 21 | 56 | 23 (solitary metastases in all cases) |
| Primary site | Colorectal (11), bladder (1), ovary (1), anal canal(1) | Colorectal (10), bladder (1), ovary (2), anal canal (1), carcinoid (1) | Colorectal (30), breast (14), sarcoma (4), lung (4), pancreas (2), renal (1), melanoma (1) | Colorectal (11), ovary (4), breast (6), kidney (1), pancreas (1) |
| Stereotactic system | In house, not specified | Precision Therapy International stereotactic frame | Leibinger, Freiburg, Germany | Stereotactic body frame (Elekta, Norcross, GA ) |
| Planning system | TMS, Helax (Nucletron BV, Veenendaal, The Netherlands) | TMS, Helax | VOXELPLAN 3D planning software | TMS, Helax |
| Ventilation control | Abdominal compression | Abdominal compression | Abdominal Plexiglas compression plate | Abdominal compression |
| Mean tumor volume, cc (range) | 70 (2–258) | 46 (2–263) | 10 (1–132) | 50 (9–516) (n = 24, included one patient with hepatocellular carcinoma) |
| Radial margins(GTV to PTV), mm | 5 | 5 | 6 | 5 |
| Craniocaudal margins (GTV to PTV), mm | 10 | 10 | 10 | 10 |
| PTV dose/no. fractions | 7.7–45 Gy/1–4 fractions | 20–45 Gy/2–4 fractions | 14–26 Gy to isocenter/ 1 fraction | 30 Gy/3 fractions (22) 28 Gy/4 fractions (1) |
| Overall treatment time | 1–72 d | 2–41 d | 1 d | Not reported |

GTV, gross tumor volume; PTV, planning target volume..

▶ TABLE 14-2 Single-institution Reports of Stereotactic Body Radiation Therapy for Liver Metastases.

| Author | Blomgren (21) | Blomgren (22) | Herfarth (26) | Wulf (28) |
|---|---|---|---|---|
| Follow-up, mo (range) Local control | 9 (1.5–23) Crude 11/17(65%) | 9.6 (1.5–24) Crude 20/21(95%) | 6 (1–26) (including 4 liver primaries) 18-mo actuarial 67% (excluding first dose cohorts, 81% at 18 mo) | 9 (2–28) 1-yr actuarial 76% (included 1 patient with hepatocellular carcinoma) |
| Overall survival | Median survival 13 mo | Mean survival 17.8 mo (range, 8–36 mo) | 1-yr actuarial 72% | 1-yr actuarial 71% |
| Toxicity | Hemorrhagic gastritis (1) | Hemorrhagic gastritis (1), duodenal ulcer (1) | 0 | 29% grade 1 or 2 acute toxicity, no acute or late grades 3 to 5 toxicity |

therefore may have been underappreciated. Four tumors disappeared completely, one decreased in size, six remained unchanged, and five increased in size at 3 to 16 months post treatment. These same authors reported their 5-year experience in larger cohort of patients but excluded patients from the first report who were inadequately treated (five patients treated in the first dose cohorts and therefore received very low doses) (22). Overall, 50 patients with 75 evaluable lung and liver tumors, who were treated between 1991 and 1996, formed the basis of this report. The mean follow-up for all patients was 12 months. Seventeen of the 50 patients had 21 hepatic metastases and the mean tumor volume was 46 cm³. Prescribed dose to the PTV varied from 20 to 40 Gy in two to four fractions. Mean total dose to the PTV ranged from 26 to 63 Gy. During a mean follow-up of 9.6 months for the liver tumors, growth arrest was observed in ten, reduction of tumor size in four, and disappearance in four (1/21 failures).

Blomgren et al. acknowledge that standard criteria for response (Response Evaluation Criteria in Solid Tumors, RECIST) (23), which are used in determining efficacy of systemic agents, are probably not applicable in this setting of aggressive local therapy, as there are likely to be residual changes on CT, especially early after treatment. Reversible CT findings after radiotherapy are further described by Gouliamos and colleagues (24), and the topic is discussed earlier in the book in the chapter regarding dose constraints in liver SBRT. A recent report of positron emission tomography (PET) as surveillance after RFA accurately identified recurrences and is likely to have similar utility in distinguishing viable tumor from scar in irradiated lesions (25).

The Heidelburg University group reported the results of a phase 1/2 study of single-fraction stereotactic radiotherapy for liver tumors (26). A comprehensive description of their stereotactic technique was described in a separate report (27). Patients were enrolled between 1997 and 1999; there were 60 liver tumors treated (56 metastases, four primary hepatic tumors) in 37 patients. Radiation dose was escalated from 14 to 26 Gy in one fraction prescribed to the

80% isodose line. Median tumor size was 10 cm³ (range, 1–132 cm³). Fifty-five evaluable tumors during a median follow-up period of 5.7 months were presented. Treatment was well tolerated with no reported cases of RILD, defined as increased alkaline phosphatase, weight gain and nonmalignant ascites. Local failure was identified in 12 (22%) of 55 and low dose was associated with eight of these (treated in earlier dose cohorts). The overall actuarial local control at 18 months for the entire group was 67%. There was a trend toward larger tumors in the uncontrolled group (mean size of 31 cm³ in the uncontrolled group versus 19 cm³ in the controlled group).

Additional experience from the University of Wuerzburg using SBRT for liver and lung tumors was reported by Wulf et al. (28). Liver metastases accounted for 23 of 51 lesions. A dose of 30 Gy in three fractions of 10 Gy was prescribed to the 65% isodose line. Median follow-up was 9 months for the liver targets and median clinical target volume (CTV) and PTV were 50 and 102 cc, respectively. Actuarial local control at 1 and 2 years, which was defined as radiographic complete response, partial response, or stable disease, was obtained in 76% and 61%, respectively. Seven patients had grade 1 or 2 acute symptoms, lasting no more than a few hours. Included were nausea, vomiting, pain, fever, and chills. There was one case of grade 2 hepatitis at 6 weeks, which resolved after several weeks of steroids. There were no grades 3 to 5 acute or late toxicity in the irradiated liver group.

## FUTURE DIRECTIONS

Adjuvant systemic therapy, either before or after local therapy for metastatic disease, is an ongoing area of investigation, predicated on the fact that patients with one or more synchronous or metachronous hepatic metastases are at high risk for harboring subclinical micro metastases, both intra- and extrahepatically. In situations where active systemic agents are available, adjuvant therapy may improve survival. Many patients referred for stereotactic liver radiotherapy will have had systemic therapy (either adjuvant at the time of their original primary diagnosis or for treatment of metastatic disease) and or will have subsequent systemic therapy planned.

The European Organization for Research and Treatment of Cancer (EORTC) is currently investigating in a phase 3 trial the role of neoadjuvant chemotherapy followed by surgical resection for patients with resectable hepatic colorectal metastases (EORTC-40983). Also ongoing is a prospective randomized study of chemotherapy alone compared with additional RFA for patients with unresectable liver metastases secondary to colorectal adenocarcinoma (EORTC-40004).

Further investigation is under way as numerous United States centers participate in an ongoing multiinstitutional phase 1/2 clinical trial of SBRT for liver metastases (coordinated by University of Colorado). The dose escalation started at 36 Gy in three fractions delivered over 5 to 10 days, and prescribed to the isodose line (70%–90%) encompassing the PTV (successive total dose escalations of 6 Gy per cohort). Accrual is ongoing, and phase 1 results are expected late in 2004.

The RTOG has been planning a phase 1/2 trial of fractionated partial liver radiation therapy for patients with unresectable primary hepatobiliary cancer and liver metastases. Patients will be stratified by disease (primary or secondary). The starting dose for phase 1 will be 30 Gy in ten fractions and dose per fraction will be increased by 0.5 Gy per dose cohort to a maximum of 50 Gy. In both studies, patients are eligible if no chemotherapy is given or planned within 2 to 4 weeks of radiotherapy. Extrahepatic disease is allowed as long as life expectancy is at least 3 months and there is no evidence of brain metastases.

In summary, liver metastases from solid tumors represent systemic, usually incurable spread of malignancy. However, in selected patients with a limited measurable burden of metastatic disease, aggressive treatment to areas of gross hepatic disease may translate into durable disease-free survivorship. SBRT for hepatic metastases is a noninvasive local therapeutic modality that has demonstrated safety and response. The most effective dose and fractionation schedule remains to be determined. However, if one to five large-dose fractions are as effective as or perhaps even more effective than ten to 30 fractions, with no increased toxicity, the overriding advantage in convenience would be substantial.

## STEREOTACTIC BODY RADIATION THERAPY FOR PRIMARY HEPATOCELLULAR CARCINOMA

### Scope of the Problem

HCC is the most frequent primary tumor of the liver in adults. It accounts for up to 6% of all human cancers (7.5% among men and 3.5% among women). This neo-plasm ranks as the fifth most common cancer in the world (564,000 cases per year) and the third most common cancer-related death (29). The incidence of HCC is increasing both in Europe and in the United States due to the increasing prevalence of hepatitis C (30), and in the next two decades, it is expected to reach levels comparable to those currently found in Japan.

HCC is a very complex malignancy for which there is limited consensus regarding prognosis and therapeutic approach. Cirrhosis underlies most cases of HCC in the West, and it is the strongest predisposition factor to this malignancy. Chronic hepatitis B (HBV) and C virus (HCV) infections are the main causes of cirrhosis. In the West, HCV is the leading cause of HCC, which usually develops in older, cirrhotic patients. In addition, individuals with alcoholic cirrhosis and hemochromatosis also harbor a high risk for HCC. In the United States, HCV-related HCC is a rapidly rising cancer.

Until more effective measures to cure viral infection are developed, early detection of HCC remains the best strategy for reducing tumor-related mortality. Ultrasonography (US) and α-fetoprotein (AFP) every 6 months is the current standard of care for screening high-risk patients. Surveillance allows for early HCC diagnosis in up to 60% to 70% of the cases, when potentially curative therapies can be used. However, only half of these patients benefit from radical interventions.

### Diagnosis and Staging

The diagnosis of HCC is generally established histologically, but recently a set of noninvasive criteria for HCC diagnosis in cirrhotic patients has been proposed (31). The diagnosis is established when two imaging techniques [ultrasound, helical CT scan, or magnetic resonance imaging (MRI)] show a coincidental nodule larger than 2 cm in diameter with arterial hypervascularization, less well seen during portal venous phase, regardless of AFP levels, or if a single positive image is associated with an AFP level above 400 ng/mL. A histologic diagnosis is mandatory in HCC smaller than 2 cm in diameter or in noncirrhotic patients. Once the diagnosis of HCC is established, a chest CT and bone scan should be obtained to rule out extrahepatic, metastatic disease.

Staging systems in HCC are still evolving, as none are widely accepted. Some of the staging systems that have been used for HCC include: American Joint Commission on Cancer Staging classification, the Okuda system, the Barcelona Clinic Liver Cancer (BCLC) system, and the Cancer of the Liver Italian Program. One of the more popular, the BCLC system (32), includes several categories: patients with very early HCC, stage A (single nodule, <2 cm, Child-Pugh class A), and early HCC (single nodule ≤5 cm or up to three nodules ≤3 cm) are considered for radical therapies, such as resection, liver transplantation, or percutaneous tumor ablation. These patients achieve 5-

year survival rates of 50% to 75%. Patients with intermediate HCC, stage B, multinodular asymptomatic tumors without vascular invasion or extrahepatic spread, are generally considered for chemoembolization. Patients with symptomatic HCC, vascular invasion or extrahepatic spread is included in the advanced disease, stage C, and have 1- and 3-year survival rates of 28% and 8%, respectively. Finally, patients with end-stage disease, stage D, are considered for supportive care only.

## Management Alternatives

Despite recent advances in early detection and diagnosis, only 30% to 40% of patients with HCC may benefit from radical therapies (i.e., liver transplantation, surgical resection, and percutaneous ablation). Liver transplantation offers the best chance for cure, particularly in patients with decompensated liver disease. The optimal candidate for liver transplantation is a patient with single HCC less than 5 cm, or with fewer than three nodules smaller than 3 cm, without extrahepatic or vascular spread. These patients have 5-year survival rates over 70% with recurrence rates of less than 15%.

Surgical resection has been considered a potentially curative option, but most patients are not candidates for resection because of tumor size, location near major intrahepatic blood vessels and bile ducts precluding a margin-negative resection, cirrhosis, or multifocality. It has been estimated that only a very small (<5%) percentage of cirrhotic patients with HCC are candidates for surgical resection. The criteria for resection include normal bilirubin level, absence of portal hypertension (defined as hepatic venous pressure gradient less than 10 mm Hg), and tumor smaller than 5 cm in diameter. Although the 5-year survival rate for this group is 60% to 70%, approximately 50% of the patients recur in 3 years. Usually, the comorbid underlying severe liver disease either precludes surgery or makes the surgical approach extremely dangerous (33).

Minimally invasive therapies are gaining attention as an alternative to standard surgical therapies in the treatment of selected nonsurgical HCC patients. Percutaneous ethanol injection is widely used for small HCCs (<3cm) (34). RFA, discussed above as an option for liver metastases, can also be considered for HCC (35).

Most patients with HCC in the West are not candidates for radical therapies and are therefore considered for palliative therapies, such as transarterial chemoembolization (TACE), lipiodol chemoembolization, external beam radiation therapy, and cryosurgery. In addition, a variety of systemic chemotherapeutic agents has been tested in HCC, none with particularly notable success. In a recent report Lee et al. showed TACE to be as effective as hepatic resection in selected patients with Child-Pugh class A and UICC stage T1-3 N0 M0 when lipiodol was compactly re-

tained within the tumor (36). However, hepatic resection continues to be the treatment of choice for patients with small resectable tumors and adequate liver function, especially in patients with serum AFP levels less than 400 ng/mL and in patients with a noncompact lipiodol. In addition, Llovet and colleagues (37) have shown improved survival when compared with conservative therapy in patients with unresectable HCC.

## Conventional External Beam Radiation Therapy for Hepatocellular Carcinoma

Radiation therapy for the treatment of unresectable HCC has been attempted for more than four decades. Early trials involved the use of low-dose whole-liver irradiation, generally in combination with intraarterial and/or intravenous chemotherapy, with reported 2-year survival rates below 10% (38,39). The use of three-dimensional conformal radiation therapy treatment planning has allowed the safe delivery of higher radiation doses to limited liver volumes.

Robertson and colleagues (40) reported results for 26 patients with primary unresectable hepatobiliary cancer treated with conformal radiation therapy and intraarterial hepatic fluorodeoxyuridine (FdUrd). The total radiation dose was titrated according to the fraction of normal liver excluded from the high-dose volume. Whole-liver radiation was administered to six patients with diffuse HCC; 11 patients with localized HCC and nine patients with cholangiocarcinoma received a radiation dose to the tumor ranging from 48 to 72.6 Gy. The median survival for patients with localized cancer was 19 months, while patients with diffuse HCC had a median survival of only 4 months. Actuarial 2-year freedom from local progression in patients with localized disease was 72%. In a later study also performed at the University of Michigan, an additional 27 patients with primary liver cancers received a median dose of 61.5 Gy (range, 28.5–90 Gy), given in twice-daily 1.5-Gy fractions, and a response rate of 45% was achieved; total dose was an important prognostic factor, with significantly longer survival among patients who received high doses (18).

Seong and colleagues (41) published clinical results for a large cohort of patients who received radiation therapy for unresectable HCC. Among the 158 patients treated, 107 received radiation plus with TACE while 51 had progressed after prior TACE. Liver cirrhosis was present in 90% of cases, and the mean tumor size was 9.0 cm. Typically, the GTV was enlarged by 2 to 3 cm to create a clinical target volume, further enlarged by 0.5 cm to create a PTV. An additional margin in the superior–inferior direction was added for respiratory motion. Total dose was adjusted according to the volume of normal liver receiving radiation, and the mean radiation dose was 48.2 Gy in daily 1.8-Gy fractions. A response rate of 67% was observed, and the overall survival rate at 2 and 5 years was 31% and 9%, respectively, from the time of diagnosis and 20% and 5%, respectively, after radiotherapy. On multivariate analysis, radiation dose was the only significant prognostic factor. A 2-year actuarial survival of 8%, 10%, and 29% was achieved after radiation doses of less than 40 Gy, 40 to 50 Gy, and above 50 GY, respectively.

RILD is an important issue for any radiation treatment of liver tumors. This topic has been discussed more thoroughly in a previous chapter. The mean dose to uninvolved liver is likely a strong predictor for the risk of RILD, given the parallel organ structure of the liver. It is not clear whether intensity-modulated radiotherapy (IMRT) would be beneficial in the setting of conventionally fractionated external beam radiotherapy. In one series a comparison of IMRT versus non-IMRT, treatment planning yielded a higher mean dose to the liver when target coverage was held constant (42).

## Stereotactic Body Radiation Therapy for Hepatocellular Carcinoma

Blomgren et al. (21) used SBRT in nine patients with HCCs, one with an intrahepatic bile duct cancer, and one with an embryonic cancer. Twenty tumors were treated in the 11 patients. The total minimum doses within the target volume varied from 14 to 45 Gy. Treatment was delivered during one to three sessions with 5 to 15 Gy per fraction (minimum dose to the target). Stable disease was observed in five tumors, reduction in size in 12 tumors, and disappearance in two at 12 months mean follow-up, for an overall 70% response rate. All patients developed fever (up to 38.5°C) and nausea for a few hours after a treatment. These symptoms could be partially prevented by pretreatment with antiemetics. One patient died 2 days after a single dose of 30 Gy to a large HCC in the left liver lobe. Autopsy was not performed. Two patients developed ascites within 3 to 6 weeks of SBRT and died (presumably from liver failure), but both patients had pretreatment cirrhosis and attribution to radiation therapy was not clearly demonstrable.

In the phase 1/2 dose-escalation study using radiosurgery-style SBRT for primary or metastatic liver tumors reported by Herfarth and colleagues (26), only four patients had a primary liver tumor; likewise, the experience reported by Wulf et al. (28) also included only a small number of HCC, rendering it difficult to draw conclusions about tumor control based on the these limited experiences. Kelsey et al. (43) addressed the question of whether the radiographic dimensions of HCC reflect the lesion size accurately. For 18 evaluable patients who underwent surgical resection of 27 primary liver tumors, preoperative imaging studies were compared to the gross pathologic specimens. The median radiographic diameter was 2.90 cm (range, 1.2–4.9 cm), and the median pathologic size was 2.50 cm (range, 1–4.8 cm). MRI and CT were equally help-

ful in estimating the gross tumor size. Overall, the clinical and pathologic sizes correlated highly. The authors concluded that in most instances, imaging by CT or MRI overestimates true gross pathologic size by a small amount. However, since treatment failures after SRBT might occur if there is underestimation of true gross tumor size by imaging, it was noted that the addition of a planning margin of 0.5 cm would have covered 93% of lesions while a margin of 1 cm would have covered 100% of lesions.

## CASE STUDIES

### Solitary Metastasis of Colon Cancer

A 45-year-old man had undergone surgical resection for a pathologic T4 N2 M0 rectosigmoid adenocarcinoma approximately 2 years before developing a solitary liver metastasis. He had undergone 6 months of adjuvant irinotecan, 5-fluorouracil (5-FU), and leucovorin chemotherapy postoperatively (no pelvic radiation). One year after his primary diagnosis, he developed a local anastomotic recurrence, which was resected, and he subsequently received postoperative adjuvant whole-pelvic radiation therapy in combination with capecitabine. His original pretreatment CEA and all subsequent CEAs have remained in the normal range.

A solitary liver metastasis was detected on routine surveillance PET scan. An MRI localized the metastasis in the posterior aspect of the medial segment of the right lobe, anterior to the portal vein (Fig. 14.1). The patient

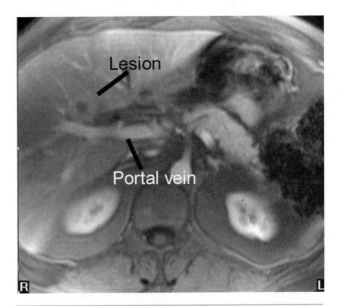

**FIGURE 14.1.** Axial magnetic resonance image demonstrating ring enhancement characteristic of metastasis and proximity to the portal vein. The lesion is located in the posterior aspect of the medial segment of the right hepatic lobe. Metastectomy would have required trisegmentectomy.

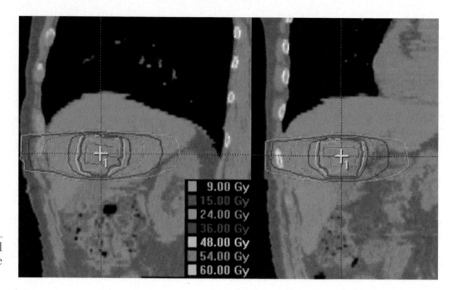

9.00 Gy
15.00 Gy
24.00 Gy
36.00 Gy
48.00 Gy
54.00 Gy
60.00 Gy

**FIGURE 14.2.** Sagittal (**left**) and coronal (**right**) views, showing total dose isodose lines.

preferred nonsurgical therapy and was therefore enrolled on a phase 1 clinical trial of stereotactic radiotherapy and was treated to a total dose of 48 Gy in three fractions of 16 Gy prescribed to the isodose line encompassing the PTV (Fig. 14.2).

### Liver Stereotactic Body Radiation Therapy after Prior Lung Stereotactic Body Radiation Therapy

A 70-year-old man developed two pulmonary metastases 1 year after undergoing preoperative radiation therapy and concurrent chemotherapy followed by low anterior resection for locally advanced rectal cancer. He underwent a course of stereotactic body radiation therapy (SBRT) to the lung, and each lesion (one in the left upper lobe and one in the left lower lobe) received a total dose of 45 Gy in three fractions, prescribed to the maximal isodose encompassing the planning target volume (PTV), followed by 5-fluorouracil–based chemotherapy.

Two months later, while receiving chemotherapy, he was found to have a liver metastasis (Fig. 14.3). The lung metastases had completely disappeared on follow-up imaging at the time of his liver recurrence; furthermore, the response was durable at 5 months. He enrolled in prospective trial of SBRT for liver metastases received 42 Gy in three fractions prescribed to the maximal isodose encompassing the PTV. Dose–volume histograms (DVHs) and pre- and post-SBRT computed tomography (CT) scans are shown in Fig. 14.4. The patient experienced no grade 2 or 3 toxicity at any time. A positron emission tomography (PET) scan obtained 2 months after radiation treatment revealed a decrease in the metabolic activity within the treated lesion (pre-SBRT specific uptake valve (SUV) 3.5, post SBRT SUV 1.9—not shown).

### Primary Hepatocellular Carcinoma

A 63-year-old woman with a history of hepatitis C was found on routine surveillance to have an elevated α-fetoprotein (AFP) level. A computed tomography (CT) scan showed an arterial phase–enhancing 3.5-cm mass in the inferior right hepatic lobe. There was a moderate amount of ascites (asymptomatic) at baseline. CT-guided biopsy confirmed grade 2 hepatocellular carcinoma (HCC) with adjacent dysplastic nodules and cirrhosis.

She was considered medically inoperable and elected to undergo stereotactic body radiation therapy (SBRT). Dose distributions are shown in Fig. 14.5. She developed a local-

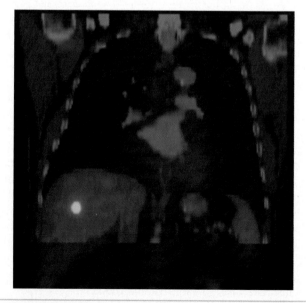

**FIGURE 14.3.** Coronal computed tomography–positron emission tomography demonstrating the solitary liver metastasis.

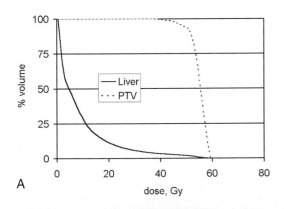

A

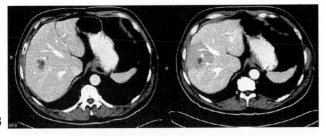

B

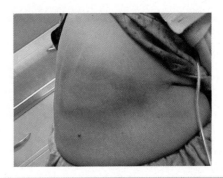

**FIGURE 14.6.** Skin reaction observed one month following completion of stereotactic body radiation therapy.

ized area of dry desquamation and hyperpigmentation involving the right posterolateral skin (Fig. 14.6); the axial isodose distribution showed that the skin received a maximum cumulative dose between 9 and 15 Gy. She also had several days of low-grade nausea, but both of these toxicities (skin and nausea) were transient. A CT scan obtained 1 month after SBRT revealed no growth in the tumor, and the AFP had already dropped by 20% compared with pre-SBRT levels.

**FIGURE 14.4.** **A:** Dose–volume histograms (DVHs) for liver planning target volume (PTV) and liver. The x-axis represents absolute dose for the total three fractions. The PTV was defined by adding 5 mm margins radially and 10 mm craniocaudally. The liver DVH is for normal uninvolved liver (total liver minus GTV). **B:** Computed tomography (CT) scan before stereotactic body radiation therapy (SBRT) (**left**). The hypodensity is located in the anterior segment of the right lobe, measuring roughly 26 mm in diameter, extending above and below this slice for several slices (not shown, estimated 3 cm in superior–inferior dimension). **Right:** CT scan performed exactly 2 months after completing SBRT. The lesion is smaller axially and now only seen well on one CT section (estimated 1 cm superior–inferior dimension). Note the subtle area of hypodensity consistent with typical radiation-related radiographic change in the normal liver in the high dose region (see Chapter 5 for additional discussion).

## REFERENCES

1. Jemal A, Murray T, Samuels A, et al. Cancer statistics, 2003. *CA Cancer J Clin* 2003;53:5–26.
2. Scheele J, Stangl R, Atendorf-Hofmann A, et al. Resection of colorectal metastases. *World J Surg* 1995;19:59–71.
3. Wood CB, Gillis CR, Blumgart LH. A retrospective study of the natural history of patients with liver metastases from colorectal cancer. *Clin Oncol* 1976;2:285–288.
4. Wagner JS, Adson MA, Van Heerden JA, et al. The natural history of hepatic metastases from colorectal cancers. *Arch Surg* 1976;111:330–334.
5. Gayowksi TJ, Iwatsuki S, Madariaga JR, et al. Experience in hepatic resection for metastatic colorectal cancer: analysis of clinical and pathological risk factors. *Surgery* 1994;116:703–711.
6. Rosen CB, Nagorney DM, Taswell HF, et al. Perioperative blood transfusion and determinants of survival after liver resection for metastatic colorectal carcinoma. *Ann Surg* 1992;216:492–505.
7. Nordlinger B, Parc R, Delva E, et al. Hepatic resection for colorectal liver metastases. *Ann Surg* 1987;205:256–263.
8. Fong Y, Cohen AM, Forter JG, et al. Liver resection for colorectal metastases. *J Clin Oncol* 1997;15:938–946.
9. Singletary AE, Walsh G, Vauthey JN, et al. A role for curative surgery in the treatment of selected patients with metastatic breast cancer. *Oncologist* 2003;8:241–251.
10. Fong Y, Fortner J, Sun RL, et al. Clinical score for predicting recurrence after hepatic resection for metastatic colorectal cancer. *Ann Surg* 1999;230:309–321.
11. Dimick J, Cowan JA, Knol JA, et al. Hepatic resection in the United States: indications, outcomes, and hospital procedural volumes from a nationally representative database. *Arch Surg* 2003;138:185–191.
12. Penna C, Nordlinger B. Colorectal metastasis (liver and lung). *Surg Clin N Am* 2002;82:1075–1090.
13. Erce C, Parks RW. Interstitial ablative techniques for hepatic tumours. *Br J Surg* 2003;90:272–289.
14. Gray B, Van Hazel G, Hope M, et al. Randomised trial of SIR-spheres plus chemotherapy vs. chemotherapy alone for treating patients with liver metastases from primary large bowel cancer. *Ann Oncol* 2001;12:1711–1120.

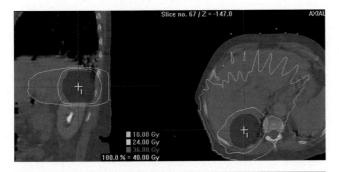

**FIGURE 14.5.** Sagittal (**left**) and axial (**right**) dose distribution for case 3. The prescription dose was 36 Gy in three fractions of 12 Gy, prescribed to the 90% isodose (absolute doses shown). Notice the proximity to the right kidney in the sagittal images.

15. Tellez C, Benson AB 3rd, Lyster MT, et al. Phase II trial of chemoembolization for the treatment of metastatic colorectal carcinoma to the liver and review of the literature. *Cancer* 1998;82:1250–1259.

16. Russell AH, Clyde C, Wasserman TH. Accelerated hyperfractionated hepatic irradiation in the management of patients with liver metastases: results of the RTOG dose-escalating protocol. *Int J Radiat Oncol Biol Phys* 1993;27:117–123.

17. Bydder S, Spry NA, Christie DR, et al. A prospective trial of short-fractionation radiotherapy for the palliation of liver metastases. *Australas Radiol* 2003;47:284–288.

18. Dawson LA, McGinn CJ, Normolle D, et al. Escalated focal liver radiation and concurrent hepatic artery fluorodeoxyuridine for unresectable intrahepatic malignancies. *J Clin Oncol* 2000;18:2210–2218.

19. Dawson LA, Normolle D, Balter J, et al. Analysis of radiation-induced liver disease using the lyman NTCP model. *Int J Radiat Oncol Biol Phys* 2002;53:810–821.

20. Lax I, Blomgren H, Naslund I, et al. Stereotactic radiotherapy of malignancies in the abdomen. *Acta Oncologica* 1994;33:677–683.

21. Blomgren H, Lax I, Naslund I, et al. Stereotactic high dose radiation therapy of extracranial tumors using an accelerator. *Acta Oncologica* 1995;34:861–870.

22. Blomgren J, Lax I, Goranson H, et al. Radiosurgery for tumors in the body: clinical experience using a new method. *J Radiosurg* 1998;1:63–74.

23. Therasse P, Arbuck SG, Eisenhauer EA, et al. New guidelines to evaluate the response to treatment in solid tumors. *J Natl Cancer Inst* 2000;92:205–216.

24. Gouliamos AD, Kotoulas C, Giannopoulo C, et al. Reversible CT findings of the liver after radiotherapy. *Radiother Oncol* 1991;21:67–68.

25. Anderson GS, Brinkmann F, Soulen MC, et al. FDG positron emission tomography in the surveillance of hepatic tumors treated with radiofrequency ablation. *Clin Nucl Med* 2003;28:192–197.

26. Herfarth KK, Debus J, Lohr F, et al. Stereotactic single-dose radiation therapy of liver tumors: results of a phase I/II trial. *J Clin Oncol* 2001;19:164–170.

27. Herfarth KK, Debus J, Lohr F, et al. Extracranial stereotactic radiation therapy: set-up accuracy of patients treated for liver metastases. *Int J Radiat Oncol Biol Phys* 2000;46:329–335.

28. Wulf J, Hadinger U, Oppitz U, et al. Stereotactic radiotherapy of targets in lung and liver. *Strahlenther Onkol* 2001;177:645–155.

29. Parkin DM, Bray F, Ferlay J, et al. Estimating the world cancer burden. GLOBOCAN 2000. *Int J Cancer* 2001;94:153–156.

30. El Serag HB, Mason AC. Rising incidence of hepatocellular carcinoma in the United States. *N Engl J Med* 1999;340:745–750.

31. Bruix J, Sherman M, Llovet JM, et al. Clinical management of hepatocellular carcinoma: conclusions of the Barcelona-2000 EASL Conference. *J Hepatol* 2001;35:421–430.

32. Llovet JM, Bru C, Bruix J. Prognosis of hepatocellular carcinoma: The BCLC staging classification. *Sem Liv Dis* 1999;19:329–338.

33. Llovet JM, Fuster J, Bruix J. Intention-to-treat analysis of surgical treatment for early hepatocellular carcinoma: resection versus transplantation. *Hepatology* 1999;39:1434–1440.

34. Arii S, Yamakoa Y, Futagawa S, et al. Results of surgical and non surgical treatment for small-sized hepatocellular carcinomas: a retrospective and nation wide survey in Japan. *Hepatology* 2000;32:1224–1229.

35. Lui L, et al. Radiofrequency ablation of liver cancers. *World J Gastroent* 2002;8: 392–399.

36. Lee HS, Kim KM, Yoon JH, et al. Therapeutic efficacy of transcatheter arterial chemoembolization as compared with hepatic resection in hepatocellular carcinoma patients with compensated liver function in a hepatitis B virus-endemic area: a prospective cohort study. *J Clin Oncol* 2002;20:4459–4465.

37. Llovet JM, Real I, Montana X, et al. Arterial embolisation or chemoembolization versus symptomatic treatment in patients with unresectable hepatocellular carcinoma: a randomized controlled trial. *Lancet* 2002;359:1734–1739.

38. Stillwagon GB, Order SE, Guse CG, et al. Hepatocellular cancers treated by radiation and chemotherapy combinations: toxicity and response: a Radiation Therapy Oncology Group (RTOG) study. *Int J Radiat Oncol Biol Phys* 1989;17:1223–1229.

39. Abrams RA, Pajak TF, Haulk TL, et al. Survival results among patients with alfa-feto protein positive, unresectable hepatocellular carcinoma: analysis of three sequential treatments of the RTOG and Johns Hopkins Oncology Center. *Cancer J Sci Am* 1998;4:178–184.

40. Robertson JM, Lawrence TS, Dworzanin LM, et al. Treatment of primary hepatobiliary cancers with conformal radiotherapy and regional chemotherapy. *J Clin Oncol* 1993;11:1286–1293.

41. Seong J, Park HC, Han KH, et al. Clinical results and prognostic factors in radiotherapy for unresectable hepatocellular carcinoma: a retrospective study of 158 patients. *Int J Radiat Oncol Biol Phys* 2003;55:329–336.

42. Cheng JC, Wu JK, Huang CM, et al. Dosimetric analysis and comparison of three-dimensional conformal radiotherapy and intensity-modulated radiation therapy for patients with hepatocellular carcinoma and radiation-induced liver disease. *Int J Radiat Oncol Biol Phys* 2003;56:229–234.

43. Kelsey CR, Schefter T, Nash R, et al. Retrospective clinicopathologic correlation of gross tumor size of hepatocellular carcinoma: implications for extracranial stereotactic radiosurgery. *Int J Radiat Oncol Biol Phys* 2003;57[Suppl 2]:S283.

## Case Study

### Case Study in Liver SBRT: Dose Optimization via Inverse Treatment Planning

William Salter and Martin Fuss

### CLINICAL PRESENTATION

A previously healthy 36-year-old man had 2 years previously undergone partial right colectomy for a pathologic T3 N1 M1 moderately differentiated adenocarcinoma of the colon. The primary tumor measured 3.5 cm grossly, and microscopically there was involvement of the subserosa and focal lymphovascular invasion. Three of 16 regional lymph nodes contained cancer, and an intraoperative liver biopsy proved the presence of metastatic disease. A postoperative computed tomography (CT) scan revealed three remaining subcentimeter lesions in the right lobe of the liver. No other site of active disease was identified.

The patient received systemic chemotherapy that included 5-fluorouracil, leucovorin, and CD 1839. Chemotherapy-related toxicity from that combination regimen prompted a change to CPT-11. Follow-up CT imaging of the upper abdomen revealed a sustained near-complete response in the known small liver lesions until a study performed 2 months prior to stereotactic body radiation therapy (SBRT), which indicated regrowth of two of the lesions to a diameter of approximately 1 cm each.

Since the patient declined surgical resection and the two liver lesions were the only sites of confirmed recurrent/persistent disease, SBRT was offered as local tumor therapy with curative intent.

### STEREOTACTIC BODY RADIATION THERAPY TREATMENT PLANNING AND DOSE DELIVERY

During simulation and treatment for SBRT at the University of Texas Health Science Center at San Antonio (UTHSCSA), the patient is immobilized using a double-vacuum whole-body immobilization system (BodyFIX; Medical Intelligence, Schwabmuenchen, Germany). Figure 14.7 depicts a patient immobilized in this manner on the CT simulator couch. The system consists of a vacuum-formed, full-body negative cast of the patient posteriorly plus a second vacuum created between a plastic top sheet, the patient, and the vacuum "cast." CT data are acquired helically and reconstructed in 3-mm slice thickness.

Target localization for hepatic lesions is facilitated by three-phase, contrast-enhanced CT scan. The respiratory motion–related component of the planning target volume (PTV) margin is quantified by real-time fluoroscopy. Treatment planning employs an inverse treatment planning intensity-modulated radiotherapy

Department of Radiation Oncology, The University of Texas Health Science Center, San Antonio, TX 78229

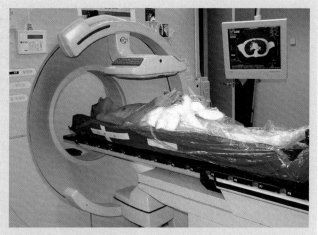

**FIGURE 14.7.** The patient was immobilized using the BodyFIX system (Medical Intelligence, Schwabmuenchen, Germany).

(IMRT) software (Corvus; Nomos, Cranberry Township, PA) in intensity-modulated radiosurgery (IMRS) mode prioritizing dose conformality over dose homogeneity. Parameters entered are the target dose prescription (typically 36 Gy in three fractions), a percentage of the target volume allowed to receive a lesser dose, the minimum dose permitted (here 3% allowed to receive a dose as low as 34 Gy), and the maximally tolerated point dose (here 200% of the prescribed target dose).

The margins for creation of a PTV from the gross tumor volume (GTV) in this particular case were 6 mm transversally and 15 mm craniocaudally, according to the established breathing amplitude. The specified pencil beam (PB) dimension was 8.5 × 10 mm (1-cm mode). The computed isodose distribution is shown in Fig. 14.8.

Treatment was delivered in three fractions separated by 48 hours using a serial tomotherapy approach and the Nomos MIMiC binary multileaf collimator (mlc) using three sequentially delivered arcs at the nominal (180-degree) couch (Varian, Palo Alto, CA) angle. Total treatment time (including control CT and setup) and beam-on time to deliver each fraction was roughly 90 and 24 minutes, respectively. Prior to delivery of each of three treatment fractions, a verification CT scan of the patient was performed in the CT simulation suite. The verification scan was then coregistered with the original treatment-planning CT to determine any correctional shifts necessary for precise targeting of the lesion. The patient was subsequently transferred via gurney, in the BodyFIX immobilized treatment position, to the linear accelerator (linac) suite for treatment.

### DISCUSSION

Acutely, the treatment delivered was well tolerated. Figure 14.9 summarizes the imaging findings in sequence of follow-up. At 12 weeks after SBRT, a sharply demarcated edema zone was documented that followed in shape the 25-Gy cumulative dose distribution (reflecting three fractions of 8.3 Gy each). At the 16-week

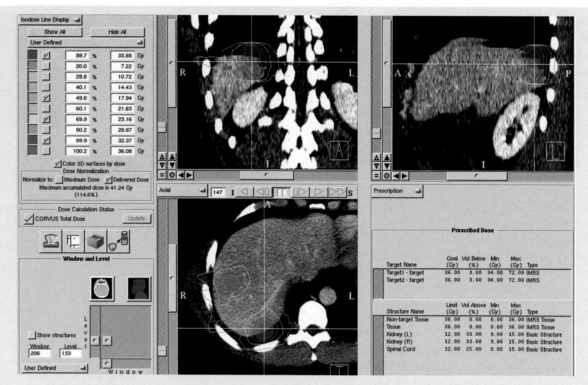

**FIGURE 14.8.** Treatment-planning system screen capture including axial, sagittal, and coronal isodose distributions. The planning target volumes (PTVs) are shaded purple and red. The prescription isodose line (36 Gy, given in three fractions) is dark blue and conforms to the PTVs closely. The red, yellow, and green lines represent the 90%, 70%, and 50% isodose lines, respectively. The right kidney is well spared.

follow-up, the edema appeared much less sharply bordered and less intense; the lesions were no longer identified. Subsequent imaging at 9 months depicts normal-appearing liver without evidence of liver edema, tumor recurrence, or new metastatic disease. Blood tests obtained during the followup period have revealed no clinically significant increase in liver function parameters.

The demonstrated case is representative of the UTHSCSA experience in treating localized malignant liver disease. Since

May 2002, 15 patients with metastatic lesions of the liver ($n = 14$ patients with 17 lesions) or small hepatocellular carcinoma ($n = 1$, solitary lesion) were treated by SBRT. The dose prescription and delivery schedule was three fractions of 12 Gy prescribed to the periphery of the PTV in small liver lesions and six fractions of 6 Gy each in large liver lesions (four patients). Treatments were delivered every other day, so that a typical treatment course was completed within a week. All patients underwent not only a verification CT procedure in the immobi-

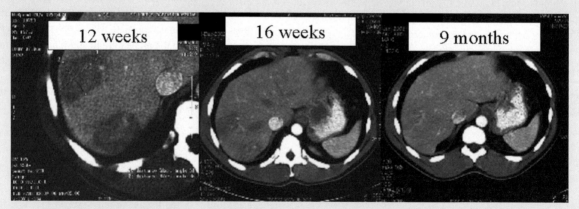

**FIGURE 14.9.** Computed tomography images of the liver at 12 weeks, 16 weeks, and 9 months after stereotactic body radiation therapy (SBRT) (see text for details). The early changes are consistent with the typical radiographic changes following SBRT to the liver discussed in Chapter 5.

lization system before delivery of each treatment fraction but also ultrasound-based image-guided targeting in treatment position using the BAT® (B-mode Acquisition and Targeting) ultrasound device (Nomos, Sewickley, Pennsylvania). Metastatic and primary liver lesions may pose difficulty for ultrasound targeting visualization, but the liver outline and intrahepatic vessels—predominantly branches of the portal vein and the venous system—can be used as guidance structures. Outcomes have been encouraging, with a crude local tumor control of 14 of 15 at median follow-up time of 6.5 months. Three of the 15 treated patients have died either as a result of progression of extrahepatic disease ($n = 2$) or local progression of hepatic disease ($n = 1$).

The use of an intensity-modulated sequential tomotherapy system is, we believe, unique to the experience at UTHSCSA. The rationale for using a rotational IMRT system over multiple three-dimensional (3D) planned static beams or static-field IMRT is our perception of an improved dose distribution, enabled by an almost 360-degree range to deliver and modulate PBs. The trade-off for this highly conformal dose distribution is the complex dose matrix and associated high number of monitor units. Since we currently treat no more than two patients by SBRT per treatment day, this machine time requirement has not been seen to represent a significant limitation of the resource.

However, we are currently exploring the relation between less complex intensity matrices and an expected related loss of treatment quality, with the intent of identifying strategies to simplify treatment delivery and reduce treatment delivery time. Such a strategy might be reasonably expected to make this treatment modality available to a higher number of patients, while maintaining the established high quality of the computed dose distributions.

A component that adds significant time to the treatment delivery is the daily imaging assessment of lesion location by both CT resimulation and ultrasound-based image guidance on the treatment table. A technologic migration to "in-room" or "on-board" CT imaging could allow a reduction in this associated time component. Despite an observation of excellent average variability of patient and target setup of less than 4 mm in the whole-body immobilization system utilized here, we will continue to adhere to a very rigid imaging control procedure. Occasionally observed, clinically relevant setup variability larger than 5 mm, especially in larger patients, requires, in our opinion, such a quality assurance imaging procedure to ensure a higher than 95% probability of full target volume coverage by the planned 100% dose distribution.

## Chapter 15

# Stereotactic Body Radiation Therapy for Renal Cell Carcinoma

*J. Peter Wersäll and Brian D. Kavanagh**

## BACKGROUND

The reported annual incidence rates of renal cell carcinoma (RCC) are quite variable according to geographic region, but the worldwide average is estimated to be approximately three per 100,000 adults (1). North America has a particularly high incidence, and more than 30,000 cases are diagnosed annually in the United States, of which nearly 40% will eventually prove to be fatal (2). Local tumor recurrence within the renal fossa after potentially curative resection is very uncommon (3), and the overwhelming majority of deaths due to RCC are thus the result of progressive metastatic disease.

Currently, interleukin-2 (IL-2) is the only agent officially endorsed by the US Food and Drug Administration (FDA) for the treatment of metastatic RCC. The initial approval was granted on the basis of a clinical trial indicating only a 14% response rate (4). A survival benefit from IL-2 in this setting has not been demonstrated, nor has IL-2 been demonstrated to improve overall or disease-free survival in the adjuvant setting following nephrectomy for RCC (5). Low-dose and high-dose IL-2 regimens yield equivalent survival outcomes, with less toxicity caused by the lower dose regimens (6). To date no combinations of IL-2 plus another systemic agent have proven to be superior to IL-2 alone. Newer agents are actively being evaluated, with minimal success thus far: In one recent clinical trial of an anti-angiogenic agent, no complete responses were observed there was only a 10% partial response rate at the highest dose evaluated (7).

Surgical resection is sometimes offered to patients with limited sites of extracranial metastatic RCC. Selection bias likely is an important factor, but the median and 4- to 5-year actuarial survivals of recent single institution

Department of General Oncology, Radiumbemmet, Karolinska University Hospital and Karolinska Institute, Stockholm, Sweden; and *Department of Radiation Oncology, University of Colorado Comprehensive Cancer Center, Aurora, CO 80010

experiences are at least as good as and often better than what is reported with the use of IL-2 alone (Table 15.1). Not surprisingly, patients who have had longer disease-free intervals prior to resection of metastatic RCC tend to fare better, perhaps because of more indolent tumor biology in those patients. However, also supporting the argument for the value of aggressively reducing the total body cancer cell burden is the result of a multiinstitutional randomized study involving more than 240 patients with metastatic RCC. Patients who underwent nephrectomy enjoyed a modest but statistically significant improvement in median survival compared with patients who received immunotherapy alone (8).

There have been few reported experiences involving stereotactic body radiation therapy (SBRT) for RCC. However, SBRT is an attractively noninvasive method for potential eradication of metastatic tumor deposits from RCC and might provide meaningful clinical benefit insofar as tumor burden reduction has been demonstrated to have very favorable clinical effect.

## RADIOBIOLOGIC CONSIDERATIONS

RCC has sometimes been loosely termed to be "radioresistant." An analysis of the *in vitro* radiosensitivity of laboratory RCC cell lines has suggested that higher cranial radiosurgery doses are required for clinical tumor control of RCC than for other tumor histologies (9). However, examination of the available clinical data does not necessarily support that hypothesis. For example, patients with brain metastases from RCC tend to fare poorly, but there is no clear proof that their survival is worse than other patients with brain metastases matched for performance status and other key prognostic factors. In modern series, the median survival of patients with brain metastases from RCC treated with whole-brain radiation therapy and/or cranial stereotactic radiosurgery has ranged broadly from 3 to 18 months (10–16). Clinical effects do

▶ **TABLE 15.1** Selected Recent Report of Surgical Resection of Renal Cell Cancer Metastases.

| Author, Year, Reference | N | Survival | Prognostic Factors |
|---|---|---|---|
| Kavolius et al., 1998 (32) | 141 | 5 y 44% | DFI,[a] solitary, age <60 |
| Friedel et al., 1999 (33) | 77 | 5 y 39% | DFI |
| Van der Poel et al., 1999 (34) | 101 | Median 28 mo | DFI |
| Csekeo et al., 2002 (35) | 52 | 5 y 35% | DFI, complete resection |
| Loizzi et al., 2003 (36) | 24 | 4 y 50% | Solitary |
| Alves et al., 2003 (37) | 14[b] | Median 26 mo | DFI |

DFI, disease-free interval
[a]Longer DFI between initial diagnosis and resection of the metastasis is usually associated with longer survival.
[b]Exclusively patients with liver metastases.

not necessarily reflect radiographic tumor response (17), and selection bias can play a role in individual institutional reports; nevertheless, overall the outcomes appear similar to large combined series of brain metastases of other histologic subtypes (18).

For the palliative treatment of extracranial sites of metastatic RCC, radiotherapy is well established as an effective therapeutic modality (19). While one retrospective analysis suggested that the degree or duration of favorable effect correlates with the biologically effective dose of radiotherapy administered (20), this relationship has not been uniformly observed (21). Preclinical studies have demonstrated that radiation and IL-2 can interact synergistically on RCC metastases (22). In a small, phase 2 study of sequential radiation and IL-2 in the treatment of patients with metastatic RCC, however, a low response rate was observed (23). A major flaw in the study methodology was that the radiation dose was only 8 Gy per fraction for two fractions. Although this dose might have some modest immunomodulatory effect, it would not be expected to have meaningful tumoricidal effect.

Ionizing radiation can excite numerous intracellular signaling pathways (24), and IL-2 is among the cytokines whose expression can be elevated after radiotherapy (25). Interestingly, spontaneous regression of metastatic RCC has been observed following radiotherapy to the primary site, with measured increase of serum IL-2 during the period of favorable clinical response (26).

Regarding tolerance of the normal renal parenchyma to radiation, the kidney itself is considered to have a parallel organ structure from a radiobiologic perspective. The most common clinical example of bilateral whole-kidney irradiation is in the setting of total body irradiation (TBI) during conditioning for bone marrow transplantation, and a fractionated dose up to around 12 Gy is usually tolerated with a very low incidence of toxicity (27); some of the multiple other agents used therapeutically with TBI can contribute to renal toxicity, making it difficult to separate out the radiation effect per se. Partial organ tolerance is assumed to be much higher, since it is

well documented from surgical series that patients who have less than one functional kidney can often maintain adequate renal function. In the Mayo Clinic series of nephron-sparing surgery for RCC in a solitary kidney, most patients underwent tumor enucleation or partial nephrectomy. Details regarding the actual volume of residual kidney remaining are not provided, but late renal insufficiency occurred in fewer than 15% of cases (28).

## CLINICAL OUTCOMES AND CASE STUDIES

SBRT emerges as a potential therapeutic option for either metastatic RCC or inoperable primary or recurrent disease within the renal fossa. Using a regimen typically involving five fractions of 8 Gy without IL-2, Qian and colleagues (29) observed a 31% response rate in a cohort of 74 patients treated for primary or metastatic RCC. At Radiumhemmet, Karolinska Hospital, 50 patients with metastatic and eight patients with inoperable primary tumor were treated with SBRT between 1997 and 2003. A more detailed report is being prepared for peer-reviewed publication (Wersäll JR, Blomgren H, Lax I, et al, Personal Communication, March 2004), but selected features of the clinical observations are summarized here.

The 58 patients treated at Karolinska Hospital had 162 individual lesions. The most common fractionation schemes were 30 to 40 Gy in two to four treatments, and the technique used involved multiple conformal, non-coplanar 6-mV beams (31). Most metastatic sites were in the lungs. Grades 1 to 2 toxicities were observed in 40% of patients. Follow-up has revealed sustained local control, defined as lack of in-field disease progression, in 90% of cases at a median follow-up time of 37 months. In 48 (30%) of 162 treated metastatic sites, a complete response was seen after 3 to 36 months. Thirty-five (22%) of 162 lesions sites showed a partial response of more than 50% after 3 to 12 months. Sixty-one metastases (38%) showed growth inhibition without a significant volume reduction.

## Case Study: Stereotactic Body Radiation Therapy for Carcinoma in a Solitary Kidney

A 55-year-old woman had had a right nephrectomy at age 2 because of a congenital malformation. She had experienced repeated renal infections in her remaining kidney throughout her early childhood until menarche. Thereafter she maintained generally good health until she presented with severe abdominal pain. A computed tomography (CT) scan of the abdomen revealed a 2-cm tumor in the left kidney.

The patient was managed conservatively initially, but a repeated CT scan 6 months later indicated that the tumor had increased in size to 3.5 cm. A positron emission tomography (PET) scan was strongly positive at the site corresponding to the tumor seen on CT scan. A core needle biopsy proved the lesion to be a grade I clear cell carcinoma. The patient declined partial nephrectomy but consented to receive SBRT as primary therapy.

Figure 15.1 illustrates the lesion as seen on the planning CT image and the isodose distributions used for the plan. Three fractions of 10 Gy were given, using a five-field beam arrangement. The dose was prescribed to the 65% isodose line, and 6-MV photons were used. Mean dose to the uninvolved portion of the left kidney was 4.6 Gy per fraction. It should be noted that a large proportion of the gross tumor volume (GTV) actually received a dose in excess of 15 Gy per fraction.

Follow-up imaging studies revealed no residual abnormality on PET scan 9 months later. The most recent CT scan, obtained 2 years and 8 months after treatment, revealed a residual irregularity in the left kidney, unchanged in size. The PET scan remained negative, and no other sites of disease have developed. Throughout the entire time from pretreatment until the most recent follow-up visit, the serum creatinine level has remained normal, and the patient has continued to feel well.

## Case Study: Repeated Stereotactic Body Radiation Therapy for First and Second Loco-Regional Recurrence of Renal Cell Carcinoma

A 70-year-old man had undergone right nephrectomy for renal cell carcinoma 7 years previously. A routine follow-up imaging study revealed a large (5 × 4 cm) tumor recurrence in the suprarenal fossa, essentially replacing the right adrenal gland, and an additional 1-cm regional lymph node. The recurrent disease was found to be unresectable in view of its relationship to nearby major blood vessels. The patient was offered SBRT as salvage therapy.

Figure 15.2 illustrates the GTV, planning target volume (PTV), and the isodose distributions used for the plan. Four fractions of 8 Gy were given, using a similar five-field beam arrangement as the previous case. The dose was likewise prescribed to a relatively low isodose line,

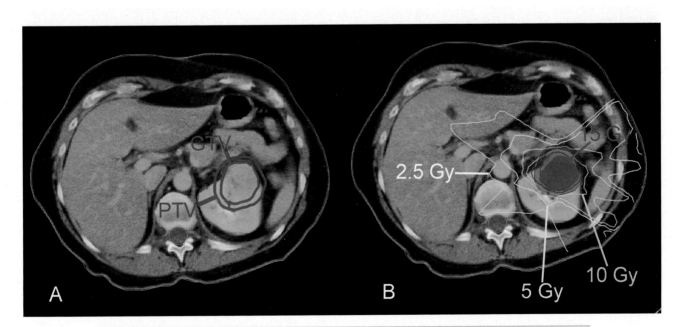

**FIGURE 15.1. A:** Axial planning computed tomography images of the gross tumor volume (GTV) and planning target volume (PTV). **B:** Isodose distribution at the same level, indicating the prescription dose per fraction, 10 Gy, and the outline of the selected other isodose contours. The PTV is shaded in blue in **B,** and the central "hotspot" region inside the PTV that received more than 15 Gy per fraction is shaded in red.

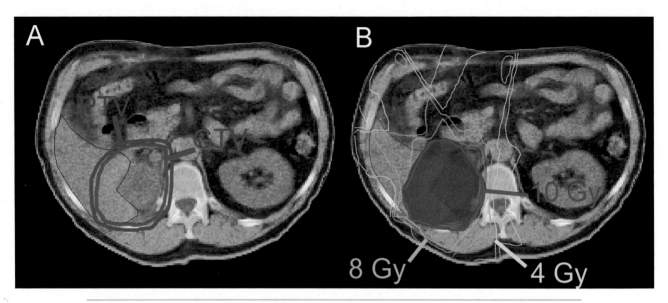

**FIGURE 15.2.** **A:** Axial planning computed tomography images of the gross tumor volume (GTV) and planning target volume (PTV). **B:** Isodose distribution at the same level, indicating the prescription dose per fraction, 8 Gy, and the outline of the selected other isodose contours. The PTV is shaded in blue in **B**, and the central "hotspot" region inside the PTV that received more than 10 Gy per fraction is shaded in red.

such that a substantial percentage of the PTV received more than 10 Gy per fraction. Less than 25% of the liver received more than 2 Gy per fraction.

The patient was followed with CT scans every 3 to 4 months. Within the first 5 years after SBRT, the volume of the radiographic abnormality decreased from the pre-treatment cross-sectional dimensions of 5 × 4 cm to 2.7 × 1.7 cm. No new sites of disease were detected. However, nearly 6 years after the SBRT, the tumor increased to a cross-sectional dimension of 5 × 2 cm. The local recur-

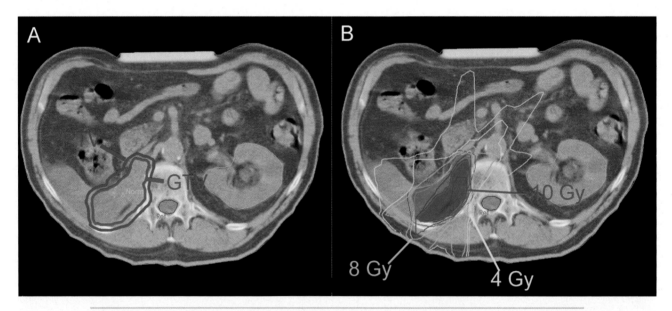

**FIGURE 15.3.** **A:** Axial planning computed tomography images of the gross tumor volume (GTV) and planning target volume (PTV) of the secondary recurrence. **B:** Isodose distribution at the same level, indicating the prescription dose per fraction, 8 Gy, and the outline of selected other isodose contours. The PTV is shaded in blue in **B,** and the central "hotspot" region inside the PTV that received more than 10 Gy per fraction is shaded in red as in the previous figure. Note that the maximum point dose to the spinal cord was less than 4 Gy per fraction during each course of stereotactic body radiation therapy.

rence within the previously irradiated volume was now enhancing with contrast on the CT scan and was clearly expanding in size rapidly. The patient was offered a second course of SBRT as salvage therapy.

Figure 15.3 illustrates the GTV, PTV, and the isodose distributions used for the plan. The reirradiation involved a similar beam arrangement and identical prescription dose schedule. Four fractions of 8 Gy were given, using a similar five-field beam arrangement as the previous case. The dose was again prescribed to an isodose line equal to approximately 65% of the maximum point dose. As indicated in the figure, most of the PTV actually received more than 10 Gy per fraction. Less than 25% of the liver received more than 2 Gy per fraction.

After the second course of SBRT, follow-up CT scans were obtained every few months. At the most recent visit, nearly 1 year after the second course of SBRT, the residual radiographic abnormality was unchanged in size. At no time has the patient experienced any side effects from SBRT despite the high cumulative total dose administered. No other sites of recurrent disease have yet emerged.

## REFERENCES

1. Pisani P, Bray F, Parkin DM. Estimates of the world-wide prevalence of cancer for 25 sites in the adult population. *Int J Cancer* 2002;97:72–81.
2. Jemal A, Murray T, Samuels A, et al. Cancer statistics, 2003. *CA Cancer J Clin* 2003;53:5–26.
3. Rabinovitch RA, Zelefsky MJ, Gaynor JJ, et al. Patterns of failure following surgical resection of renal cell carcinoma: implications for adjuvant local and systemic therapy. *J Clin Oncol* 1994;12:206–212.
4. Fyfe G, Fisher RI, Rosenberg SA, et al. Results of treatment of 255 patients with metastatic renal cell carcinoma who received high-dose recombinant interleukin-2 therapy. *J Clin Oncol* 1995;13:688–696.
5. Clark JI, Atkins MB, Urba WJ, et al. Adjuvant high-dose bolus interleukin-2 for patients with high-risk renal cell carcinoma: a cytokine working group randomized trial. *J Clin Oncol* 2003;21:3133–3140.
6. Yang JC, Sherry RM, Steinberg SM, et al. Randomized study of high-dose and low-dose interleukin-2 in patients with metastatic renal cancer. *J Clin Oncol* 2003;21:3127–3132.
7. Yang JC, Haworth L, Sherry RM, et al. A randomized trial of bevacizumab, an anti-vascular endothelial growth factor antibody, for metastatic renal cancer. *N Engl J Med* 2003;349:427–434.
8. Flanigan RC, Salmon SE, Blumenstein BA, et al. Nephrectomy followed by interferon alfa-2b compared with interferon alfa-2b alone for metastatic renal-cell cancer. *N Engl J Med* 2001;345:1655–1659.
9. Leith JT, Cook S, Chougule P, et al. Intrinsic and extrinsic characteristics of human tumors relevant to radiosurgery: comparative cellular radiosensitivity and hypoxic percentages. *Acta Neurochir Suppl (Wien)* 1994;62:18–27.
10. Schoggl A, Kitz K, Ertl A, et al. Gamma-knife radiosurgery for brain metastases of renal cell carcinoma: results in 23 patients. *Acta Neurochir (Wien)* 1998;140:549–555..
11. Lagerwaard FJ, Levendag PC, Nowak PJ, et al. Identification of prognostic factors in patients with brain metastases: a review of 1292 patients. *Int J Radiat Oncol Biol Phys* 1999;43:795–803.
12. Amendola BE, Wolf AL, Coy SR, et al. Brain metastases in renal cell carcinoma: management with gamma knife radiosurgery. *Cancer J* 2000;6:372–376.
13. Goyal LK, Suh JH, Reddy CA, et al. The role of whole brain radiotherapy and stereotactic radiosurgery on brain metastases from renal cell carcinoma. *Int J Radiat Oncol Biol Phys* 2000;47:1007–1012.
14. Brown PD, Brown CA, Pollock BE, et al. Stereotactic radiosurgery for patients with "radioresistant" brain metastases. *Neurosurgery* 2002;51:656–665.
15. Sheehan JP, Sun MH, Kondziolka D, et al. Radiosurgery in patients with renal cell carcinoma metastasis to the brain: long-term outcomes and prognostic factors influencing survival and local tumor control. *J Neurosurg* 2003;98:342–329.
16. Cannady SB, Cavanaugh KA, Lee SY, et al. Results of whole brain radiotherapy and recursive partitioning analysis in patients with brain metastases from renal cell carcinoma: a retrospective study. *Int J Radiat Oncol Biol Phys* 2004;58:253–258.
17. Culine S, Bekradda M, Kramar A, et al. Prognostic factors for survival in patients with brain metastases from renal cell carcinoma. *Cancer* 1998;83:2548–2553.
18. Gaspar L, Scott C, Rotman M, et al. Recursive partitioning analysis (RPA) of prognostic factors in three Radiation Therapy Oncology Group (RTOG) brain metastases trials. *Int J Radiat Oncol Biol Phys* 1997;37:745–751.
19. Huguenin PU, Kieser S, Glanzmann C, et al. Radiotherapy for metastatic carcinomas of the kidney or melanomas: an analysis using palliative end points. *Int J Radiat Oncol Biol Phys* 1998;41:401–405.
20. DiBiase SJ, Valicenti RK, Schultz D, et al. Palliative irradiation for focally symptomatic metastatic renal cell carcinoma: support for dose escalation based on a biological model. *J Urol* 1997;158[Pt 1]:746–749.
21. Wilson D, Hiller L, Gray L, et al. The effect of biological effective dose on time to symptom progression in metastatic renal cell carcinoma. *Clin Oncol (R Coll Radiol)* 2003;15:400–407.
22. Chakrabarty A, Hillman GG, Maughan RL, et al. Radiation therapy enhances the therapeutic effect of immunotherapy on pulmonary metastases in a murine renal adenocarcinoma model. *In Vivo* 1994;8:25–31.
23. Redman BG, Hillman GG, Flaherty L, et al. Phase II trial of sequential radiation and interleukin 2 in the treatment of patients with metastatic renal cell carcinoma. *Clin Cancer Res* 1998;4:283–286.
24. Dent P, Yacoub A, Contessa J, et al. Stress and radiation-induced activation of multiple intracellular signaling pathways. *Radiat Res* 2003;159:283–300.
25. Indaram AV, Visvalingam V, Locke M, et al. Mucosal cytokine production in radiation-induced proctosigmoiditis compared with inflammatory bowel disease. *Am J Gastroenterol* 2000;95:1221–1225.
26. MacManus MP, Harte RJ, Stranex S. Spontaneous regression of metastatic renal cell carcinoma following palliative irradiation of the primary tumour. *Ir J Med Sci* 1994;163:461–463.
27. Borg M, Hughes T, Horvath N, et al. Renal toxicity after total body irradiation. *Int J Radiat Oncol Biol Phys* 2002;54:1165–1173.
28. Ghavamian R, Cheville JC, Lohse CM, et al. Renal cell carcinoma in the solitary kidney: an analysis of complications and outcome after nephron sparing surgery. *J Urol* 2002;168:454–459.
29. Qian G, Lowry J, Silverman P, et al. Stereotactic extra-cranial radiosurgery for renal cell carcinoma. *Int J Radiat Oncol Biol Phys* 2003;57[Suppl 2]:S283.
30. Lax I, Blomgren H, Naslund I, et al. Stereotactic radiotherapy of malignancies in the abdomen: methodological aspects. *Acta Oncol* 1994;33:677–683.
31. Kavolius JP, Mastorakos DP, Pavlovich C, et al. Resection of metastatic renal cell carcinoma. *J Clin Oncol* 1998;16:2261–2266.
32. Friedel G, Hurtgen M, Penzenstadler M, et al. Resection of pulmonary metastases from renal cell carcinoma. *Anticancer Res* 1999;19:1593–1596.
33. van der Poel HG, Roukema JA, Horenblas S, et al. Metastasectomy in renal cell carcinoma: a multicenter retrospective analysis. *Eur Urol* 1999;35:197–203.
34. Csekeo A, Fawzi Sel-T. Surgical treatment for metastatic renal cell tumors of the lung [in Hungarian]. *Magy Seb* 2002;55:73–76.
35. Loizzi M, Sollitto F, Sardelli P, et al. Endothoracic nodules in patients who under-went nephrectomy for renal cell carcinoma: results of surgical resection. *Minerva Med* 2003;94:103–110.
36. Alves A, Adam R, Majno P, et al. Hepatic resection for metastatic renal tumors: is it worthwhile? *Ann Surg Oncol* 2003;10:705–710.

# Stereotactic Body Radiation Therapy for Retroperitoneal and Pelvic Tumors

*John M. Buatti, Sanford L. Meeks, Terese L. Howes*

## INTRODUCTION

High-precision extracranial radiation delivery is challenging, because the target position can shift relative to bony anatomy between the time of image acquisition and the time of treatment. Our group at the University of Iowa has investigated and implemented the use of optically guided three-dimensional (3D) ultrasound for high-precision radiation delivery to extracranial sites (1–3). We present here illustrative cases for which the system was used in the treatment of tumors in the retroperitoneum and pelvis.

## Case Example 1: Metastatic Melanoma in the Psoas Muscle

An 80-year-old hypertensive man with a history of prostate cancer status post prostatectomy and squamous cell skin cancer at the left elbow was diagnosed with a T4 N0 M0 amelanotic melanoma on his right back region. After surgical resection and sentinel lymph node biopsy of the right inguinal node, he received interferon therapy for 6 months with two breaks and subsequent discontinuation secondary to toxicity. Metastatic disease was noted 2 years after diagnosis via an abnormal positron emission tomography (PET) scan. The PET scan revealed two areas of concern; one in the left upper lung lobe and the second in the left posterior abdominal region. Computed tomography (CT) scan of the chest, abdomen, and pelvis confirmed the presence of a lung nodule and a ring-enhancing lesion within the left psoas muscle. A biopsy of the lesion within the psoas muscle was attempted, but was nondiagnostic. Therefore, the patient underwent resection of the left upper lobe lung lesion via thoracoscopic apical segmentectomy, and the tumor proved to be a ma-

Department of Radiation Oncology, Carver College of Medicine, University of Iowa, Iowa City, IA 52242

lignant spindle cell neoplasm consistent with metastatic disease of his skin primary.

The patient had no further treatment for 2 months and then returned for a repeated CT scan of the chest, abdomen, and pelvis. The lung lesion was no longer present, consistent with surgical removal. However, the lesion within the left psoas muscle had increased in size to $2.0 \times 2.0$ cm. Salvage options were discussed including standard external beam radiation therapy versus stereotactic body radiation therapy (SBRT), and the patient elected to receive the latter.

## Case Example 2: Recurrent Sacral Chordoma

An 82-year-old man with a medical history including atrial fibrillation, neurogenic bladder with recurrent urosepsis, and hypothyroidism presented nearly 5 years previously with lower back pain. Magnetic resonance imaging (MRI) imaging revealed a bulky soft-tissue mass involving the lower sacrum from S-2 to the coccyx with encasement of several sacral nerves on the left and displacement of sacral nerves on the right. Biopsies revealed a dedifferentiated chordoma. Resection was then performed, and postoperative radiation therapy to a dose of 70 Gy provided.

Tumor recurrence was noted with a second surgery performed 6 months after the initial surgery. Five months after the second surgery, the mass had recurred and measured $3 \times 9 \times 14$ cm. The patient underwent multiple direct puncture ablations with ethanol and phenol under CT guidance, and a partial response was noted via MRI imaging. However, regrowth occurred, and the patient was then referred to our institution.

The patient desired palliation of his severe pelvic pain, which required high doses of narcotic analgesics. On examination, the patient was bedridden, and any movement resulted in severe pain. He was incontinent of both bladder and bowel. Minimal strength of the lower extremities was noted, however, examination was difficult due to the patient's pain level. Due to the patient's previous history of radiation in this area, his multiple resection procedures, and his refractory pain, the option of SBRT was discussed. The risks of treatment-related injury to the surrounding organs and nerves were acknowledged, and the patient elected to receive treatment.

## METHODS OF TREATMENT SETUP AND DELIVERY

### Ultrasound- and Optical-guided Localization

While the initial stereotactic systems for optical-guided radiotherapy provide submillimeter localization accuracy, they were limited to intracranial therapy (5–7). Outside of the cranium, soft-tissue targets can move relative to rigid fixation points (e.g., bone structures) between the times of image acquisition, treatment planning, and treatment delivery. Therefore, real-time imaging is required to establish extracranial stereotactic localization of the lesion at the time of treatment delivery. We have developed a system for 3D ultrasound guidance (SonArray; Zmed, Ashland, MA) to correct for these misalignments at the time of treatment.

Ultrasound was chosen because it is an inexpensive yet flexible imaging modality that can easily be adapted for use in a radiation therapy treatment room. The interpretation of two-dimensional (2D) ultrasound images is difficult, however, and can be highly dependent on the skill and expertise of the operator in manipulating the transducer and mentally transforming the 2D images into a 3D tissue structure. Much of this difficulty results from using a spatially flexible 2D imaging technique to view 3D anatomy.

Three-dimensional ultrasound reconstruction helps overcome this limitation. The position and angulation of the ultrasound probe in any arbitrary orientation is determined using an array of four infrared light-emitting diodes (IRLEDs) attached to the probe (Fig. 16.1). Similar to our system for intracranial optic guidance, charged couple device (CCD) cameras are used to determine the positions of the IRLEDs, and this information is input to the computer workstation. The position of each ultrasound pixel can then be determined using the IRLEDs, and an ultrasound volume can be reconstructed by coupling the position information with the raw ultrasound data.

In addition to building the 3D image volume, optical guidance is used to determine the absolute position of the ultrasound volume in the treatment room coordinate system. Because the relative positions of the ultrasound volume and the ultrasound probe are fixed, the knowledge of the probe position in the treatment room at the time of data acquisition is sufficient to determine the position of the image volume relative to the linear accelerator

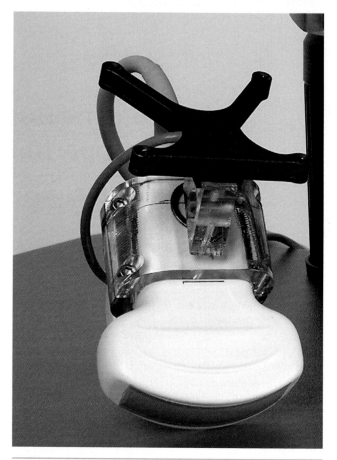

**FIGURE 16.1.** Three-dimensional ultrasound probe with attached infrared light-emitting diodes.

(linac) isocenter. The determination of the relative position of the image and probe corresponds to a calibration step that is performed at the time of system installation and at regular quality assurance testing (1).

The system used at the University of Iowa was originally developed at the University of Florida (1–5,9) and is commercially available under the trade name RadioCameras (Zmed). This system uses the Polaris position sensor unit (Northern Digital, Waterloo, Ontario, Canada) to track optically the position of either active or passive infrared markers arranged in an array to form a rigid body. Optical tracking systems have native coordinate systems that are most often located at the center of the detector. In the RadioCameras system, the Polaris is mounted in the ceiling above the linac. Therefore, the origin for the camera system is located at the ceiling of the treatment room and the axes of the coordinate system are dependent on the camera's orientation. The most logical origin for clinical use in radiotherapy is the machine isocenter, with the coordinate axes located parallel to the vertical, lateral, and longitudinal couch motions. A calibration procedure is required to transform the coordinate system from the Polaris's native coordinate system to the linac's coordinate system. This calibration uses a calibration apparatus that places passive markers at known coordinates relative to the machine isocenter. An optical measurement of the apparatus is obtained, thereby establishing a transformation matrix from camera coordinates to room coordinates. After this calibration, the position of any infrared marker in the room may be determined relative to the isocenter.

## Preclinical Testing

The accuracy of optical guided 3D ultrasound for extracranial radiosurgery patient positioning was tested using a specially designed absolute ultrasound phantom (1,3). This phantom consists of 15 echoic spheres imbedded in a tissue-equivalent nonechoic medium. The spheres are arranged in sets of five located at three different depths: 30, 60, and 130 mm. A CT scan (0.51 × 0.51 × 1.25 mm) of the phantom was acquired with a passive infrared tracking array attached to it. An infrared array was used to track the position of the phantom in the room coordinate system. Then, the ultrasound phantom was placed in the treatment vault and the ultrasound probe was fixed on top of the phantom. Coupling of the probe and the phantom was achieved with a thin layer of water. Next, a sphere within the phantom was selected as the target sphere and positioned at the room isocenter on the basis of the CT–optical tracking of the phantom.

The localization of the target sphere was then determined using our 3D ultrasound guidance system. The 3D ultrasound volume of the sphere was acquired using optical tracking as described above. The 3D ultrasound–based position of the target sphere was determined by finding the center of the sphere in the image using a circle tool placed on each of the three orthogonal ultrasound views. The target localization accuracy using the 3D ultrasound optic-guided system was thus determined by comparing its experimentally determined position to the position of the target sphere as determined from the CT scan. Complete details regarding preclinical testing, commissioning, and quality assurance of the optically guided ultrasound system can be found in the literature (1,3,8).

## Simulation and Treatment Planning

The patient is immobilized using a custom vacuum cushion as is commonly used in radiation therapy (Vac-Loc; Med-Tec, Orange City, IA). The CT is then acquired with the patient immobilized in the same position that will be used during the radiotherapy treatment in order to maintain a generally consistent position of mobile anatomy. The CT images are transferred to our 3D treatment planning system (Pinnacle3; ADAC, Milipitas, CA) where the tumor volume and normal structures of interest are delineated. A treatment plan is then designed to conform the prescription dose closely to the planning target volume (PTV),

while minimizing the dose to the nearby normal structures, typically with maximally separated noncoplanar beams.

Due to possible collisions of the gantry with the patient or the treatment couch, the available geometry for beam entrance is much more limited in SBRT planning than that for conventional radiotherapy. When the treatment couch is at its home position (0 degrees, International Electrotechnical Commission (IEC) angle convention), the gantry is capable of full rotation about the patient. As the couch is moved away from its home position, the gantry is capable of rotating approximately (±) 30 degrees from vertical, creating a cone of possible beam entrances above the patient. As a starting point, the gantry and treatment table angles are chosen to achieve maximal beam separation within this limited space of achievable treatment geometries. The planner then inspects the beam's eye views (BEVs) for each of these beams and modifies the gantry and table angles to avoid critical structures and/or minimize the projection of the PTV. Each beam is shaped to match the BEV projection of the planning target volume using a multileaf collimator (mlc) that has a 5-mm leaf resolution at isocenter (Millennium MLC-120; Varian Oncology Systems, Palo Alto, CA). The field shapes are designed with zero margin added to the BEV projection of the planning target volume, and mlc leaves at the edge of the target.

## Treatment Delivery

The day of the treatment, the patient is placed in the same immobilization cushion that was used during CT scanning. The patient is initially set up relative to isocenter using conventional laser alignment. A 3D ultrasound volume is then acquired and reconstructed in the computer workstation. The target volume and critical structure outlines, as delineated on the planning CT scans, are overlaid on the acquired ultrasound volume in relation to isocenter. The contours determined from the CT scans are then manipulated until they align with the anatomic structures on the ultrasound images. The amount of movement required to align the contours with the ultrasound images determines the magnitude of the target misregistration with isocenter based on conventional setup techniques. The target is then placed at the isocenter by tracking an infrared array attached to the treatment couch, which allows precise translation from the initial position to the 3D ultrasound–determined position. Once all of the setup information has been verified using repeated ultrasound acquisition and coregistration, treatment proceeds as planned.

## Clinical Follow-up of Example Cases

The patient with metastatic melanoma received SBRT to the left iliopsoas region. A single fraction, radiosurgery-like regimen was used to provide a dose of 24 Gy, pre-

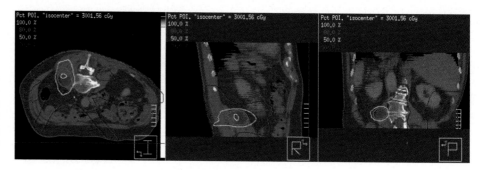

**FIGURE 16.2.** Treatment with extracranial stereotactic radiation therapy to treat metastatic disease within the left psoas muscle using an 11-field plan prescribed to the 80% isodose shell.

scribed to the 80% isodose shell (Fig. 16.2). The treatment was provided with an 11-field technique.

The patient tolerated the treatment without difficulty. Follow-up CT imaging performed 2 months after treatment delivery revealed resolution of the lesion with the left psoas muscle (Fig. 16.3). Subsequent imaging studies performed 7 months after treatment showed no evidence of recurrence within the psoas muscle. The patient later developed other sites of metastatic disease, for which both chemotherapy and palliative conventionally fractionated external beam radiotherapy were provided. He died 3 years after the initial diagnosis.

The patient with recurrent sacral chordoma received a single fraction of 15 Gy prescribed to the 88% isodose shell. Treatment was provided with an 8-field technique composed of 6- and 18-mV photon beams (Fig. 16.4). Six days after radiation therapy, the patient underwent implantation of a morphine pump and intrathecal catheter. The patient has been seen in follow-up with a vast improvement in pain control, although the relative contributions to pain control from the radiotherapy and morphine pump cannot be determined.

## DISCUSSION

SBRT is a natural extension of high-precision intracranial stereotactic radiosurgery, but it is more complex because

motion of soft-tissue targets relative to bony references between the time of image acquisition and treatment delivery is unavoidable. We have developed a system that relies on 3D ultrasound optical guidance to precisely correct for internal organ motion, and adjust the position of the target at the isocenter of the treatment. Because our image-guided system uses 3D images, it has the ability to quantify the patient's alignment in the 6 *df*. This method provides easy and precise feedback regarding the patient position based on the 3D image localization, very similar to optical systems already used for intracranial targets.

Our clinical observations illustrated by the patient vignettes treated with single-fraction SBRT to the pelvis and retroperitoneal regions reported here are demonstrative of the feasibility and acute safety of this approach. However, target movement relative to fixed bony landmarks proves to be a challenging technical aspect of treatment delivery. When PTV misalignments are corrected, one must be concerned that the high dose regions may move closer to organs at risk, hence decreasing the amount of normal-tissue sparing. This issue should be monitored clinically but can only be adequately addressed with future integration of treatment planning systems with image-guided delivery systems.

Another concern can arise with the accuracy of ultrasound localization. Our institution has investigated the question of user variability in 3D ultrasound image registration for daily prostate localization. Image registration

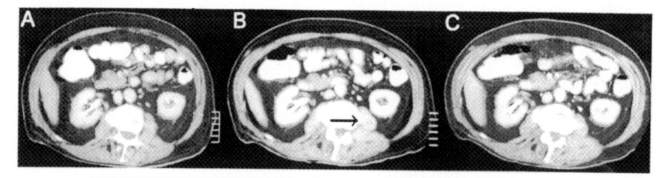

**FIGURE 16.3.** **A:** Initial computed tomography (CT) scan at time of positive positron emission tomography (PET) scan showing subtle irregularity in left psoas of uncertain significance. **B:** CT scan 2 months later, showing unequivocal enhancing lesion (*arrow*), at which time the decision was made to proceed with stereotactic body radiation therapy (SBRT). **C:** Follow-up image 2 months after SBRT showing regressing lesion in the treated volume.

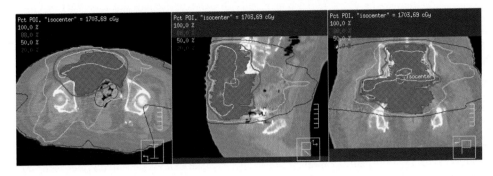

*FIGURE 16.4.* Treatment with extracranial stereotactic radiation therapy for a recurrent sacral chordoma previously treated with multiple resections and standard external beam radiation therapy. Treatment plan uses an 8-field plan prescribed to the 88% isodose shell.

was tested and compared between trained, experienced users of ultrasound with greater than 100 hours of experience to relatively inexperienced users who had received instruction in the use of ultrasound, but had less than 10 hours of experience. The standard deviation of the shift for the experienced users was 1.2 mm, 0.9 mm, and 1.4 mm in the anteroposterior, lateral, and axial directions, respectively. The standard deviation of the shift for the inexperienced users in the anteroposterior, lateral, and axial directions was 3.6 mm, 1.5 mm, and 2.9 mm, respectively. Therefore, an average difference of approximately 1.5 mm was detected when comparing trained, experienced radiation therapy users of daily ultrasound with less experienced radiation therapists. Clearly, these results indicate that appropriate therapist training is critical in the clinical implementation of image-guided radiotherapy technologies.

Methods that automate the process may alleviate some of these problems. Automated image registration algorithms have proven beneficial for multimodality image registration. Although these algorithms hold some promise for autoregistration of ultrasound to CT, ultrasound imaging's poor signal-to-noise ratio may limit their applicability. To avoid errors related to user variability, our image selection and registration process for the treatment of extracranial stereotactic radiation therapy is a collaborative effort between the radiation therapist, radiation oncologist, and physicist.

Considering the currently available technology, the degree of accuracy achieved using this technique is acceptable in properly selected patients and provides a noninvasive treatment alternative with a high level of patient satisfaction. Further investigation is required, but this technique currently offers the potential for rapid, effective treatment with low morbidity. Future improvements of the system include the ability to gate the radiation beam on the basis of internal target motion as perceived from real-time ultrasound imaging.

The application of this system has potential in treating previously irradiated volumes as well as potential as a boost therapy to areas receiving conventional radiation therapy. Eventual optimal clinical application of SBRT will undoubtedly, like intracranial radiosurgery, not only address accuracy but also require significant attention to patient selection, long-term patient follow-up, and outcome.

## REFERENCES

1. Bouchet LG, Meeks SL, Goodchild G, et al. Calibration of three-dimensional ultrasound images for image-guided radiation therapy. *Phys Med Biol* 2001;46:559–577.
2. Ryken TC, Meeks SL, Buatti JM, et al. Ultrasonic guidance for spinal extracranial radiosurgery: technique and application for metastatic spinal lesions. *Neurosurg Focus* 2001;11:1–6.
3. Bouchet LG, Meeks SL, Bova FJ, et al. 3D ultrasound image guidance for high precision extracranial radiosurgery and radiotherapy. *Radiosurgery* 2002;4:262–278.
4. Bova FJ, Buatti JM, Friedman WA, et al. The University of Florida frameless high-precision stereotactic radiotherapy system. *Int J Radiat Oncol Biol Phys* 1997;38:875–882.
5. Buatti JM, Bova FJ, Friedman WA, et al. Preliminary experience with frameless stereotactic radiotherapy. *Int J Radiat Oncol Biol Phys* 1998;42:591–599.
6. Meeks SL, Bova FJ, Wagner TH, et al. Image localization for frameless stereotactic radiotherapy. *Int J Radiat Oncol Biol Phys* 2000;46:1291–1299.
7. Ryken TC, Meeks SL, Pennington EC, et al. Initial experience with frameless stereotactic radiosurgery. *Int J Radiat Oncol Biol Phys* 2001;51:1152–1158.
8. Tome WA, Meeks SL, Orton NP, et al. Commissioning and quality assurance of an optically guided 3D ultrasound target localization system for radiotherapy. *Med Phys* 2002;29:1781–1788.
9. Tome WA, Meeks SL, Buatti JM, et al. A high-precision system for conformal intracranial radiotherapy. *Int J Radiat Oncol Biol Phys* 2000;47:1137–1143.

# Case Study

## Case Study in Prostate SBRT: The SHARP Protocol

Berit L. Madsen and Laura Jeanne Esagui

### CLINICAL PRESENTATION

A healthy 77-year-old man was noted to have a prostate-specific antigen (PSA) level of 7.2 ng/mL. A genitourinary system review revealed an International Prostate Symptom Score (IPSS) of 8/35, indicating mild obstructive symptoms, and an International Index of Erectile Function (IIEF) score of 23/25, consistent with good sexual function. Physical examination revealed no palpable abnormality in the prostate gland, and an ultrasound-guided prostate biopsy was performed. No hypoechoic areas were noted within the prostate, which was estimated to have a volume of 34 cc. Needle biopsies revealed Gleason 3+3 adenocarcinoma in 20% of cores obtained from the right lateral and right base only, representing 20% of each core. For a clinical T1c low-risk prostate cancer, the patient declined watchful waiting and desired potentially curative therapy. He was offered a choice of brachytherapy, conventionally fractionated external beam radiotherapy, or enrollment in an institutional review board (IRB)–approved clinical trial of stereotactic hypofractionated accurate radiotherapy of the prostate (SHARP). He elected to participate in the SHARP trial.

### SBRT TREATMENT PLANNING AND DOSE DELIVERY

The SHARP trial is a phase 1/2 trial of stereotactic body radiation therapy (SBRT) for prostate cancer initiated in 2000 at the Virginia Mason Medical Center. The scientific rationale for the trial is based on the estimated low $\alpha/\beta$ ratio for prostate cancer of approximately 1.5 Gy (1–3), which favors a hypofractionated schedule. The trial is offered to patients with prostate cancer with low risk of extracapsular extension by the Partin criteria (4). The five-fraction hypofractionated regimen used in this protocol is designed to achieve a biologically equivalent dose (BED) to the cancer of 78 Gy given in 2-Gy fractions. The BED to be delivered in five fractions is calculated according to a standard formula, neglecting a proliferation component:

$$BED = (nd) + \left( \frac{nd^2}{\alpha/\beta} \right)$$

where $n$ is the number of fractions and $d$ is the dose per fraction.

Assuming $\alpha/\beta = 1.5$, the $BED_{Gy1.5}$ for 78 Gy (2 Gy $\times$ 39 fractions) is $182_{Gy1.5}$. The daily dose for an equivalent course delivered in five fractions is obtained by substituting these values into the equation above:

Section of Radiation Oncology, Virginia Mason Medical Center, Seattle, WA
    98101

$$182 = (5d) + \left( \frac{5d^2}{1.5} \right)$$

The nonnegative solution for $d$ is 6.7 Gy, and patients enrolled on this trial are therefore treated with five fractions of 6.7 Gy for a total dose of 33.5 Gy.

The $\alpha/\beta$ ratio for acute effects is estimated to be approximately 10 Gy. From the general BED equation above, if two courses of treatment, each involving $n_i$ fractions of $d_i$ Gy/fraction, provide the identical BED for a given $\alpha/\beta$ ratio, then the following condition is true:

$$n_1 d_1 \left( \frac{1 + d_1}{\alpha/\beta} \right) = n_2 d_2 \left( 1 + \frac{d_2}{\alpha/\beta} \right)$$

To determine the equivalent total dose in 2-Gy fractions that provides the same acute effects in $BED_{Gy10}$, let $n_1 = 5$, $d_1 = 6.7$, and $d_2 = 2$. The resulting solution for $n_2 d_2$ is 46.6 Gy. Thus, the hypofractionated course should allow us to deliver the equivalent of a tumor dose of 78 Gy and early-responding normal tissue dose of 46.6 Gy given in conventional fractions. The significant reduction in the volume irradiated with the stereotactic technique might also reduce acute and late toxicity.

Before simulation, patients have three nonradioactive gold markers implanted into the prostate under transrectal ultrasound guidance with a standard 17-gauge biopsy needle. The cylindrical markers measure 1.2-mm diameter by 3-mm length and are placed at the apex, mid gland, and base. The position of the markers is recorded with regard to the ultrasound image of the prostate gland. To minimize prostate motion due to bowel distention, patients are instructed to follow a prescribed minimum residue diet and to take an antiflatulent medication (Phazyme 166 Maximum strength tablet) after each meal for 4 days prior and during simulation and treatment.

Patients are simulated and treated in a flex–prone position with the pelvis raised on a specially designed cushion (Fig. 16.5).

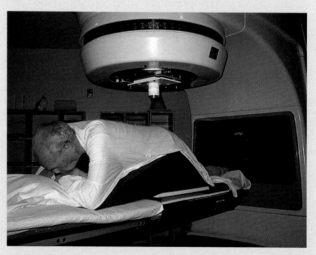

**FIGURE 16.5.** Patient treatment position on special cushion with custom cerrobend cone in place.

▶ **TABLE 16-1** Standard Field Arrangements for Stereotactic Hypofractionated Accurate Radiotherapy of the Prostate

| Beam No. | 1 | 2 | 3 | 4 | 5 | 6 |
|---|---|---|---|---|---|---|
| Gantry angle (degrees) | 70 | 290 | 110 | 210 | 250 | 150 |
| Couch angle (degrees) | 180 | 180 | 220 | 220 | 140 | 140 |
| Fractional dose at isocenter (cGy) | 134 | 134 | 134 | 67 | 134 | 67 |

SHARP, stereotactic hypofractionated accurate radiotherapy of the prostate

Following the anteroposterior (AP) and lateral scout images, a helical computed tomography (CT) scanner is used to acquire axial 10-mm slices from 300 to 30 mm superior to the most cranial gold fiducial marker. Subsequently, 3-mm-thick slices are acquired from 30 mm superior to the most cranial marker to 30 mm inferior to the most caudal marker. Finally, additional axial images are acquired at 10-mm spacing from 30 to 300 mm inferior to the most caudal marker in the prostate. In this way, the coarser images are used to define the body, while the finer images define the target. The entire scan uses a pitch of 1 and a 48- to 50-cm field of view (FOV).

Magnetic resonance imaging (MRI) can be used for target definition and fused with the CT scan based on the marker locations in the two studies. In most cases, MRI images of the prostate provide better definition of the prostate/rectum interface as well as the lateral borders of the gland. It is our policy, whenever possible, to acquire both an MRI and CT. MRI of the pelvis is acquired with a Siemens Symphony 1.5-T scanner with quantum gradients (Munich, Germany). The body phased-array coil is used with the patient in the flex–prone position on the special cushion. The sequence for the scan is a three-dimensional (3D) medic $T_2$ axial with a matrix of 256 × 205. Forty-eight slices are acquired with an 18-cm FOV and 2 -mm slice thicknesses. The MRI and CT images are easily fused on the basis of the location of the fiducial markers and bony landmarks seen in both imaging modalities.

Stereotactic treatment planning is performed with the pReference treatment planning system (Northwest Medical Physics Equipment, Lynnwood WA). Using CT and MRI images, the radiation oncologist defines the prostate, considered the clinical

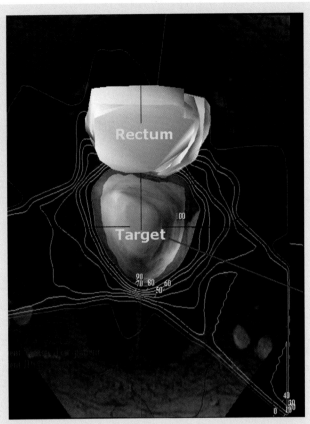

**FIGURE 16.6.** Representative isodose distribution for stereotactic hypofractionated accurate radiotherapy of the prostate.

target volume (CTV). The flex–prone position allows a set of noncoplanar beams directed in a quasi-coronal plane. A standard six-field noncoplanar beam arrangement has been developed; couch and beam angles are described in Table 16.1. A 3- to 4-mm margin is added in all directions to the block edge. Custom small-field collimators are manufactured. Dose is prescribed at the isocenter. Typical isodose distributions are illustrated in Fig. 16.6. Dose–volume histograms of rectal dose for ten recent plans are depicted in Fig. 16.7 and Table 16.2.

To ensure proper patient setup on the treatment machine, the CT coordinates of the three gold fiducial markers are entered into the Isoloc 5.2 computer program (Northwest Medical

▶ **TABLE 16-2** Dose–Volume Histogram for Rectal Volume, Ten Patients Treated with SHARP[a].

| Patient | 100% volume (cc) | 90% volume (cc) | 80% volume (cc) | 50% volume (cc) | 30% volume (cc) |
|---|---|---|---|---|---|
| Mean | 0.90 | 4.29 | 6.04 | 11.5 | 18.16 |
| SD | 1.18 | 3.15 | 3.93 | 6.83 | 11.5 |

SHARP, stereotactic hypofractionated accurate radiotherapy of the prostate.
[a] Rectal volume is defined as the anterior half of the solid organ from the anus to the bottom of the sacroiliac joint.

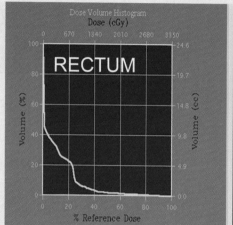 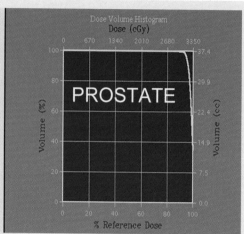

**FIGURE 16.3.** Typical dose–volume histogram for prostate and rectum.

Physics Equipment). Isoloc translates the position of fiducial markers from one coordinate system to another (for example CT system to linear accelerator system). Prior to each treatment, a verification simulation on the linear accelerator is performed. Orthogonal portal images are acquired and used to analyze the position of the fiducial markers. The marker locations are compared with their expected location with reference to the isocenter, and the necessary treatment table shifts are determined and accomplished to ensure proper beam orientations. A typical stereotactic treatment with standard port films takes approximately 60 minutes. With electronic portal imaging, treatment time can be reduced to 20 to 40 minutes.

## DISCUSSION

The patient tolerated SHARP well. He experienced mild urinary urgency and dysuria within 2 weeks of treatment that resolved completely soon thereafter. He has had no rectal complaints and continues to have erections. Nine months after treatment, the PSA level decreased to 0.4 ng/mL.

We have documented intrafraction movement with the SHARP technique by studying patients on a standard fluoroscopy simulator at 6-minute intervals and by evaluating marker position on portal images prior and subsequent to treatment (5). Analysis of portal images revealed a mean absolute prostate movement of 2.0 mm (superior/inferior), 1.9 mm (anterior/posterior), and 1.4 mm (right/left) with maximum standard deviation of 2.0. Analysis of radiographs at 6-minute intervals showed the greatest average prostate motion between 0 and 6 minutes: 1.5 mm (superior/inferior), 1.4 mm (anterior/posterior), and 0.4 mm (right/left). Beyond 6 minutes, the movements decreased to 0.4, 0.9, and 0.8 mm, respectively. Bony landmark

motion averaged 0.9 mm (superior/inferior), 0.9 mm (anterior/posterior), and 0.4 mm (right/left) between 0 and 6 minutes, decreasing to less than 0.5 mm in any direction beyond 6 minutes. Because most patient and organ movement occurs early after patients are positioned, a settling-in period is advisable prior to simulation and treatment.

Thirty-six patients have been treated on the ongoing SHARP protocol. The average age is 69 years, median follow-up is 12 months. We have seen an average rise in American Urologic Association symptom scale score of 5 patients during the first month of follow-up with return to baseline within 3 months after treatment. There has been no late urinary toxicity. We have seen less than 3% grade 2 late gastrointestinal toxicity. Preliminary analysis of the PSA responses has been very encouraging; however, longer follow-up is required to assess the durability of the tumor control effect.

## References

1. Duchesne GM, Peters LJ. What is the $\alpha/\beta$ ratio for prostate cancer? Rationale for hypofractionated high-dose rate brachytherapy. *Int J Radiat Oncol Biol Phys* 1999;44:747–748.
2. Fowler J, Chapell R, Ritter M. Is $\alpha/\beta$ for prostate tumors really low? *Int J Radiat Oncol Biol Phys* 2001;50:1021–1031.
3. Brenner DJ, Hall EJ. Fractionation and protraction for radiotherapy of prostate carcinoma. *Int J Radiat Oncol Biol Phys* 1999;43:1095–1101.
4. Partin AW, Kazan MW, Subong EN, et al. Combination of prostate specific antigen, clinical stage, and Gleason score to predict pathologic stage of localized prostate cancer; a multi-institutional update. *JAMA* 1997;277:1445–1451.
5. Madsen B, Hsi A, Pham H, et al. Intrafractional stability of the prostate using a stereotactic radiotherapy technique. *Intl J Radiat Oncol Biol Phys* 2003; 57(5):1285–1291.

# Stereotactic Body Radiation Therapy for Paraspinal Tumors

*Yoshiya Yamada and *Michael Lovelock*

## INTRODUCTION

Tumors of the spine and paraspinal region are among the most common clinical problems in oncology. Primary tumors of the spine are rare, and the vast majority of paraspinal malignancies are metastases (1). Approximately 95% of spinal metastases are extradural. In a study of 2,000 patients with bony metastases, nearly 70% had vertebral body metastases (2). Approximately 18,000 new cases of spinal metastases are diagnosed in North America every year (3), affecting more than 100,000 patients per year (4).

Paraspinal tumors are typically symptomatic. Prominent pain is present in 90% of patients (5). Motor weakness, paraesthesia, and myelopathy are also significant problems associated with spinal tumors. Despite the enormity of the clinical problem associated with these lesions, there is no consensus for management. A recently presented abstract outlining a randomized trial of standard radiotherapy with or without decompressive surgery found a significant palliative benefit for surgery followed by radiation (6). However, patients will often present after having failed multiple therapies including, surgery, radiation, and chemotherapy. Patients who for medical or other reasons are not candidates for surgery are also common problems for the radiation oncologist when the spinal cord is in close proximity to the lesion(s). In some cases, incomplete resections leaving behind gross residual disease require radiation doses higher than thought safe for the spinal cord to absorb. In the case of primary extradural spinal malignancies with gross disease, typical histologies such as sarcomas often require radiation doses higher than the tolerance of the spinal cord.

Whether recurrent primary or metastatic disease, these patients present a common and vexing dilemma.

## SPINAL CORD TOLERANCE TO RADIOTHERAPY

Radiation-induced myelitis is one of the most dreaded complications related to radiation therapy. The true tolerance of the spinal cord to radiation is not known. The TD 5/5 (the dose at which there is a 5% probability of myelitis necrosis at 5 years from treatment) for 5-cm, 10-cm, and 20-cm lengths of the spinal cord in standard fractionation has been estimated by Emami et al. (7) as 5,000 cGy, 5,000 cGy, and 4,700 cGy, respectively. The TD 50/5 (dose at which there is a 50% probability of myelitis necrosis at 5 years) is 7,000 cGy in standard fractionation for 5- and 10-cm segments of the cord (7). These dose levels are estimates based upon extrapolations of data sets that stretch back to 1948 (8). Despite the inexact science behind the derivation of the dose tolerances suggested by Emami et al. (7), these estimations have been widely adopted in clinical practice. To minimize the risk of spinal cord necrosis, the radiation tolerance with standard fractionation has been traditionally stated to be 45 to 50 Gy.

A survey of the medical literature suggests that the TD 5/5 of 45 Gy is likely a conservative estimate of cord tolerance. The University of Florida has reported that out of 1,112 evaluable cases, only two patients (0.18%) experienced myelitis. Patients who received 40 to 45 Gy ($N = 471$) to the cord did not develop myelitis. However, in the 45- to 50-Gy cohort, ($N = 14$) two patients developed myelitis, even though the dose to the cord was calculated to be less than 180 cGy per fraction. In patients who received 50 to 55 Gy ($N = 75$) to the cord, no patients developed myelitis.

Lindstadt et al. (9) reported no cases of myelitis when patients with primary brainstem gliomas were irradiated to a median dose of 7,200 cGy using 100 cGy twice a day

Departments of Radiation Oncology and *Medical Physics, Memorial Sloan Kettering Cancer Center, New York, NY 10021

hyperfractionation, suggesting that smaller fraction sizes may increase cord tolerance. Five cases of myelitis were reported in the analysis of Macbeth et al. (10) of 1,048 patients in the United Kingdom Medical Research Council Randomized Control Trials (UK MRC RCT) of lung cancer. For patients given significantly hypofractionated dose schedules of 10 Gy × 1 or 8.5 Gy × 2, three cases of myelitis were found (N = 524 patients). Two cases of myelitis were noted in the cohort treated with one of the following schedules: 4.5 Gy × 6, 5 Gy × 6, 3 Gy × 10, 3 Gy × 13 (N = 153 patients) (10). In a report of 144 cases in which the cord dose exceeded 56 Gy, one patient developed myelitis (60 Gy/30 to an 8-cm segment) (11). A retrospective review of patients treated at the Princess Margaret Hospital between 1955 and 1985 found 35 patients who developed radiation myelitis. All patients who experienced myelopathy had at least 8 cm of cord irradiated. Twenty-four patients developed myelitis after their initial course of treatment, 11 had repeated radiotherapy, and four patients had received hyperfractionation. No case of radiation myelopathy was observed over a period of 30 years (over 6,000 treatments), when up to 50 Gy was administered to the cord in daily single (1.8–2 Gy) fractions (12).

Animal data indicate that the spinal cord repairs radiation-induced damage over time. Ang et al. (13) repeated radiation of the spinal cord in 56 Rhesus monkeys. All the animals initially were irradiated to 44 Gy in 11 fractions. The animals were further irradiated 1 or 2 years later with 57.2 Gy in 26 fractions or 66 Gy in 30 fractions. Of the 16 animals who received 101.2 Gy in total over 1 year, two developed myelopathy. One of 24 animals that received 101 to 110 Gy over a 2-year period developed myelopathy. Of the 16 animals who were reirradiated after a 3-year interval, only one developed myelopathy. In a preliminary study, three of 16 animals that received 70.4 Gy developed myelitis, while three of the six animals that received 77 Gy and seven of eight animals that received 83.6 Gy developed myelitis. On the basis of these data, the authors concluded that 76%, 85%, and 101% of the radiation damage induced by the initial radiation had undergone repair at 1, 2, and 3 years after the initial radiation had been administered. The authors of this paper suggest that if the initial cord dose was 45 Gy, then repeated doses up to 66 to 68 Gy in 2-Gy fractions to the cord would be safely tolerated, provided sufficient time for repair of radiation effects (13). Observations in repeatedly irradiated rat spinal cords also support the ability of the spinal cord to repair radiation-induced injury over time (14,15).

After performing an exhaustive review of the medical literature, Schultheiss et al. (16) suggest that the actual 5% risk of myelopathy likely lies between 57 and 60 Gy in standard fractionation (Table 17.1.). Clinical factors such as the consequences of underdosing a tumor near the spinal cord must also be taken into account when determining an acceptable dose to the cord. At our institution,

▶ **TABLE 17.1** Reported Incidence of Myelopathy.

| Authors (Reference No.) | Dose | Incidence |
|---|---|---|
| Eichhorn 1972 (29) | 2.45 Gy × 27 | 8/46 |
| | 2.45 Gy × 18 + 3.16 Gy × 9 | 5/22 |
| | 7.6 Gy × 1 + 2.9 Gy × 9 | 2/22 |
| Choi 1980 (30) | 3 Gy × 15 | 0/16 |
| Hazra 1974 (31) | 3 Gy × 15 | 0/75 |
| Abramson 1973 (32) | 4 Gy × 10 | 4/103 |
| Fitzgerald 1982 (33) | 4 Gy × 10 | 6/45 |
| Miller 1977 (34) | 4 Gy × 10 | 4/97 |
| Madden 1979 (35) | 4 Gy × 10 | 1/43 |
| Guthrie 1973 (36) | 4 Gy × 10 | 0/42 |
| | 3 Gy × 20 | 0/32 |
| Dische 1981 (37) | 5.8 Gy × 6 | 8/71 |
| Hatlevoll 1983 (38) | 6 Gy × 3 + 4 Gy × 5 | 43% |

From Schultheiss TE, Kun LE, Ang KK, et al. Radiation response of the central nervous system. *Int J Radiat Oncol Biol Phys* 1995;31: 1093–1112, with permission.

we have set the maximum cord dose to be 54 Gy in standard fractionation, in the absence of chemotherapy or a history of radiation. In terms of single-fraction therapy, we recommend that the maximum cord dose be kept below 10 Gy. We do not assume radiation repair when repeating radiation over the spinal cord. Although these dose limits are likely conservative estimates of true cord tolerance, given the catastrophic nature of myelitis, we recommend caution in irradiating the spinal cord above these levels.

## PATIENT SETUP AND IMMOBILIZATION

An essential requirement for sparing the spinal cord is reliable and accurate setup. A variety of approaches has been used to setup and immobilize paraspinal patients. Hamilton et al. (17) adopted an approach similar to that used for intracranial stereotactic radiosurgery in which an external reference system is rigidly attached to the patient's bony anatomy. Patients undergo a procedure using either general or local anesthesia to affix two clamps to the spinous processes of vertebral segments just above and below the involved segment. A 2-cm incision is required for each clamp. The patient, lying prone in the stereotactic body frame, is immobilized by attaching the two clamps to rigid arms that form part of the frame. The patient undergoes computed tomography (CT) scanning the frame, the target is delineated, and the isocenter is located within the coordinate system of the frame. The still-immobilized patient is treated by transferring the frame to the linear accelerator (linac) couch. With careful alignment of the frame at the CT unit and the linac, the overall treatment accuracy is 1.4 to 2 mm. Radiographs of the bone and clamps taken before and after treatment show that the system effectively immobilizes the target during treatment.

A noninvasive stereotactic body frame developed by Lax et al. (18) to treat a variety of sites may also be used to treat paraspinal tumors. The frame, which is U-shaped in cross-section, extends from above the patient's head to the thighs. It has fiducial systems that can be visualized in CT or magnetic resonance imaging (MRI) scans, and scales along the principal axes that facilitate setup using the room lasers. Patient setup and immobilization are achieved with a vacuum pillow that is held in place by the frame and is formed to the patient's body contours over a large area. The patient lies supine on the vacuum cushion with the arms placed above the head. For paraspinal sites, the initial method of use of the body frame was stereotactic in that the bony target was located in the frame's coordinate system, and the setup at the linac based on the isocenter's frame coordinates. The reproducibility of the target in the stereotactic coordinates was measured using repeat CT scans. For a variety of target types, including soft tissue, the target position was within 5 mm of the planned position in the transverse direction over 95% of the time (19). In the longitudinal direction, the target was within 8 mm over 89% of the time, although this would have been influenced by the 10-mm CT slice thickness used. Others have used this type of frame (20), and other body frames are in use (21), as it is further discussed in Chapters 7 and 9.

At Memorial Sloan Kettering Cancer Center (MSKCC), the Memorial Stereotactic Body Frame (MSBF) (22) was developed that uses a different method to constrain the patient, especially in the lateral direction. In addition to a 210-cm-long U-shaped frame equipped with a CT fiducial system and used to support a vacuum cushion, four pressure plates, each 10 cm in the anteroposterior direction and 5-cm in the superoinferior direction, can be positioned by varying their lateral insertion depth. The plates are adjusted during the initial patient setup such that they press firmly on the patient's bony anatomy, such as the lateral pelvic bones, and the lateral ribs under the arms. Additional fixation is provided by an arch that attaches to the MSBF and has two vertical pressure plates. These are positioned to press firmly on the anterior aspect of the hips. The MSBF is used with a tilt table that allows patients to quickly and easily step into the MSBF, which is then returned to its horizontal position. The pressure plates and hip-restraining arch are all set to the positions recorded during the initial setup. Setup for treatment takes only a few minutes. Patients are scanned before each treatment on a CT unit that has been installed in the same room as the linac. This facilitates a simple, rapid couch-to-couch transfer of the MSBF and patient. In 33 pretreatment scans of six patients, the mean positioning error, the systematic error, and the random error of a bony target in the lateral, anteroposterior, and superoin-

ferior directions were found to be (in mm) $2.3 \pm 1.6 \pm 1.6$, $0.1 \pm 2.0 \pm 0.$, and $0.2 \pm 2.4 \pm 1.8$, respectively.

When used in a purely stereotactic fashion, the use of a noninvasive body frame cannot guarantee that the target is positioned within the tight tolerances required to avoid cord irradiation. As noted, outliers occur, which are unacceptable in single- or hypofractionated treatments. For this reason, image guidance is advisable at the time of treatment. When using the MSBF, the pretreatment CT scan is sent via digital imaging and communication in medicine (DICOM) to a CT–CT registration program. The setup error of the patient's bony anatomy with respect to the body frame is determined automatically using the mutual information maximization method. If the shift of the bony anatomy is greater than 2 mm in any direction, a couch correction is implemented.

Several specialized treatment machines are now available that greatly simplify achieving a precise setup. The Novalis (BrainLAB, Westchester, IL), a 6-mV linac that comes equipped with a micromultileaf collimator, uses dual in-room x-ray units and amorphous silicon imagers to verify isocenter position in real time by providing orthogonal radiographs of patients in the treatment position. Registration software capable of automatically generating digitally reconstructed radiographs (DRRs) makes it possible to achieve an accurate initial setup. The CyberKnife (Accuray, Sunnyvale, CA) includes a system based on a miniature linac mounted on a robotic arm also features in-room x-ray units. Using fiducial markers implanted into the spine, this unit can potentially track the marker positions as a patient breathes. This novel approach may eventually make patient immobilization unnecessary, at least during regular breathing. Tomotherapy, provided by a linac mounted in a fashion similar to a CT scanner, with its ability to acquire three-dimensional (3D) pretreatment images of the bony anatomy is potentially well suited for precise setup.

In parallel with the development of new machines have been improvements to linacs that are more conventional and CT scanners. Faster CT scanners have made possible CT studies with slice spacing of 2 mm or less. This allows DRRs of sufficient quality to allow resolution of vertebral bodies and intervertebral spaces. Amorphous silicon portal imagers, and their associated image processing software, have made it possible to create portal images in which individual vertebral bodies can be resolved, even in the largest of patients (Fig. 17.1). What remains is to provide a means of immobilizing patients in the position in which they were initially scanned. At MSKCC, an immobilization cradle (the memorial body cradle [MBC]) was developed expressly for image-guided setup using orthogonal portal images (Fig. 17.2). It was designed specifically to facilitate the rapid setup and immobilization of paraspinal patients to a setup error tolerance of 2 mm or less. Other than the scales along the three principal direc-

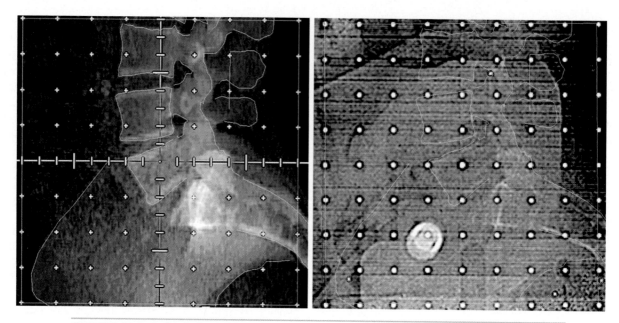

**FIGURE 17.1.** **Left:** The lateral digitally reconstructed radiograph of an obese patient. The computed tomography image thickness and slice spacing were set to 2 mm to improve longitudinal resolution, allowing good resolution of each vertebra. The blue and yellow lines are drawn on separate layers in the image. They are used to determine the setup error by separately overlaying the blue and yellow outlines on the grid and anatomical features respectively seen in the portal image. **Right:** The corresponding portal image. The yellow outlines have been manually shifted until they best match the image. The software reported a required isocenter shift of 1 mm in the anterior direction.

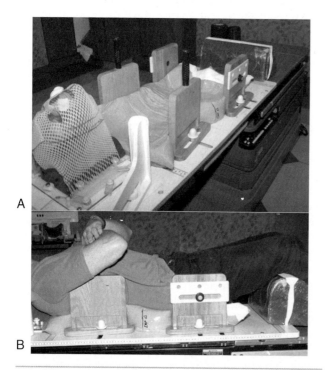

**FIGURE 17.2.** **A and B:** The immobilization cradle used for paraspinal treatment. The four paddles are positioned to press firmly against the patient's ribs and hips. For cervical and upper thoracic sites, a face mask is also used. The alpha-cradle cushion forms to the patient's body shape, and locks itself into position around the four paddles. It helps to improve patient comfort, and superior–inferior reproducibility.

tions, it has no internal fiducial system. Patients are positioned in the cradle by checking the position of alignment tattoos in the cradle coordinate system using the room lasers. Setup of the patient to a tolerance of 2 mm averages between 12 and 15 minutes, including the time to acquire and register the portal images. Registration with the reference DRRs is done manually with the assistance of imaging software. Immobilization performance has been assessed by taking an additional orthogonal portal image pair after treatment and comparing with the first. From 45 anterior pre-postportal image pairs, the mean and standard deviation of the observed patient shift from beginning to end of treatment was 0.1 ± 0.7 mm laterally, and 0.2 ± 0.8 mm in the superior–inferior direction, and from 28 lateral portal images, the shift in the anteroposterior direction was 0.1 ± 0.7 mm.

The best setup accuracy that can be achieved must be viewed in context with all dose delivery uncertainties. For two-dimensional (2D) image-guided setup, such sources of uncertainty include the following: CT scanner resolution—about 1 mm in the transverse directions and perhaps 2 mm longitudinally; dose calculation grid spacing—usually about 2 mm, and the resolution of the dose kernels themselves—about 2 mm, the resolution of the detector used to commission the accelerator—unless a stereotactic diode or similar was used, the planning system will not accurately compute the step dose gradients adjacent to the spinal cord; the positional tolerance on the device used by the imager to determine field position, the jaws or the grid tray—about 1 mm, and the ability to implement a small correction with couch translations (execution error)—perhaps 1 mm. For these reasons, the setup error tolerance used in our clinic is 2 mm. There are diminishing returns on effort expended in trying to reduce setup error much beyond 2 mm. In effect, the final dose delivery error would be dominated by other sources, and so little reduced.

## TREATMENT PLANNING ISSUES

At MSKCC, dose distributions are planned using an in-house inverse treatment planning system. Treatments are delivered using a linac equipped with a 120 leaf multileaf collimator (mlc) whose leaf widths project to 5 mm at isocenter using a dynamic sliding-window technique. Although in sites such as the liver, a sharp dose falloff in all directions is best achieved with noncoplanar beams, the direction of the steep dose gradients in paraspinal cases is largely determined by the geometry of the cord, thus in many cases a coplanar arrangement of five to nine beams is optimum. Noncoplanar beams are especially useful if there are other structures to be avoided such as a kidney. In general, 15-mV beam or a combination of 6- and 15-mV beams are used. When the total monitor units (MUs) are high, as required for a 20-Gy fraction for example, the dose rate is increased to 600 MU/min.

Although case-dependent, the maximum dose gradient that can be achieved with the dynamic multileaf collimation (DMLC) technique is approximately 10% per millimeter. Thus, keeping the maximum cord dose below tolerance may result in a cold spot to part of the target if it lies close to or abuts the cord. In critical cases, cord blocks are used in addition to DMLC to further reduce cord dose. Given that a patient setup and immobilization method has been clinically evaluated, practical setup tolerances will have been decided upon, and their effect on the dose delivered to the target can be taken into account. If, for example, the setup error tolerance is 2 mm, moving the isocenter 2 mm directly toward the cord, and recalculating the dose distribution will yield an estimate of what the cord might actually receive. Alternatively, an ancillary structure that extends the cord contour by 2 mm on each slice and has the same maximum dose constraint as the cord can be created. Optimization with this additional constraint will generate a dose distribution that can safely be delivered given the possible setup errors.

Dose painting is a new technique that utilizes inverse treatment planning and intensity-modulated radiation therapy (IMRT) (23). It enables the delivery of optimized, tightly conformal dose distributions that can be tailored to meet the oncologic characteristics of the target. Multiple dose constraints are placed on the different target re-

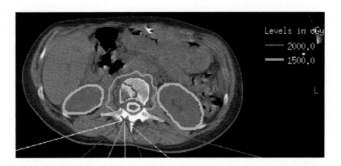

**FIGURE 17.3.** Dose painting. The left and right kidneys are outlined in green, the cord in yellow, the gross tumor volume (GTV) in blue, and the vertebral body [clinical tumor volume (CTV)] in purple. The orange 15-Gy isodose contour line encloses the CTV, and the red 20-Gy line almost completely encloses the CTV.

gions to create a dose distribution that may feature more than two or more dose levels while keeping dose to critical structures to a minimum. For example, in Fig. 17.3, the gross tumor volume (GTV) outlined in light blue, and the clinical target volume (CTV), in this case the vertebral body, were planned to receive 20 Gy and 15 Gy, respectively, in a single fraction, while the maximum point dose to the spinal cord was less than 10 Gy.

## CLINICAL EXPERIENCE

A relative paucity of clinical data exists concerning stereotactic and image-guided radiosurgery for paraspinal malignancies. The first report of stereotactic radiosurgery for spinal lesions used a stereotactic fixation system that was directly attached to the vertebral spinous processes. Nine patients were treated in the prone position to a median dose of 10 Gy in a single fraction, prescribed to the 80% isodose line. Cord doses ranged from 800 cGy to 1,500 cGy. All patients had previously undergone radiation therapy. With a median follow up of 6 months, all patients were controlled at the sites of treatment (24,25). Although it was reliable within 2 mm in the transverse plane and 4 mm in the longitudinal plane, the invasive nature of the system precluded widespread use.

A linac mounted on a robotic arm was used to treat 16 patients with a variety of benign and malignant paraspinal lesions. Doses between 1,100 and 2,500 cGy were given in one to five fractions, and the maximum cord dose allowed for extramedullary lesions was 800 cGy. Although follow up was limited, no significant toxicity was noted for any of the patients treated, with over 6 months' follow-up. No radiographic evidence of tumor progression was seen (26). One hundred twenty-five metastatic lesions in 115 patients were treated with a similar system, using radiosurgical cones for beam shaping. A mean tumor dose

▶ TABLE 17.2  Dose–Volume Histogram Analysis Mean Values for Patients Treated For Primary Spine Malignancies.

| Prescribed dose (cGy) | 7,000 | 5940–7000 |
|---|---|---|
| Planned target volume (mL) | 153 | 86–316 |
| % Planned target volume | 90% | 83–100% |
| Cord maximum | 68% | 14–75% |
| Cord average | 31% | 7–66% |

▶ TABLE 17.4  Palliation Achieved with Paraspinal Intensity-modulated Radiation Therapy.

| Symptom | Pretreatment (N) | After Treatment (N) | % Palliation |
|---|---|---|---|
| Paraesthesia | 12 | 1/12 | 92 |
| Pain | 23 | 2/23 | 91 |
| Strength | 10 | 1/10 | 90 |

of 14 Gy (range, 12–20 Gy) prescribed to the 80% isodose line was delivered in a single fraction. Seventy-four of 79 patients who had presented with pain reported reduction in levels of pain. No acute radiation toxicity or neurologic deficit was observed (27).

Ten patients who received 25 Gy in ten fractions via standard external beam radiotherapy underwent a single image-guided beam shaped spinal radiosurgery boost (6–8 Gy), prescribed to the 90% isodose line, using a gantry-mounted linear accelerator with dynamic intensity modulation. These patients were immobilized with vacuum bag positioning devices. Nine of ten patients experienced significant pain relief. With a mean follow up of 6 months, no patient exhibited acute radiation toxicity (28).

At MSKCC, 35 patients (14 primary and 21 secondary malignancies) have received treatment for paraspinal malignancies with either the MSBF or MBC. All treated lesions were solid tumors. Of the primary lesions,11 cases of recurrent primary sarcoma (six cases of osteogenic sarcoma) and three cases of chordoma were treated. Of the secondary lesions, the most common histology was renal cell carcinoma ($N = 6$). One patient died of acute subarachnoid hemorrhage and did not complete treatment. This patient is not included in the analysis. The dosimetric data for these cohorts are summarized in Tables 17.2 and 17.3. All patients have been followed with MRI scans at 3- to 4-month intervals. The median follow up for the entire group is 11 months (range, 1–42 months). For patients treated for primary lesions of the spine, the median follow up is 15 months (range, 2–30 months). Patients

treated for metastatic disease to the spine had a median follow up of 7 months (range, 1–24 months). Median survival from the time of treatment for patients with primary and metastatic disease was found to be 15 months and 7 months, respectively. No patient has been lost to followup. When patients with less than 3 months' follow-up were excluded, 90% of patients (median follow-up, 12 months) were found to have excellent palliation of symptoms. Thirty-four of 35 patients reported palliation of symptoms at 3 months' follow-up after treatment. One patient with renal cell carcinoma experienced worsening of symptoms during radiation therapy and demonstrated radiographic evidence of disease progression. Clinical outcomes are summarized in Tables 17.4 and 17.5.

Two patients have reported Radiation Therapy Oncology Group (RTOG) mucositis up to grade 2 when cervical lesions have been treated. Mucositis has resolved within 6 weeks of completing radiation therapy in both cases. One patient was diagnosed with idiopathic vasculitis 3 months after completion of radiation and has had no evidence of active cancer in subsequent follow-up visits. Otherwise, no significant toxicity has been observed. One patient has exhibited mild skin hyperpigmentation [7,000 cGy to the planning target volume (PTV)]. No significant late toxicity, including neuropathy or myelopathy, has been encountered. Patients have consistently reported a significant durable palliative benefit with treatment. Pain has returned in only patients who have experienced recurrence of their tumor.

At the time of last follow-up, 90% of patients treated for metastatic disease and 86% of patients treated for primary spine tumors have not exhibited radiographic progression. The mean time to failure for patients ($N = 2$) with primary

▶ TABLE 17-3  Dose–Volume Histogram Analysis Mean Values for Patients Treated for Metastatic Malignancies[a].

| Prior radiation therapy | 3,000 cGy/10 | 2,000–4,500 cGy |
|---|---|---|
| Prescribed dose | 2,000 cGy/5 | 2,000–3,000 cGy |
| Planning target volume, mL | 187 | 47–316 |
| % Planning target volume | 88% | 68–98% |
| Cord maximum, % | 34% | 13–60% |
| Cord average, % | 14% | 4–81% |

[a]All had prior radiation therapy to the same site.

▶ TABLE 17-5  Mean Reduction in Symptoms in Patients with Median 12-months Follow-up.

| | Pretherapy | After therapy | P |
|---|---|---|---|
| Pain/10 | 6.6 | 1.5 | >0.0001 |
| Weakness/5 | 4.2 | 4.8 | 0.004 |
| Numbness/5 | 4.5 | 4.9 | 0.02 |

lesions was 18.5 months (range, 15–22 months). For patients treated for metastatic tumors ($N = 2$), the mean time to failure was 5.5 months (range, 3–9 months). Figures 17.4 and 17.5 (see Case Study) demonstrate actuarial local control rates of 75% and 81% for primary and secondary tumors, respectively. Although follow-up is not mature, the clinical results have been encouraging.

## SUMMARY

Although paraspinal SBRT is still a maturing field, the preliminary clinical experience from multiple institutions has been encouraging. The incorporation of innovations such as IMRT and improvements in imaging and computer-based 3D dosimetry with exact immobilization and image-guided systems have greatly increased the accuracy of radiotherapy near the spinal cord. This has allowed extension of the intracranial radiosurgery paradigm to the paraspinal arena. The availability of this technology has given oncologists a powerful tool in their armamentarium in treating these clinically difficult lesions.

## REFERENCES

1. Ortiz GJ. The incidence of vertebral body metastases. *Int Orthop* 1955;19:309–311.
2. Clain A. Secondary malignant disease of bone. *Br J Cancer* 1965;19:15–29.
3. Gokaslan ZL, York JE, Walsh GL, et al. Transthoracic vertebrectomy for metastatic spinal tumors. *J Neurosurg* 1998;89:599–609.
4. Black P. Spinal metastasis: current status and recommended guidelines for management. *Neurosurg* 1979;5:726–746.
5. Sorensen S, Helweg-Larson S, Mouridsen H, et al. Effect of high-dose dexamethasone in carcinamatous metastatic spinal cord compression treated with radiotherapy: a randomized trial. *Eur J Cancer* 1994;30A:22–27.
6. Regine WF, Tibbs PA, Young A, et al. Metastatic spinal cord compression: A randomized trial of direct decompressive surgical resection plus radiotherapy vs. radiotherapy alone. *Int J Radiat Oncol Biol Phys* 2003;57[Suppl 1]: S125.
7. Emami B, Lyman J, Brown A, et al. Tolerance of normal tissue to therapeutic irradiation. *Int J Radiat Oncol Biol Phys* 1991;21:109–122.
8. Boden G. Radiation myelitis of the cervical spinal cord. *Br J Radiol* 1948;21:464–469.
9. Linstadt DE, Edwards M, Prados M, et al. Hyperfractionated irradiation for adults with brainstem gliomas. *Int J Radiat Oncol Biol Phys* 1991;20:757–760.
10. Macbeth FR, Wheldon TE, Girling DJ, et al. Radiation myelopathy: estimates of risk in 1048 patients in three randomized trials of palliative radiotherapy for non-small cell lung cancer: the Medical Research Council Lung Cancer Working Party. *Clin Oncol (R Coll Radiol)* 1996;8:176–181.
11. McCunniff AJ, Liang MJ. Radiation tolerance of the cervical spinal cord. *Int J Radiat Oncol Biol Phys* 1989;16:675–678.
12. Wong CS, Van Dyk J, Milosevic M, et al. Radiation myelopathy following single courses of radiotherapy and retreatment. *Int J Radiat Oncol Biol Phys* 1994;30:575–581.
13. Ang KK, Jiang GL, Feng Y, et al. Extent and kinetics of recovery of occult spinal cord injury. *Int J Radiat Oncol Biol Phys* 2001;50:1013–1020.

14. Wong CS, Minkin S, Hill RP. Re-irradiation tolerance of rat spinal cord to fractionated x-ray doses. *Radiother Oncol* 1993;28:197–202.
15. Wong CS, Hao Y. Long-term recovery kinetics of radiation damage in rat spinal cord. *Int J Radiat Oncol Biol Phys* 1997;37:171–179.
16. Schultheiss TE, Kun LE, Ang KK, et al. Radiation response of the central nervous system. *Int J Radiat Oncol Biol Phys* 1995;31:1093–1112.
17. Hamilton AJ, Lulu BA, Fosmire H, et al. Linac-based spinal stereotactic radiosurgery. *Stereotact Funct Neurosurg* 1996;66:1–9.
18. Lax I, Blomgren H, Naslund I, et al. Stereotactic radiotherapy of malignancies in the abdomen: methodological aspects. *Acta Oncol* 1994;33:677–683.
19. Blomgren H, Lax I, Naslund I, et al. Stereotactic high dose fraction radiation therapy of extracranial tumors using an accelerator: clinical experience of the first thirty-one patients. *Acta Oncol* 1995;34:861–870.
20. Wulf J, Hadinger U, Oppitz U, et al. Stereotactic radiotherapy of extracranial targets: CT-simulation and accuracy of treatment in the stereotactic body frame. *Radiother Oncol* 2000;57:225–236.
21. Lohr F, Debus J, Frank C, et al. Noninvasive patient fixation for extracranial stereotactic radiotherapy. *Int J Radiat Oncol Biol Phys* 1999; 45:521–527.
22. Yenice KM, Lovelock DM, Hunt MA, et al. CT image-guided intensity-modulated therapy for paraspinal tumors using stereotactic immobilization. *Int J Radiat Oncol Biol Phys* 2003;55:583–593.
23. Ling CC, Humm J, Larson S, et al. Towards multidimensional radiotherapy (MDCRT): biological imaging and biological conformality. *Int J Radiat Oncol Biol Phys* 2000;47:551–560.
24. Hamilton AJ, Lulu BA, Fosmire H, et al. Preliminary clinical experience with linear accelerator-based spinal stereotactic radiosurgery. *Neurosurgery* 1995;36:311–319.
25. Hamilton AJ, Lulu BA. A prototype device for linear accelerator-based extracranial radiosurgery. *Acta Neurochir Suppl (Wien)* 1995;63:40–43.
26. Ryu SI, Chang SD, Kim DH, et al. Image-guided hypo-fractionated stereotactic radiosurgery to spinal lesions. *Neurosurgery* 2001;49:838–846.
27. Gerszten PC, Ozhasoglu C, Burton SA, et al. Evaluation of CyberKnife frameless real-time image-guided stereotactic radiosurgery for spinal lesions. *Stereotact Funct Neurosurg* 2003;81:84–89.
28. Ryu S, Fang Yin F, Rock J, et al. Image-guided and intensity-modulated radiosurgery for patients with spinal metastasis. *Cancer* 2003;97:2013-2018.
29. Eichhorn HJ, Lessel A, Rotte KH. Einfuss verschiedener Bestrahlungsrhythmen auf Tumor- und Normalgewebe *in vivo*. *Strahlentheraphie* 1972;146:614–629.
30. Choi NC, Grillo HC, Gardiello M, Scannell HG and Wilkins EW. Basis for new strategies in postoperative radiotherapy of bronchogenic carcinoma. *Int J Radiat Oncol Biol Phys* 1980;6:31–35.
31. Hazra TA, Chandrasekaran MS, Colman M, Prempree T, Inalsignh M. Survival in carcinoma of the lung after a split course of radiotherapy. *Br J Radiol* 1974;47:464–466.
32. Abramson N, Cavanaugh PJ. Short-course radiation therapy in carcinoma of the lung. *Radiology* 1973;108:685–687.
33. Fitzgerald RH, Marks RD, Wallace KM. Chronic radiation myelitis. *Radiology* 1982;144:609–612.
34. Miller RC, Aristizabal SA, Leith JT, Manning MR. Radiation myelitis following split-course therapy for unresectable lung cancer. *Int J Radiat Onco. Biol Phys* 1977;2:179.
35. Madden FJ, English J, Moore AK, Newton KA. Split course radiation in inoperable carcinoma of the bronchus. *Eur J Cancer* 1979;15:1175–1177.
36. Guthrie RT, Ptacek JJ, HjassAC. Comparative analysis of two regimens of split course radiation in carcinoma of the lung. *Am J Roentgenol* 1973;117:605–608.
37. Dische S, Martin WM, Anderson P. Radiation myelopathy in patients treated for carcinoma of the bronchus using a six fraction regime of radiotherapy. *Br J Radiol* 1981;54:29–35.
38. Hatlevoll R, Host H, Kaalhus O. Myelopathy following radiotherapy of bronchial carcinoma with large single fractions: A retrospective study. *Int J Radiat Oncol Biol Phys* 1983;9:41–44

## Case Study

### Case Study of Spinal SRBT: Radiosurgery for Vertebral Metastasis

Samuel Ryu, Fang-Fang Yin, and Jack Rock

### CLINICAL PRESENTATION

A 60-year-old man had undergone radical prostatectomy for cancer nearly 5 years ago. He had subsequently developed a prostate-specific antigen (PSA) level recurrence of cancer, for which he received hormonal therapy. Four years after his initial diagnosis, he developed multiple painful bone metastases, particularly to the lumbosacral region. He received conventionally fractionated palliative radiation therapy, 30 Gy in ten fractions, to fields covering L-4 through the sacroiliac joints.

Ten months later, he presented with lower extremity weakness and sensory changes. Magnetic resonance imaging (MRI) showed compression fracture in the L-5 and S-1 vertebral bodies with epidural thecal sac compression by a soft tissue mass. He underwent surgical resection of the soft-tissue mass at L-5 to S-1. While recuperating from the surgery, new symptoms developed, including pain in the lower lumbar region with radiculopathy. There were associated sensory and motor changes. Decreased pinprick and numbness were noted in the lateral aspect of the left foot and muscle weakness (2/5) of the dorsi- and plantar flexion with dropfoot gait. He also developed an increased tenderness at the lower thoracic region. Repeated MRI revealed signal changes at T-10 consistent with a new isolated metastatic involvement as well as an L-5 to S-1 lesion with progressive thecal sac compression.

Single-fraction stereotactic body radiation therapy (SBRT) (sometimes called extracranial radiosurgery) was offered in an effort to relieve symptoms associated with the T-10 and L-5 to S-1 lesions.

### TREATMENT PLANNING AND DOSE DELIVERY

Immobilization was achieved in supine position by using vacuum body fixation device. Computed tomography (CT) simulation (3-mm slice thickness) was performed with intravenous (IV) contrast. During the simulation, infrared markers were placed on the patient's skin. The simulation images were sent to a BrainScan planning computer (BrainLAB, Heimstetten, Germany) for treatment planning. Both the clinical target volume (CTV) and the critical organs were identified for planning. The planning target volume (PTV) was defined with an additional 2 to 3 mm to that of the CTV to accommodate positioning variations. Most of our treatment plans for spinal radiosurgery involved multiple intensity-modulated beams (range, 5–9 beams) to achieve conformal radiation

Departments of Radiation Oncology and Neurosurgery, Henry Ford Hospital, Detroit, MI 48201

distribution to the spine and minimize radiation to the spinal cord or other critical structures (1,2). Dose–volume histograms (DVHs) were used to identify appropriate doses for target and critical organs and to evaluate treatment plans. Each slice of the target volume was reviewed for radiation dose distribution. Every effort was made, mainly by using radiation intensity modulation, to limit cord dose below 10 Gy to the 10% partial cord volume.

The patient was treated with a single high-dose fraction to each site: 16 Gy to T-10 and 14 Gy to L-5 to S-1, including the epidural soft-tissue mass. The dose was prescribed to the 90% isodose line at the periphery of the involved spines. Radiosurgery treatment of T-10 is illustrated in Fig. 17.4 with a DVH and cross-sectional image of the isodose distribution.

Repositioning of the patient was performed by image fusion between the digitally reconstructed simulation CT image and the orthogonal image taken at the time of treatment and infrared marker. The picture of patient setup is shown in Fig. 17.5. Steroids were not used, and the patient did not require hospitalization for any part of the treatment planning and dose delivery.

### DISCUSSION

The patient improved symptomatically and functionally after treatment. At the 1-month follow-up visit, he reported no pain. There was no tenderness over the spine and no any pain on external or internal rotation of the hip. His sensory examination was normal to light touch and pinprick. Functionally, the patient was able to walk 10 feet with minimal assistance, but a dropfoot gait was stable. Follow-up MRI scan showed shrinkage of the epidural soft tissue mass at L-5 to S-1. This case presentation shows two scenarios of using spinal radiosurgery: for treatment of spinal metastasis as a primary treatment and for recurrent lesion that was treated previously.

Among the extracranial target locations for SBRT, the spinal cord and vertebrae are the structures with the least breathing-related movement and, therefore, are particularly well suited for stereotactic radiosurgery. We have conducted a clinical feasibility study to determine the accuracy and precision of targeting. The isocenter location was found to be within 1.36 ± 0.11mm of intended location, as measured by image fusion of the digitally reconstructed image from the CT simulation and the port film (3). There was a rapid dose falloff toward the spinal cord; the distance from 90% to 50% isodose line averaged 5 mm. In general, less than 10% of the anterior spinal cord volume was included in the 80% isodose region of the prescribed dose (3,4).

A subsequent study to determine the optimum spine radiosurgery dose is ongoing at the Henry Ford Hospital (5). An analysis was performed in 49 patients with 61 lesions. Most patients had back pain as the presenting symptom. The involved spine was treated with a single fraction of 10 to 16 Gy. The median time to pain relief was 14 days. The earliest pain relief was seen within 24 hours. The median duration of pain relief was 13 months. Complete pain relief was achieved in 38%, with partial pain relief in 48% of the lesions. Relapse of the pain at the

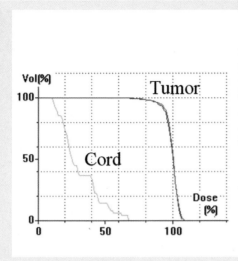
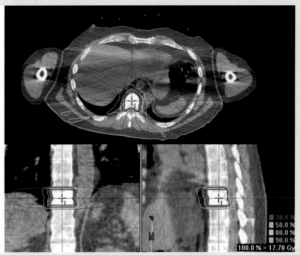

FIGURE 17.4. **Left:** Intensity-modulated radiosurgery treatment plan with integral dose–volume histogram of normal and target volumes. **Right:** Radiation isodose curves shown on the cross-sectional image at the isocenter of radiosurgery for T-10.

treated site was seen only in 7%. We have observed neurologic improvement from cord compression and radiographic tumor control. Only 5% developed progressive metastasis in the adjacent spines on the radiologic studies. There was no acute or subacute radiation toxicity detected clinically during the maximum follow-up of 24 months.

Single-fraction SBRT can be used for patients with single or multiple isolated spinal metastases. The procedure is image-guided and noninvasive, and patient tolerance has been excellent. Because treatment is given in a single outpatient hospital visit this treatment added more convenience to the patient. Surgery should be considered for patients with neurologic symptoms from frank cord compression (6), but further studies are needed for a better understanding of proper patient selection to determine which patients would be well served by radiosurgery alone or as an adjunct to surgery or conventionally fractionated external beam radiotherapy.

## References

1. Yin F-F, Ryu S, Ajlouni M, et al. A technique of intensity-modulated radiosurgery (IMRS) for spinal tumors. *Med Phys* 2002;29:2815–2822.
2. Yin F-F, Zhu J, Hui Y, et al. Dosimetric characteristics of Novalis shaped beam surgery unit. *Med Phys* 2002;29:1729–1738.
3. Ryu S, Yin FF, Rock J, et al. Image-guided intensity-modulated radiosurgery for spinal metastasis. *Cancer* 2003;97:2013–2018.
4. Ryu S, Sharif A, Yin FF, et al. *Tolerance of human spinal cord to single dose radiosurgery: Proceedings of International Congress of Radiation Research, August 17–22, Brisbane, Australia 2003*
5. Ryu S, Rock J, Yin FF, et al. Image-guided Single dose radiosurgery for single spinal metastasis. In: Program and abstracts of the 40th meeting of the Amercian Society of Clinical Oncologists; June 5–8, 2004; New Orleans, LA. Abstract 1268.
6. Regine WF, Tibbs PA, Young A, et al. Metastatic spinal cord compression: a randomized trial of direct decompressive surgical resection plus radiotherapy vs. radiotherapy alone. *Int J Radiat Oncol Biol Phys* 2003;57[Suppl 2]:S125.

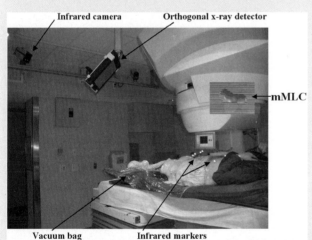

FIGURE 17.5. Photo of patient setup. Patient is positioned and immobilized in a vacuum device and bag. Infrared markers on the skin and reference position are seen as well as orthogonal x-ray detectors.

# INDEX

*Page numbers followed by f indicate figures; page numbers followed by t indicate tables.*